Protein-Based NANOCOMPOSITES FOR TISSUE ENGINEERING

Woodhead Publishing Series in Biomaterials

Protein-Based NANOCOMPOSITES FOR TISSUE ENGINEERING

Edited by

SHOWKAT AHMAD BHAWANI

Department of Chemistry, Faculty of Resource Science and Technology, UNIMAS, Kota Samarahan, Malaysia

ZOHEB KARIM

MoRe Research Ornskoldsvik AB, Ornskoldsvik, Sweden

MOHAMMAD JAWAID

Department of Chemical and Petroleum Engineering, College of Engineering, United Arab Emirates University, Al Ain, United Arab Emirates

ELSEVIER

WP WOODHEAD PUBLISHING

An imprint of Elsevier

Woodhead Publishing is an imprint of Elsevier
50 Hampshire Street, 5th Floor, Cambridge, MA 02139, United States
125 London Wall, London EC2Y 5AS, United Kingdom

ISBN: 978-0-323-99357-9

For information on all Woodhead Publishing publications visit our website at https://www.elsevier.com/books-and-journals

Publisher: Matthew Deans
Acquisitions Editor: Sabrina Webber
Editorial Project Manager: Sara Greco
Production Project Manager: Surya Narayanan Jayachandran
Cover Designer: Mark Rogers

Typeset by TNQ Technologies

Dedication

Dedication to Late Ziaur Rahman (Father of Prof (Dr.) Mohammad Jawaid)

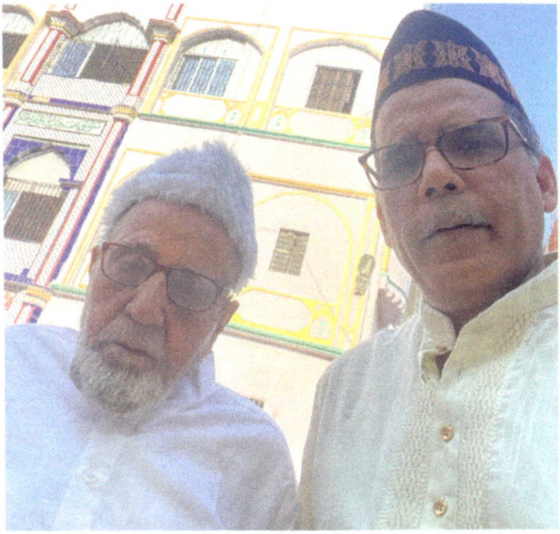

This is my last photo with my father on 11th April, 2024.

My father passed away on 29th April, 2024, at 2:30 PM IST at home, Gaya, Bihar (India).
Inna lillahi wa inna ilayhi **raji**'un إِنَّا لِلّٰهِ وَإِنَّا إِلَيْهِ رَاجِعُونَ..
"To God we belong and to Him we return."
I pray to Allah Subhanutallah to forgive his small and big sins and give him a high place in Paradise (Jannatul Firdous).

He was my mentor and guide and without his support and guidance, it would have been very difficult to achieve my success.

Contents

Contributors

Nasir Adamu
Science Laboratory Technology, Federal Polytechnic Daura, Daura, Katsina State, Nigeria

Rohana Adnan
School of Chemical Sciences, Universiti Sains Malaysia, Penang, Malaysia

Hilal Ahmad
Interdisciplinary Research Center for Membranes and Water Security, King Fahd University of Petroleum & Minerals (KFUPM), Dhahran, Saudi Arabia

Khalid M. Alotaibi
Department of Chemistry, College of Science, King Saud University, Riyadh, Saudi Arabia

Mohd Saquib Ansari
Department of Biomedical Sciences, Shaheed Rajguru College of Applied Sciences for Women, University of Delhi, Delhi, New Delhi, India

Yasser Azim
Department of Applied Chemistry, Zakir Husain College of Engineering & Technology, Faculty of Engineering and Technology, Aligarh Muslim University, Aligarh, Uttar Pradesh, India

Basree
Department of Applied Chemistry, Zakir Husain College of Engineering & Technology, Faculty of Engineering and Technology, Aligarh Muslim University, Aligarh, Uttar Pradesh, India

Anant Narayan Bhatt
Institute of Nuclear Medicine and Allied Sciences, Defence Research and Development Organization, Delhi, New Delhi, India

Showkat Ahmad Bhawani
Faculty of Resource Science and Technology, Universiti Malaysia Sarawak (UNIMAS), Kota Samarahan, Sarawak, Malaysia

Jacelyn Mohana Das
School of Chemical Sciences, Universiti Sains Malaysia, Penang, Malaysia

H. Fadlullah
Chemistry Education Department, Universitas Sultan Ageng Tirtayasa, Banten, Indonesia

Homa Fatma
Molecular Cancer Genetics & Translational Research Laboratory, Section of Genetics, Department of Zoology, Aligarh Muslim University, Aligarh, Uttar Pradesh, India

M. Hazwan Hussin
School of Chemical Sciences, Universiti Sains Malaysia, Penang, Malaysia

Mohamad Nasir Mohamad Ibrahim
School of Chemical Sciences, Universiti Sains Malaysia, Penang, Malaysia

Nur Farhana Jaafar
School of Chemical Sciences, Universiti Sains Malaysia, Penang, Malaysia

Mohd Jameel
Molecular Cancer Genetics & Translational Research Laboratory, Section of Genetics, Department of Zoology, Aligarh Muslim University, Aligarh, Uttar Pradesh, India

Hayfa Alajilani Abraheem Jamjoum
School of Chemical Sciences, Universiti Sains Malaysia, Penang, Malaysia; Department of Chemistry, Faculty of Science, University of Sabratha, Sabratah, Libya

Jayanudin
Department of Chemical Engineering, Universitas Sultan Ageng Tirtayasa, Banten, Indonesia

Sakshi Kapoor
Nanoscale Research Facility, Indian Institute of Technology Delhi, New Delhi, India

Noor Haida Mohd Kaus
School of Chemical Sciences, Universiti Sains Malaysia, Penang, Malaysia

Abhishek Kumar
Department of Biomedical Sciences, Shaheed Rajguru College of Applied Sciences for Women, University of Delhi, Delhi, New Delhi, India; Institute of Nuclear Medicine and Allied Sciences, Defence Research and Development Organization, Delhi, New Delhi, India

Ilham Maulana
Department of Chemistry, Faculty of Mathematics and Natural Sciences, Universitas Syiah Kuala, Banda Aceh, Indonesia

Abdul Moheman
Department of Chemistry, Gandhi Faiz-E-Aam College, Shahjahanpur, Uttar Pradesh, India

Mohammad Mushaf
Institute of Eminence Teaching Fellow, Talent Development Center, Indian Institute of Science, Challakere, Karnataka, India

Nahid Nishat
Department of Chemistry, Faculty of Science, Jamia Millia Islamia (Central University), New Delhi, India

Rakesh Pandey
Institute of Nuclear Medicine and Allied Sciences, Defence Research and Development Organization, Delhi, New Delhi, India

Tabassum Parveen
Department of Botany, Aligarh Muslim University, Aligarh, Uttar Pradesh, India

Mohammad Amir Qureshi
Department of Chemistry, Faculty of Science, Jamia Millia Islamia (Central University), New Delhi, India; Department of Applied Sciences and Humanities, KCC Institute of Technology and Management, Knowledge Park III, Greater Noida, Uttar Pradesh, India

Rani Rahat
College of Dentistry, University of Illinois, Chicago, IL, United States

Mohd R. Razali
School of Chemical Sciences, Universiti Sains Malaysia, Penang, Malaysia

Mohammad Shahadat
School of Chemical Sciences, Universiti Sains Malaysia USM, Penang, Malaysia; Department of Textile and Fiber Engineering, Indian Institute of Technology, New Delhi, India

Hifzur R. Siddique
Molecular Cancer Genetics & Translational Research Laboratory, Section of Genetics, Department of Zoology, Aligarh Muslim University, Aligarh, Uttar Pradesh, India

Khairi Suhud
Department of Chemistry, Faculty of Mathematics and Natural Sciences, Universitas Syiah Kuala, Banda Aceh, Indonesia

Abu Tariq
Department of Chemistry, Aligarh Muslim University, Aligarh, Uttar Pradesh, India

Khalid Umar
School of Chemical Sciences, Universiti Sains Malaysia, Penang, Malaysia; Materials Technology Research Group, School of Chemical Sciences, Universiti Sains Malaysia, Minden, Penang, Malaysia

Sadiq Umar
College of Dentistry, University of Illinois, Chicago, IL, United States

About the editors

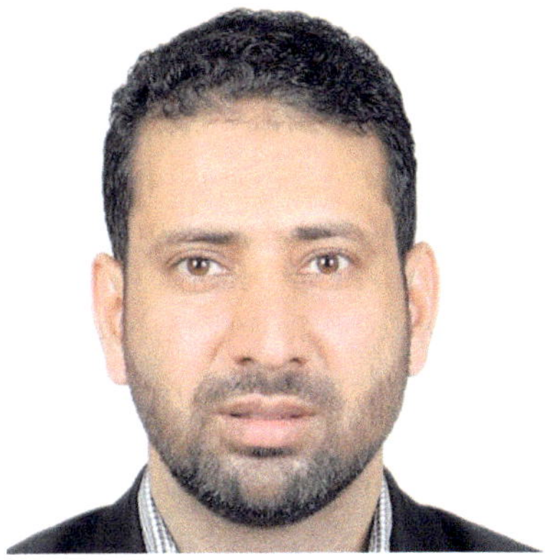

Dr. Showkat Ahmad Bhawani is presently working as an Associate Professor at the Department of Chemistry, Faculty of Resource Science and Technology, Universiti Malaysia Sarawak. In addition to this, he has a teaching experience of 2 years from King Abdulaziz University, North Jeddah and a postdoctoral experience of 3 years from the Universiti Sains Malaysia, Malaysia. He has received his MSc in Analytical Chemistry and PhD in Applied Analytical Chemistry from Aligarh Muslim University, Aligarh, India. He is working on the synthesis of molecular imprinting polymers for the removal/extraction of dyes, fungicides, and various natural products from environmental and biological samples. He is also developing new test methods and determining standard conditions for the analysis of various analytes from environmental and biological samples. He is a member of the American Chemical Society and life member of Asian Polymer Association and editorial board member of several journals.

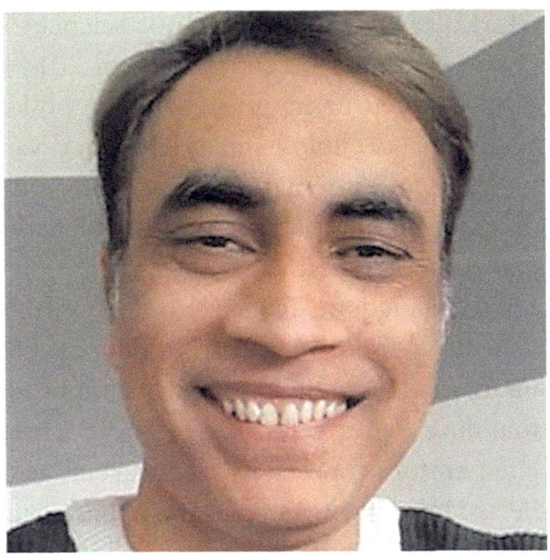

Dr. Zoheb Karim is presently working as Head R&D, Alfa Laval A/S, Denmark. He is leading a team of six people and his main activity is related to the innovation of polymeric membranes for separation science. He did his PhD from Lulea University of Technology, Sweden, in Materials Science. He has more than 60 publications, 15 book chapters, and he has also guided PhD and master students within time. Furthermore, he was invited by various reputed universities, research institutes, and companies for lecturer. He has also presented his research work in very reputed universities like Oxford University, IIT Delhi, IIT Chennai, IIT Kanpur, Denmark Technical University, Delhi University, etc.

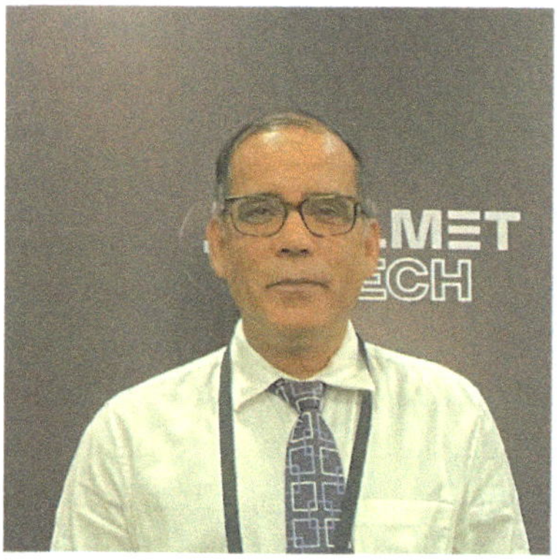

Dr. Mohammad Jawaid is currently working as a Distinguished Professor at Chemical and Petroleum Engineering Department, United Arab Emirates University, UAE. He has more than 25 years of experience in teaching, research, and industries. His areas of research interests include hybrid composites, lignocellulosic reinforced/filled polymer composites, advance materials: graphene/nanoclay/fire retardant, modification and treatment of lignocellulosic fibers and solid wood, biopolymers and biopolymers for packaging applications, nanocomposites and nanocellulose fibers, and polymer blends. So far, he has published 90 books, 95 book chapters, more than 500 peer-reviewed international journal papers, and several published review papers under top 25 hot articles in ScienceDirect during 2013–20. He has also obtained 6 patents and 6 copyrights/industrial design. H-index and citation in Scopus are 95 and 38,177 and in Google scholar, H-index and citation are 113 and 51,512; H-index =82 (Web of Science). 40 PhD and 17 master's students graduated under his supervision in 2014–24 in the fields of hybrid composites, green composites, nanocomposites, natural fiber-reinforced composites, nanocellulose, etc. He secured various research grants at university, national, and international levels on polymer composites of around USD 2.1 million. He has also delivered plenary and invited talks in international conferences related to composites in India, Turkey, Malaysia, Thailand, the United Kingdom, France, Saudi Arabia, Egypt, Spain, and China. Besides that, he is also a member of technical committees of several national and international conferences on composites and materials science. He is founding Series Editor of Springer Three Book Series. He worked as a guest editor of special issues of several peer-reviewed journals. Besides that, he is also a reviewer of several high-impact international peer-reviewed journals of Elsevier, Springer, Wiley, Saga, ACS, RSC, Frontiers, etc. Dr.

Mohammad Jawaid also received several awards at national and international levels. He is also the Winner of Newton-Ungku Omar Coordination Fund: UK-Malaysia Research and Innovation Bridges Competition 2015. He is also Professional membership of ACS, SPE, APA, MySET, etc. He is a Fellow and Chartered Scientist of the Institute of Materials, Minerals & Mining (IOM3), UK. He is also among the 1% highly cited researchers according to Clarivate 2023.

CHAPTER 1

Protein-based nanocomposites: An overview

Showkat Ahmad Bhawani[1], Abdul Moheman[2], Abu Tariq[3] and Khalid M. Alotaibi[4]

[1]Faculty of Resource Science and Technology, Universiti Malaysia Sarawak (UNIMAS), Kota Samarahan, Sarawak, Malaysia; [2]Department of Chemistry, Gandhi Faiz-E-Aam College, Shahjahanpur, Uttar Pradesh, India; [3]Department of Chemistry, Aligarh Muslim University, Aligarh, Uttar Pradesh, India; [4]Department of Chemistry, College of Science, King Saud University, Riyadh, Saudi Arabia

1. Introduction

Twenty distinct amino acids combine to form proteins, which are extremely complicated polymers. The components are joined by substituted amide. Primary, secondary, tertiary, and quaternary are the four stages of protein structures that are present in proteins. Proteins have a variety of functional qualities, including solubility, emulsification, gelation, elasticity, and cohesion-adhesion, because of the complexity of their structure and composition [1,2]. Because of their excellent biocompatibility, amphiphilicity, simple degradability, digestibility, edibleness, and nontoxicity, proteins are employed to create nanocarriers [3]. Because of the diversity of their structural design, proteins are not only manufactured into numerous types of nanocarriers to fulfill varied application needs, but they can also scavenge free radicals to prevent oxidative degradation of bioactive compounds [4]. Furthermore, proteins can easily construct nanocarriers by interacting with various biopolymers and offering a multitude of functional groups. This can greatly enhance the solubility, biocompatibility, and bioavailability of bioactive compounds [5]. It is clear from this that protein nanocarriers have a lot of promise and prospective uses in the transport of bioactive materials. To self-assemble into three-dimensional spatial nanostructures or interact with a wide range of nanomaterials, proteins are typically used as precursors in the construction of smart photonic networks. The variety of synthesizing approaches has

Protein-Based Nanocomposites for Tissue Engineering
ISBN 978-0-323-99357-9
https://doi.org/10.1016/B978-0-323-99357-9.00006-5

provided fresh insights into the creation of protein-based systems including nanowires [6], nanotubes [7], nanoflowers [8], nanosheets [9], and nanocages [10]. When proteins interact with various inorganic nanomaterials, they acquire distinct physicochemical characteristics [11,12]. Some reported state-of-the-art protein-based systems showed excellent biocompatibility for the increased capabilities. Furthermore, additional features are needed under certain applicable situations, including the requirement for water solubility [13], high selectivity [14], cell-penetrating ability [15], good stability [16], capacity to mimic enzyme characteristics [3,17,18], and other skills for rapid signal expression [19]. As a result, to meet the specified needs, certain proteins with particular functionalities are used. Protein-based systems modified by antibody proteins are typically utilized to create innovative immunosensors or high-specificity immunoassays [14,20].

New protein-based material designs for a wide range of applications are proliferating in the literature [21−25]. The use of proteins in a variety of biomaterial applications has become attractive due to the ease with which researchers may program the production of any protein [26]. Protein-based materials have several appealing characteristics, including accessibility and participation in a circular economy of source materials, as well as biocompatibility and biodegradability [27]. Moreover, a large number of structural proteins are extremely manipulable due to their polymeric nature, which is based on discrete repeats of amino acid sequences [28]. It is frequently possible to fuse an amino acid sequence that is found to impart desirable properties with another protein, combining the desirable aspects of both; for instance, fusing the sequence that gives a protein its strength with the sequence that gives it its elasticity can result in a strong, yet stretchy, material. Natural proteins like collagen, keratin, elastin, resilin, and silk are the focus of research because of their inherent elasticity and strength [26]. Furthermore, a number of biomaterial applications are showing promise for composite materials that mimic silk, elastin, resilin, collagen, or keratin, or any mix of these, or that include inorganic components [26]. Since proteins are amphoteric molecules, they have the ability to spontaneously migrate to interfaces between oil and water or air and water. Proteins can interact with nearby molecules at the interface to create a robust cohesive, viscoelastic layer that is resistant to both mechanical and thermal forces [29]. As a result, proteins are typically utilized in coatings and adhesives that are edible. Though they are occasionally not completely hydrophobic or slowly disintegrating, protein films have shown superior gas barrier qualities and reduced water vapor penetration when compared to starch [30]. Proteins demonstrate the benefits of these characteristics in the creation of biomaterial packaging. As a result, industrial applications have long made use of different proteins' capacity to create films [31].

2. Protein-based composites

A very few important protein-based composites are discussed in this section.

2.1 Milk protein-based composites

Casein and whey proteins make up the majority of the 33 g/L of protein found in milk [31]. The utilization of milk proteins in the creation of bio-nanocomposite formation is highly appealing due to its high nutritional quality, water solubility, and emulsification capacity. The main protein in milk is casein. About 94% of casein is made up of protein, and the remaining 6% is made up of low-molecular-weight molecules. Casein micelles are large colloidal particles produced by casein and calcium phosphate proteins that have long been of interest. These spherical micelles have a hydrophilic coating of casein kappa covering their hydrophobic inner surface. This layer stabilizes the micelles and causes both spatial and electrostatic discharge between the molecules. Consequently, copolymers of blocks with an average hydrodynamic radius of 250 nm and strong inclinations to self-regulate micelles between 50 and 500 nm are produced by dual proteins [32]. As natural nanocarriers, casein micelles in milk actually transfer calcium phosphate and amino acids from mother to infant [33]. These micelles exhibit remarkable stability and retain their structural integrity across a range of dairy product preparation techniques. The use of casein/copolymer micelles to transfer hydrophobic charges via other polymers has recently been demonstrated to be an efficient way to block saturated fatty acids that are saturated with vitamin D, omega-3, and beta-carotene (a precursor to vitamin A) [34].

Twenty percent of milk proteins are made up of whey proteins, which are soluble at pH 4.6 [35,36]. As a by-product of making cheese, liquid whey is produced in huge amounts, with an annual production that keeps increasing. Because so much of this whey is not used, there are significant issues with waste disposal. Thus, there is a great deal of interest in discovering novel applications for whey proteins, like bio-nanocomposites.

One can utilize either solution intercalation or solvent-casting to make milk protein-based bio-nanocomposites. First, separate preparations of clay solutions and milk proteins are made. The milk proteins are dissolved in a solvent that has been mixed with high shear, and the same solvent that was used to create the film-forming solution is first used to swell and disperse layered nanoclay particles. The mixture is treated with ultrasonic treatment and high-shear mixing to accomplish the intercalation of the solvent into the stacked layers [37–39]. Next, a dropwise addition of the clay solution is made to the milk protein solution. After undergoing another round of high-shear mixing and ultrasonic treatment, the slurry is poured onto a glass plate. To create a free-standing film, the solution is allowed to cure at room temperature or at a higher temperature. The most crucial stage in this method for creating a milk protein-based bio-nanocomposite is the intercalation or exfoliation of nanoclay particles in a polymer matrix. The fabrication of whey-protein-isolate/poly(vinylidene pyrrolidone)-coated montmorillonite (MMT) composite films was reported to have a filler content of 0–4.8 vol.% [40]. A partial exfoliation of the nanoparticles was observed by transmission electron microscopy. Because of the high aspect ratio of the nanoparticle aggregates, the geometrical impedance factor rose noticeably as the filler quantity increased.

2.2 Soybean protein-based composites

Compared with cereal grains, which have a protein content of 8%–15%, soybeans have a protein content of 38%–44% [41]. Soybean protein can be categorized mostly as globulin. Several other functional features of soybean protein, including cohesiveness, adhesiveness, water and fat absorption, emulsification, dough and fiber formation, texturizing ability, and whippability, have also been reported, in addition to its film-forming ability [42]. A soybean protein-based film can be created by partially denaturing polypeptide chains with the use of heat, a solvent, an electrolyte to create cross-linking, or a pH change. In addition, composite films of soybean protein isolate (SPI) and several clays (organic MMT, bentonite, talc powder, and zeolite) have been synthesized [43]. The clay mineral sample was added to a glycerol and distilled water mixture, well mixed, and then sonicated to create the clay suspension. After that, SPI was heated and dissolved in the clay suspension before being cast and allowed to dry. In comparison with the traditional SPI film, the resulting soybean protein/clays bionanocomposites exhibited a considerable ($P < .05$) improvement in tensile strength, but a significant ($P < .05$) loss in water vapor permeability and water solubility [43].

Dean and Yu [38] synthesized films of soybean protein-based nanocomposite materials and evaluated their mechanical and microstructural characteristics. The nanocomposite film was created by mixing glycerol and water, adding Cloisite Na+, then treating the mixture with ultrasound for an hour. Soybean protein isolates and the Cloisite Na+ suspension were mixed together in a high-speed mixer and then extruded at 140°C using a twin screw extruder [38]. Elastic modulus exhibited the greatest improvement, according to the data. Tensile strength of nanocomposite films rose by 23% and 47%, respectively, with and without ultrasonic treatment [38]. The creation of rectorite/SPI biodegradable nanocomposite sheets was also documented [44]. According to this study, rectorite was extensively exfoliated and intercalated in the SPI matrix, based on the unique structures of both SPI and rectorite, as well as the molecular chain's capacity to move due to solution mixing and melting compression. Simultaneously, the exfoliated rectorite lamellae improved the strength and modulus of SPI polymers, potentially mitigating the plasticization deficit. The maximum strength was attained at 12.92 MPa, nearly twice as strong as pure SPI plastics, with 12 weight percent rectorite loading [44].

2.3 Gelatin-based composites

Collagen extracted from animal bones and skin is thermally denaturated with extremely diluted acid to create gelatin. Moreover, fish skins can also be used to extract it. The conversion of collagen to gelatin happens in two stages, which includes (1) heat denaturation, which breaks down hydrogen and electrostatic links at about 40°C, and (2) hydrolytic breakdown of covalent bonds [45].

It has been observed that when gelatin is casted from aqueous solutions containing a plasticizer, like sorbitol or glycerin, the films become transparent, flexible, strong, and oxygen-impermeable. Gelatin is used in the food and pharmaceutical, such as in microencapsulation and the creation of coatings for tablets and capsules. In an effort to enhance the mechanical and water resistance characteristics of the polymer, gelatin is also investigated for the creation of a bio-nanocomposite using layered silicate, such as MMT [46]. Using an electrospinning technique, the synthesis of hydroxyapatite (HA) precipitate/gelatin matrix nanocomposites as promising bone-regenerating materials was investigated [47]. When compared to the pure gelatin counterpart, these nanocomposite fibers greatly increased the bone-derived cellular activity [47]. In another study, researchers investigated nano-hydroxyapatite/gelatin composites to ensure optimal bone tissue integration and biocompatibility. These polymer/nano-hydroxyapatite composites demonstrated favorable biocompatibility and biodegradable properties that could make them valuable as constituents in tissue replacement material [48].

2.4 Albumin-based composites

A family of proteins called albumins is present in the bodies of many different species, including humans. Ovalbumin, bovine serum albumin, and human serum albumin are just a few of the several varieties of albumin [49,50]. Therapy relies heavily on regulated drug release, which is made possible by its capacity to selectively bind and transport different molecules [51–53]. Significantly lowering the danger of immunological responses, albumin demonstrates biodegradability and biocompatibility, which is essential given its possible use as a drug carrier [54,55]. The development of nanoscale drug delivery systems comprising albumin is crucial to regulate the size of particles and aggregation processes [56]. The aforementioned factors could impact albumin's therapeutic effectiveness and bioavailability. To create carriers with optimal drug delivery capabilities, it is important to investigate and monitor the size and shape of the nanocarriers during the synthesis process [57,58]. Numerous investigations have demonstrated albumin's affinity for biodistribution within cancer cells and the uptake of this protein by these cells [59,60]. As a result, numerous research studies have been undertaken to create albumin-containing chemotherapeutic drug carriers that will enable precise drug accumulation at the affected site [61–68]. The nanocomposites made of oxidized Arabic gum and bovine serum albumin were examined [69]. Following the loading of these materials with piperine, the medication exhibited analgesic, antifungal, and antibacterial properties. In another study, researchers carried out investigations on albumin-based nanocomposites combined with N5,N6-Bis(2 fluorophenyl)[1,2,**5**]oxadiazolo[3,4- b]pyrazine-5,6-diamine (BAM15), an active chemical that may prevent obesity and its potential symptoms. The conducted trials showcased the exceptional biocompatibility of the produced carriers together with their capacity to target the liver, potentially because of the albumin included in their structure.

2.5 Collagen based composites

The most prevalent structural protein in the tissues of mammals is collagen. Three α-helical chains make up the basic structure, and they can join as homo- or hetero-trimers [70]. These trimers come together to form increasingly intricate supramolecular structures, such as networks, hexagonal networks, anchoring fibrils, beaded filaments, and fibrils [70]. Glycine-X-Y repetitions, in which X is typically hydroxyproline and Y is proline, make up the majority of the basic structure of collagen [71]. Collagen's thermostability is believed to be influenced by the presence of hydroxyproline; mutations that eliminate hydroxyproline at different locations in the collagen sequence dramatically lower the material's thermal denaturation temperature [72]. In conclusion, collagen and materials derived from collagen have been employed in several fields, such as corneal implants, where they have proven to be highly effective [73]. A porous gel containing collagen that encourages tissue regrowth has been utilized for tissue grafts [74]. Different mixing ratios of collagen-elastin were produced in thin films [75]. Whereas the elastin component offered resilience, the collagen components sustained the tensile strength of the regenerated tissues. For artificial blood vessels, researchers produced electrospun collagen-elastin nanofiber meshes from aqueous solutions [76]. The shape of the fibers was controlled by adjustments to the flow velocity, applied electric field, collecting distance, and beginning solution composition. The fiber diameter increased from 220 to 600 nm with an increase in elastin content [77]. A method for creating multilamellar vascular grafts from a recombinant elastin-like protein reinforced with collagen microfibers was developed [78]. Control over collagen microfiber density and orientation was made possible by this method. In addition, collagen-elastin matrices were clinically investigated as a dermal alternative for the treatment of severe burns [79]. These native, structurally intact collagen fibrils are covered with elastin to assist skin regeneration, and together they form these 1 mm thick protein three-dimensional matrices. Effective clinical trials proved the usefulness of these systems, showing that all patients recovered to full range of motion without experiencing any allergic reactions or infections [80].

2.6 Elastin-based composites

Blood vessels, lung epithelium, skin, and other tissues all contain elastin, a significant structural protein found in mammals [81]. Structure-wise, elastin is constructed of tandem tetra-, penta-, and hexa-repeats of distinct peptide sequences that are primarily hydrophobic residues like proline, glycine, valine, and alanine. Repeats of lysine and alanine are abundant in these hydrophilic domains, which are scattered across these sequences [82]. Most tissues, including blood vessels and the dermis, need elastin proteins to create elastic fibers [83,84]. Animal tissues like skin can yield various elastin protein networks, but another source is recombinant human tropoelastin (full-length 60 kDa), which is the soluble precursor of elastin [84]. The hydrophilic domains of elastin have a high lysine content and are important in elastin cross-linking [83,84], which helps to stabilize the structure. The hydrophobic domains of elastin are rich in nonpolar amino acids and have common repeat motifs like [GVGVP]n.

2.7 Resilin-based composites

Resilin (superelastic rubbers) are present in the flying and jumping organs of insects, where the animals must repeatedly extend and retract their appendages millions of times over their lives [85,86]. Insects are able to jump and fly with efficiency because of resilin which stores mechanical energy [87]. Three domains make up Resilin: an N-terminal domain (exon I) that contains 18 11-amino acid repeats, a middle chitin-binding domain (exon II), and a C-terminal region (exon III) that has 11 13-amino acid repeats. The N-and C-terminal repeat-containing regions appear to be essential for the special qualities of the protein. Because cross-linked resilin (via tyrosines) has over 300% elongation before breaking [85] and shows excellent resilience up to 95% under high-frequency elastic motions [85,86], it offers opportunities for biomaterial applications. Hydrogels containing resilin and resilin-based materials have been developed with the aim of applying them in tissue engineering [85]. The existence of unique tyrosine-tyrosine cross-links is a crucial component of the structure of resilin. These can be added via the enzyme transglutamase or chemical oxidation to recombinant resilin components. Recombinant resilin has been used to make hydrogels, which replicate the elastic properties of the subendothelial layer of the vascular system and offer a potential material for long-term cell attachment and vascular tissue regeneration [88].

2.8 Keratin-based composites

Another large class of insoluble proteins, keratin proteins [89,90], are found in the cytoplasmic epithelia and epidermal appendage structures (hairs, nails, wools, hooves, etc.) as intermediate filaments. Both "soft" hair keratins and "hard" epithelial keratins are made up of two protein chains, types I and II, that differ in their molecular weights and compositions but share a core alpha-helical domain [89]. "Soft" hair keratins have a larger cysteine concentration in the nonhelical domains and, as a result, produce harder and more lasting structures through the creation of intermolecular disulfide bonds, despite the fact that different keratins are closely related in secondary structures [89]. Keratin is especially appealing for use in biomaterial applications because of its insolubility and prevalence in agricultural waste materials like chicken feathers and inappropriate wool [91].The ability of keratin to function as a matrix for cell development is further enhanced by the inclusion of the cell adhesion sequences leucine-aspartic acid-valine and arginine glycine-aspartic acid in its native sequence [91]. Wool, or keratin, is readily functionalized by chlorination to yield a halamine-charged substance [91]. Halamine-charged keratin, found in textiles, films, and nanofibers, has antibacterial properties [91]. Moreover, even after several washings, these materials retain their effectiveness. In the production of materials for a variety of uses, halamine-charged keratin may play a significant role [91].

3. Conclusions

A new class of polymers called nanocomposites is permeating every part of human existence. As completely new kinds of materials based on plant, animal, and other natural components, they exhibit significant promise for possible applications as high-performance biodegradable materials. These materials have a bright future ahead of them, but their high costs and current low manufacturing level prevent them from being used in many different applications. Reducing the cost of biodegradable polymers and enhancing their mechanical strength and water resistance are crucial elements in the development of renewable plastics-based industries. To enable a broad spectrum of applications for bio-nanocomposites based on renewable polymers, more research and formulation work on the bio-nanocomposite is needed to enable easy manipulation of mechanical and other properties based on end-user requirements. Protein-based materials provide a wealth of options for customizing a material's macroscopic characteristics through modifications to the protein sequences used in their synthesis or processing techniques. Composite biomaterials based on proteins can be shaped into a variety of biomaterials with adjustable characteristics, such as the ability to regulate cell reactions. To meet the expanding range of medical material and device needs, biomaterials generally have made significant progress due to the capacity to customize or adjust the mechanical, surface, and regeneration properties. These composites' inherent biocompatibility, biodegradability, and natural abundance, along with their special natural properties (mechanical, optical, electrical, chemical, and thermal), have shown promise for producing the next generation of functionalized biomaterials. Comprehending the molecular-level interactions among these proteins will facilitate the development of the upcoming generation of multifunctional protein composite biomaterials, which will possess improved characteristics and functions tailored to particularly address regenerative medicine needs. Evaluation of cell interactions for the variety of composite materials produced can be employed as in vivo screens of material degradation profiles and inflammatory responses, as well as to comprehend linkages between the protein composites and biological responses. With immediate application to tissue regeneration, nanomedicine, and disease treatments, the results of these investigations will offer a novel biomaterials platform that will address a critical need in the field of biomedical science.

Acknowledgments

The authors acknowledged the financial support from the Tun Zaidi Chair through the Research Grant F07/TZC/2160/2021.

References

[1] Zhang W, Xu SY, et al. Food chemistry. 3rd ed. Beijing: China Light Industry Press; 2003. p. 267–302.
[2] Damodaran S. Protein functionality in food system. New York: Marcel Dekker; 1994. p. 1–38.
[3] Rajendran CK, Udenigwe SRC, Yada R. Nanochemistry of protein-based delivery agents. Front Chem 2016;31:1–9.
[4] Samaranayaka AG, Li-Chan EC. Food-derived peptidic antioxidants: a review of their production, assessment, and potential applications. J Funct Food 2011;3:229–54.
[5] Elzoghby AO, Samy WM, Elgindy NA. Protein-based nanocarriers as promising drug and gene delivery systems. J Contr Release 2012;161:38–49.
[6] Sun H, Zhang X, Miao L, Zhao L, Luo Q, Xu J, Liu J. Micelle-induced self-assembling protein nanowires: versatile supramolecular scaffolds for designing the light-harvesting system. ACS Nano 2016;10(1):421–8.
[7] Luo Y, Song Y, Wang M, Jian T, Ding S, Mu P, Liao Z, Shi Q, Cai X, Jin H, Du D, Dong W-J, Chen C-L, Lin Y. Bioinspired peptoid nanotubes for targeted tumor cell imaging and chemo-photodynamic therapy. Small 2019;15:1902485.
[8] Song Y, Wang M, Li S, Jin H, Cai X, Du D, Li H, Chen C-L, Lin Y. Efficient cytosolic delivery using crystalline nanoflowers assembled from fluorinated peptoids. Small 2018;14:1803544.
[9] Kim JH, Kim SC, Kline MA, Grzincic EM, Tresca BW, Cardiel J, Karbaschi M, Dehigaspitiya DC, Chen Y, Udumula V, Jian T, Murray DJ, Yun L, Connolly MD, Liu J, Ren G, Chen C-L, Kirshenbaum K, Abate AR, Zuckermann RN. Discovery of stable and selective antibody mimetics from combinatorial libraries of polyvalent, loop-functionalized peptoid nanosheets. ACS Nano 2019;14(1):185–95.

[10] Huang X, Chisholm J, Zhuang J, Xiao Y, Duncan G, Chen X, Suk JS, Hanes J. Protein nanocages that penetrate airway mucus and tumor tissue. Proc Natl Acad Sci U S A August 8, 2017;114(32):E6595−602.
[11] Zhang N, Mei K, Guan P, Hu X, Zhao YL. Protein-based artificial nanosystems in cancer therapy. Small 2020;16:1907256.
[12] Ruan X, Liu D, Niu X, Wang Y, Simpson CD, Cheng N, Du D, Lin Y. 2D graphene oxide/Fe-mof nanozyme nest with superior peroxidase-like activity and its application for detection of woodsmoke exposure biomarker. Anal Chem 2019;91(21):13847−54.
[13] Bhaskar S, Lim S. Engineering protein nanocages as carriers for biomedical applications. NPG Asia Mater 2017;9(4):e371.
[14] Cheng N, Yang S, Shi Q, Du D, Dong L, Luo Y, Xu W, Lin Y. Au@Pd nanopopcorn and aptamer nanoflower assisted lateral flow strip for thermal detection of exosomes. Anal Chem 2019;91(21):13986−93.
[15] Ding S, Khan AI, Cai X, Yang S, Lyu Z, Du D, Dutta P, Lin Y. Overcoming blood−brain barrier transport: advances in nanoparticle-based drug delivery strategies. Mater Today 2020;37:112−25.
[16] Tang Z, Wu H, Cort JR, Buchko GW, Zhang Y, Shao Y, Aksay IA, Liu J, Lin Y. Constraint of DNA on functionalized graphene improves its biostability and specificity†. Small 2010;6:1205−9.
[17] Wang H, Chao Y, Liu J, Zhu W, Wang G, Xu L, Liu Z. Photosensitizer-crosslinked in-situ polymerization on catalase for tumor hypoxia modulation and enhanced photodynamic therapy. Biomaterials 2018;181:310−7.
[18] Jiao L, Yan H, Wu Y, et al. When nanozymes meet single-atom catalysis. Angew Chem Int Ed 2020;132(7):2585−96.
[19] Li H, Yan X, Kong D, Jin R, Sun C, Du D, Lin Y, Lu G. Recent advances in carbon dots for bioimaging application. Nanoscale Horiz 2020;5:218−34.
[20] Fu Q, Wu Z, Du D, Zhu C, Lin Y, Tang Y. Versatile barometer biosensor based on Au@Pt core/shell nanoparticle probe. ACS Sens June 23, 2017;2(6):789−95.
[21] Zhao R, Torley P, Halley PJ. Emerging biodegradable materials: starch- and protein-based bio-nanocomposites. J Mater Sci 2008;43:3058−71.
[22] Aljabali AA, Rezigue M, Alsharedeh RH, Obeid MA, Mishra V, Serrano-Aroca Á, Tambuwala MM. Protein-based nanomaterials: a new tool for targeted drug delivery. Ther Deliv 2022;13(6):321−38.
[23] Hu X, Cebe P, Weiss AS, Omenetto F, Kaplan DL. Protein-based composite materials. Mater Today 2012;15:208−15.
[24] Abascal NC, Regan L. The past, present and future of protein-based materials. Open Biol. 2018;8:180113.
[25] Ding S, Zhang N, Lyu Z, Zhu W, Chang Y-C, Hu X, Du D, Lin Y. Protein-based nanomaterials and nanosystems for biomedical applications: a review. Mater Today 2021;43:166−84.
[26] Desai MS, Lee SW. Protein-based functional nanomaterial design for bioengineering applications. Wiley Interdiscip Rev Nanomed Nanobiotechnol. 2015;7:69−97.
[27] Lin CY, Liu JC. Modular protein domains: an engineering approach toward functional biomaterials. Curr Opin Biotechnol 2016;40:56−63.
[28] Freeman R, Boekhoven J, Dickerson MB, Naik RR, Stupp SI. Biopolymers and supramolecular polymers as biomaterials for biomedical applications. MRS Bull 2015;40:1089−101.
[29] Phillips MC. Protein conformation at liquid interfaces and its role in stabilizing emulsions and foams. Food Technol 1981;35:50.
[30] Miller KS, Krochta JM. Oxygen and aroma barrier properties of edible films: a review. Trend Food Sci Technol 1997;8:228−37.

[31] Dalgleish DG, Kinsella JE, et al. Food proteins. Champagne: American Oil Chemists Society; 1989. p. 155–78.
[32] Molino NM, Wang S-W. Caged protein nanoparticles for drug delivery. Curr Opin Biotechnol 2014;28:75–82.
[33] Porcaro F, Roudeau S, Carmona A, Ortega R. Advances in element speciation analysis of biomedical samples using synchrotron-based techniques, vol 104; 2018. p. 22–41.
[34] Kumagai PS, Araujo APU, Lopes JLS. Going deep into protein secondary structure with synchrotron radiation circular dichroism spectroscopy. Biophys Rev 2017;9(5):517–27.
[35] Yew SP, Tang HY, Sudesh K. –Photocatalytic activity and biodegradation of polyhydroxybutyrate films containing titanium dioxide|| Polymer Degradation and Stability, vol 91; 2006. p. 1800–7.
[36] Brunner JR, Whitaker JR, et al. Food proteins. Westport: AVI Publishers, Inc.; 1977. p. 175–208.
[37] Krochta JM. In: Gennadios A, editor. Protein-based films and coatings. Boca Raton: CRC Press; 2002. p. 1–41.
[38] Dean K, Yu L. In: Smith R, editor. Biodegradable polymers for industrial application. Boca Raton: CRC Press; 2005. p. 289–309.
[39] Graveland-Bikker JF, de Kruif CG. Unique milk protein based nanotubes: food and nanotechnology meet. Trend Food Sci Technol 2006;17:196–203.
[40] Hedenqvist MS, Backman A, Gällstedt M, et al. Morphology and diffusion properties of whey/montmorillonite nanocomposites. Compos Sci Technol 2006;66(13):2350–9.
[41] Snyder HE, Kwon TW. Soybean utilization. New York: Van Nostrand Reinhold Company, Inc.; 1987.
[42] Krochta JM, Baldwin EA, et al. Edible coatings and films to improve food quality. Lancaster: Technomic Publishing Company Inc.; 1994. p. 213–58.
[43] Rhim JW, Lee JH, Kwak HS. Mechanical and water barrier properties of soy protein and clay mineral composite films. Food Sci Biotechnol 2005;14:112–6.
[44] Huang J, Cui GJ, Wei M, Huang J. Facile exfoliation of rectorite nanoplatelets in soy protein matrix and reinforced bionanocomposites thereof. J Appl Polym Sci 2007;104:3367–77.
[45] Eastoe JE, Leach AA. The science and technology of gelatin. New York: Academic Press, Inc.; 1977. p. 73–107.
[46] Zheng JP, Li P, Ma YL, Yao KD. Gelatin/montmorillonite hybrid nanocomposite. I. Preparation and properties. J Appl Polym Sci 2002;86:1189–94.
[47] Kim H-W, Song J-H, Kim H-E. Nanofiber generation of gelatin–hydroxyapatite biomimetics for guided tissue regeneration. Adv Funct Mater 2005;15:1988–94.
[48] Li J, Chen YP, Yin Y, et al. Modulation of nano-hydroxyapatite size via formation on chitosan–gelatin network film in situ. Biomaterials 2007;28(5):781–90.
[49] Hutapea TPH, Madurani KA, Syahputra MY, Hudha MN, Asriana AN, Suprapto, Kurniawan F. Albumin: source, preparation, determination, applications, and prospects. J Sci Adv Mater Dev 2023;8:100549.
[50] Tiwari R, Sethiya NK, Gulbake AS, Mehra NK, Murty USN, Gulbake A. A review on albumin as a biomaterial for ocular drug delivery. Int J Biol Macromol 2021;191:591–9.
[51] Pompili E, Zaccherini G, Baldassarre M, Iannone G, Caraceni P. Albumin administration in internal medicine: a journey between effectiveness and futility. Eur J Intern Med 2023;117:28–37.
[52] Mishra V, Heath RJ. Structural and biochemical features of human serum albumin essential for eukaryotic cell culture. Int J Mol Sci 2021;22:8411.

[53] Wouw J, Joles JA. Albumin is an interface between blood plasma and cell membrane, and not just a sponge. Clin Kidney J 2022;15:624–34.
[54] Xu X, Jinyu Hu J, Xue H, Hu Y, Liu Y, Lin G, Liu L, Xu R. Applications of human and bovine serum albumins in biomedical engineering: a review. Int J Biol Macromol 2023;253:126914.
[55] Spada A, Emami J, Tuszynski JA, Lavasanifar A. The uniqueness of albumin as a carrier in nanodrug delivery. Mol Pharm 2021;18:1862–94.
[56] Madeira PP, Rocha ILD, Rosa ME, Freire MG, Coutinho JAP. On the aggregation of bovine serum albumin. J Mol Liq 2022;349:118183.
[57] Karimi M, Bahrami S, Ravari SB, Zangabad PS, Mirshekari H, Bozorgomid M, Shahreza S, Sori M, Hamblin MR. Albumin nanostructures as advanced drug delivery systems. Expet Opin Drug Deliv 2016;13:1609–23.
[58] Larsen MT, Kuhlmann M, Hvam ML, Howard KA. Albumin-based drug delivery: harnessing nature to cure disease. Mol Cell Ther 2016;4:3.
[59] Wang Y, Iqbal H, Ur-Rehman U, Zhai L, Yuan Z, Razzaq A, Lv M, Wei H, Ning X, Xin J, et al. Albumin-based nanodevices for breast cancer diagnosis and therapy. J Drug Deliv Sci Technol 2023;79:104072.
[60] Hoogenboezem EN, Duvall CL. Harnessing albumin as a carrier for cancer therapies. Adv Drug Deliv Rev 2018;130:73–89.
[61] Ma N, Liu J, He W, Li Z, Luan Y, Song Y, Garg S. Folic acid-grafted bovine serum albumin decorated graphene oxide: an efficient drug carrier for targeted cancer therapy. J Colloid Interface Sci 2017;490:598–607.
[62] Akbal O, Vural T, Malekghasemi S, Bozdŏgan B, Denkbąs EB. Saponin loaded montmorillonite-human serum albumin nanocomposites as drug delivery system in colorectal cancer therapy. Appl Clay Sci 2018;166:214–22.
[63] Yu X, Xu Z, Wang X, Xu Q, Chen J. Bactrian camel serum albumins-based nanocomposite as versatile biocargo for drug delivery, biocatalysis and detection of hydrogen peroxide. Mater Sci Eng C 2020;109:110627.
[64] Elgohary MM, Helmy MW, Abdelfattah EA, Ragab DM, Mortada SM, Fang J, Elzoghby AO. Targeting sialic acid residues on lung cancer cells by inhalable boronic acid-decorated albumin nanocomposites for combined chemo/herbal therapy. J Contr Release 2018;285:230–43.
[65] Chen Z, Hong G, Liu Z, Yang D, Kankala RK, Wu W. Synergistic antitumor efficacy of doxorubicin and gambogic acid-encapsulated albumin nanocomposites. Coll Surf, B 2020;196:111286.
[66] Liu Z, Wang X, Zhang C, Lin K, Yang J, Yi Zhang Y, Hao J, Tian F. Folic acid-coupled bovine serum albuminmodified magnetic nanocomposites from quantum-sized Fe_3O_4 and layered double hydroxide for actively targeted delivery of 5-fluorouracil. Int J Biol Macromol 2024;256:128385.
[67] Xinyu Y, Adilijiang X, Qilan X, Azhati Z, Yiyan S, Ling C, Jin C. GSH-responsive curcumin/doxorubicin encapsulated Bactrian camel serum albumin nanocomposites with synergistic effect against lung cancer cells. J Biomed Sci 2020;34:54–66.
[68] Bardania H, Jafari F, Baneshi M, Mahmoudi R, Ardakani MT, Safari F, Barmak MJ. Folic acid-functionalized albumin/graphene oxide nanocomposite to simultaneously deliver curcumin and 5-fluorouracil into human colorectal cancer cells: an in vitro study. BioMed Res Int 2023;2023:8334102.
[69] Jalali ES, Shojaosadati SA, Hamedi S. Green synthesis of bovine serum albumin/oxidized gum Arabic nanocomposite as pH-responsive carrier for controlled release of piperine and the molecular docking study. Int J Biol Macromol 2023;225:51–62.
[70] Ricard-Blum S. The collagen family. Cold Spring Harbor Perspect Biol 2011;3:a004978.

[71] Shoulders MD, Raines RT. Collagen structure and stability. Annu Rev Biochem 2009;78:929–58.
[72] Fallas JA, O'Leary LE, Hartgerink JD. Synthetic collagen mimics: self-assembly of homotrimers, heterotrimers and higher order structures. Chem Soc Rev 2010;39:3510–27.
[73] Fagerholm P, et al. A biosynthetic alternative to human donor tissue for inducing corneal regeneration: 24-month follow-up of a phase 1 clinical study. Sci Transl Med 2010;2:46ra61.
[74] Milthorpe BK. Xenografts for tendon and ligament repair. Biomaterials 1994;15:745–52.
[75] Pulkkinen HJ, Tiitu V, Valonen P, Jurvelin JS, Lammi MJ, Kiviranta I. Engineering of cartilage in recombinant human type II collagen gel in nude mouse model in vivo. Osteoarthr Cartil 2010;18:1077–87.
[76] McDaniel JR, Radford DC, Chilkoti A. A unified model for de novo design of elastin-like polypeptides with tunable inverse transition temperatures. Biomacromolecules 2013;14:2866–72.
[77] Grove TZ, Osuji CO, Forster JD, Dufresne ER, Regan L. Stimuli-responsive smart gels realized via modular protein design. J Am Chem Soc 2010;132:14 024.
[78] Pena-Francesch A, Jung H, Hickner MA, Tyagi M, Allen BD, Demirel MC. Programmable proton conduction in stretchable and self-healing proteins. Chem Mater 2018;30:898–905.
[79] Jin E, Reddy N, Zhu Z, Yang Y. Graft polymerization of native chicken feathers for thermoplastic applications. J Agric Food Chem 2011;59:1729–38.
[80] Qiu W, Teng W, Cappello J, Wu X. Wetspinning of recombinant silk-elastin-like protein polymer fibers with high tensile strength and high deformability. Biomacromolecules 2009;10:602–8.
[81] Wise SG, Mithieux SM, Weiss AS. Engineered tropoelastin and elastin-based biomaterials. In: McPherson A, editor. Advances in protein chemistry and structural biology, vol 78. New York, NY: Academic Press; 2009. p. 1–24.
[82] Vrhovski B, Weiss AS. Biochemistry of tropoelastin. Eur J Biochem 1998;258:1–18.
[83] Jessica FA, Bax DV, Mithieux SM, Nivison-Smith L, Rnjak J, Anna W, Wisea SG, Weiss AS. Elastin-based materials. Chem Soc Rev 2010;39:3371–9.
[84] Wise SG, Mithieux S, Weiss AS. Engineered tropoelastin and elastin-based biomaterials. Adv Prot Chem Struct Biol 2009;78(1).
[85] Elvin CM, Carr A, Huson M, et al. Synthesis and properties of crosslinked recombinant pro-resilin. Nature 2005;437:999–1002.
[86] Qin G, Lapidot S, Numat K, Hu X, Meirovitch S, Dekel M, Podoler I, Shoseyov O, Expression DLK. Cross-linking, and characterization of recombinant chitin binding resilin. Biomacromolecules 2009;10(12):3227–34.
[87] Wong DC, Pearson RD, Elvin CM, Merritt DJ. Expression of the rubber-like protein, resilin, in developing and functional insect cuticle determined using a Drosophila anti-rec 1 resilin antibody. Dev Dynam 2012;241:333–9.
[88] Kim Y, Gill EE, Liu JC. Enzymatic cross-linking of resilin-based proteins for vascular tissue engineering applications. Biomacromolecules 2016;17:2530–9.
[89] Rouse JG, Van Dyke ME. A review of keratin-based biomaterials for biomedical applications. Materials 2010;3:999–1014.
[90] Reichl S, Borrelli M, Geerling G. Keratin films for ocular surface reconstruction. Biomaterials 2011;32:3375–86.
[91] Dickerson MB, Sierra AA, Bedford NM, Lyon WJ, Gruner WE, Mirau PA, Naik RR. Keratin-based antimicrobial textiles, films, and nanofibers. J Biomed Mater Res B Appl Biomater 2013;1:5505–14.

Further reading

[1] Cuq B, Gontard N, Guilbert S. Proteins as agricultural polymers for packaging production. Cereal Chem 1998a;75:1–9.

[2] Jing W, Jiang M, Fu X, Yang J, Chen L, Leng F, Xu P, Huang W, Yang CYZ. Self-assembly drug-albumin nanocomposites for nonalcoholic fatty liver disease treatment. Int J Biol Macromol 2022;214:697–707.

CHAPTER 2

Types, stability, biocompatibility, and toxicity of protein-based nanocomposites

Mohd Jameel[1], Homa Fatma[1], Khalid Umar[2] and Hifzur R. Siddique[1]

[1]Molecular Cancer Genetics & Translational Research Laboratory, Section of Genetics, Department of Zoology, Aligarh Muslim University, Aligarh, Uttar Pradesh, India; [2]Materials Technology Research Group, School of Chemical Sciences, Universiti Sains Malaysia, Minden, Penang, Malaysia

1. Introduction

One of the major healthcare concerns is tissue and organ failure due to various injuries, diseases, and developmental defects. Although organ donation is one of the alternatives for organ failure patients, the shortage of organ donors, immune rejection of organs, and increasing number of transplant waiting lists suggest that organ donation is not a practical approach [1]. To meet the ever-growing demand for organ donation and to overcome the shortcoming of organ transplantation, one of the promising options is tissue engineering and regenerative medicine, which combines various fields to create therapies and products that help in the replacement, repairment, and retainment of damaged tissues [1]. Tissue engineering requires scaffolds that help to grow new cells and their proliferation. The introduction of growth factors can direct the cell toward the desired behavior and process, which leads to the development of fully functional tissue or organ that can be implanted in the patient. Moreover, tissue engineering is also exploited in developing the 2D- and 3D-microenvironments that mimic the tumor niche's biomechanical properties [2]. However, tissue engineering faces an important limitation: not all materials can mimic the properties of natural materials or behave in a desired way inside biological fluids. To overcome this roadblock, customized nanoparticle engineering is being considered where the material and nano-level properties can solve this problem [3].

Protein-Based Nanocomposites for Tissue Engineering
ISBN 978-0-323-99357-9
https://doi.org/10.1016/B978-0-323-99357-9.00012-0

Nanotechnology is the branch of applied science that studies materials' properties and molecular and atomic scale usage. Nanomaterials range from 1 to 100 nm and have a high surface-to-volume ratio leading to a variety of exceptional properties that are not found in bulk materials. Nanomaterials can be classified based on dimensions, such as one-dimensional nanowires, two-dimensional nanoplates, and three-dimensional quantum dots, etc. [4]. Nanoparticles that are composed of numerous phases with at least one phase having one, two, or all three dimensions are in nanometer size. Nanocomposites include nanoparticles, nanofibers, and nanoclays. Nanocomposites have better optical and mechanical properties (high ductility, strength, and scratch resistance). Nanocomposites are composed of metallic, nonmetallic, and polymeric material, which helps overcome the defects of present characteristics and provides additional advantages over the primary features [5]. When these nanocomposites of a particular size, geometry, and surface chemistry are mixed with biopolymers, they are known as bio-nanocomposites. Compared with normal polymers, the bio-nanocomposites showed improved mechanical properties, dimensional stability, and solvent or gas resistance. Moreover, bio-nanocomposites can be polysaccharides-based or protein-based, depending upon the polymers used in developing nanocomposites. In addition, various inorganic nanoparticles are also employed in the nanocomposite as additives to improve the performance of polymers [6].

Protein nanocomposites are promising nanoparticles combining proteins' unique structure and properties with synthetic nanomaterials, enhancing functionality. Protein-based nanocomposites are helpful in environmental remediation, biomedicine, photonics, and biosensors due to advanced renewability, abundance, and ambient processability [7]. The biomimetic nanocomposite formed by the coprecipitation of $CaCO_3$ and soy protein isolates showed improved mechanical and thermal properties and better tensile strength. Due to nanosize and strong interface interaction [8]. One of the mandatory requirements for the clinical use of nanocomposites is biocompatibility, which ensures that the nanocomposites are nontoxic and do not produce any injurious effects on the biological systems. The nanocomposites are first validated for their structural specificity via FTIR, SEM, etc., and then, the biological efficacy is tested in vitro and preclinical setups before going for clinical trials. Once the nanocomposites are deemed safe during clinical trials, they are produced commercially (Fig. 2.1; [9]). Once the nanocomposites enter a biological environment, a protein "corona" is formed over it, that is, the formation of layers of proteins. The uncontrolled

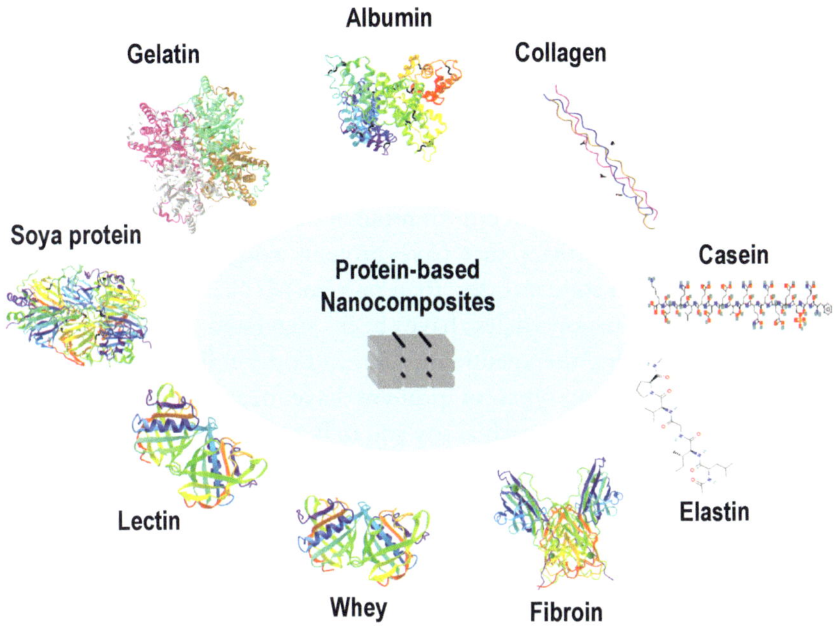

Figure 2.1 ***Schematic diagram showing the different types of protein-based nanoparticles.*** Protein-based nanocomposites can be produced using different animal and plant protein types such as collagen, albumin, gelatin, lectin, whey, casein, fibroin, elastin, and soy protein.

nanoparticle–protein interaction may lead to the inefficient release of nanoparticles in the system, which may prove fatal [10]. Casein-based nanocomposite conjugated with reinforcing material, organized montmorillonite, and cross-linking agent, ethylene glycol diglycidyl ether showed better physical properties, thermal stability, and mechanical properties combined with lower selling ratio, biodegradation rate, and high biocompatibility [11]. It has also been reported that the development of bovine serum albumin (BSA) with a black phosphorous-based-γ-Fe_2O_3 nanocomposite has shown excellent biocompatibility with colon cancer cell lines [10]. The successful development of BSA-immobilized nanocomposites has opened the door for interaction studies for various other proteins such as HAS. GB/T 16886.5-2003 (ISO 10993-5: 1999) has recommended that any polymeric biomaterial showing more than 75% cell viability can be used in biomedical applications. The chitosan-grafted fish gelatin bio-nanocomposite has been shown [12]. This chapter focuses primarily on protein-based nanocomposites, biocompatibility, and toxicity.

2. Types of protein-based nanocomposites

Proteins are widely abundant in nature; thus, protein-based nanocomposites are biodegradable, biocompatible, cost-effective, and relatively easy to prepare as it involves simple protocols. Protein-based nanocomposites can be broadly divided into classes-protein nanoparticles (nanoparticles that are prepared from proteins only) and protein-conjugated nanoparticles (nanoparticles that have proteins conjugated to the nanoparticles made from sources other than proteins) [13].

Protein-based nanoparticles have been suggested as an alternative method for delivering therapeutic proteins and offer unique advantages for this purpose. Different types of proteins have been utilized in protein nanoparticle formulations, such as soy and milk proteins that are commonly consumed on a daily basis. Animal proteins such as gelatin, albumin, collagen, casein, and elastin are being used to prepare nanoparticles based on their biodegradability and biocompatibility. Moreover, many plant proteins are also used to generate nanoparticles such as Zein and whey (Fig. 2.2; [14]). Gelatin NPs have been shown to have a high degree of biocompatibility and biodegradability, making them well-suited for use in biomedical applications. In addition, the ability of gelatin NPs to cross the blood—brain barrier makes it a promising option for the treatment of brain disorders. Another advantage of using gelatin NPs is their ability to target macrophages to treat various diseases. In tissue engineering, it is used to create 3D scaffolds to produce bio-artificial tissues and organs. The wide range of applications and easy preparation make gelatin nanoparticles an attractive option for various biomedical applications [15]. Albumin-based drug delivery systems are already in the market for arthritis, diabetes, hepatitis, etc. Albumin-based nanoparticles give more control over the drug release in the biological system. Also, the small size of albumin and its ability

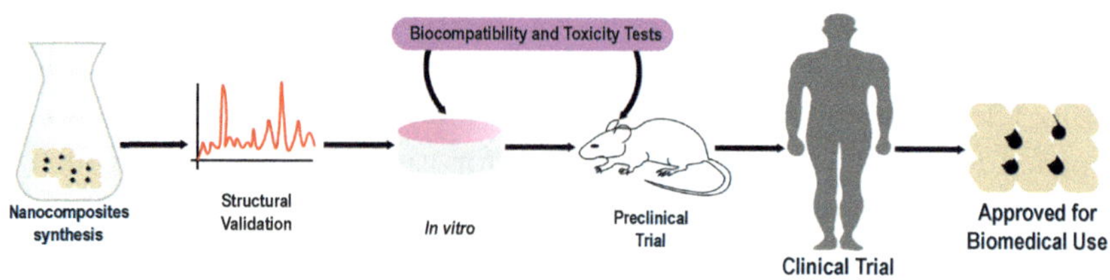

Figure 2.2 ***Schematic diagram showing the steps followed in the commercial approval of nanocomposites.*** The structures of synthesized nanoparticles are often validated by resonance and SEM. After structural validation, the biocompatibility and toxicity of nanocomposites are tested in different in vitro and in vivo settings.

to remain in circulation for a prolonged period makes it an effective carrier for delivering drugs to tumor tissues. In addition, using the EPR mechanism, which takes advantage of the enhanced permeability and retention of drugs in tumor tissue, can further increase the accumulation of drugs at the target site. This makes albumin an attractive option for targeted drug delivery in cancer therapy [15].

Collagen-based nanocomposites are widely used in bone tissue engineering. Although pure collagen is natural and biocompatible, however; it lacks osteoinductive, osteoimmunomodulatory, and antibacterial activities. Doping collagen with bioactive minerals such as $SrCrO_3$ or Ag_3PO_4 can increase in vitro cell proliferation, antibacterial activity, and tissue compatibility. Furthermore, it increases osteogenesis and osteogenic differentiation in rat bone marrow mesenchymal cells [16]. Superparamagnetic iron oxide/casein/silk fibroin nanocomposite is a tissue engineering scaffold. It has been observed that mouse embryonic cardiac cells that were seeded on the scaffold have elongated morphologies, upregulated genetic expression of GATA-4, troponin, α-myosin heavy chain, and increased cardiac cell differentiation [17]. The small size of nanocomposites and their ability to remain in circulation for an extended period makes them effective carriers for drug delivery to tumor tissues. In addition, using the EPR mechanism, which takes advantage of the enhanced permeability and retention of drugs in tumor tissue, can further increase the accumulation of drugs at the target site. This makes protein-based nanocomposites an attractive option for targeted drug delivery in cancer therapy.

3. Stabilizing agent in biological systems

Once the nanoparticles are formed, they often bind to each other, form microparticles, and lose their functional properties. To maintain their functional relevance, nanoparticles are usually prepared with stabilizers that cap the nanoparticle at the interface of nanoparticles and medium. It has been well noted that various polymeric ligands are available to stabilize the nanoparticle in aqueous dispersion [18].

3.1 PEG coating of plasmonic NPs

Polyethylene glycol (PEG) is a well-investigated and commonly used polymer in nanotechnology as it reduces protein adsorption. The pharmacokinetic studies conducted in vivo have shown that PEGylation of nanoparticles can result in an elongated circulation half-life [19]. This is typically attributed to decreased adsorption of opsonizing/serum proteins and enhanced stability of nanoparticles in blood/serum. The study has also been carried out to see a localized surface plasmon resonance (LSPR) phenomenon-based optical fiber sensor (OFS) to detect the level of dopamine. It has been well noted that dopamine plays a crucial role in the human system by acting as a neurotransmitter and hormone. The tapered fiber probe was fixed in place using silver nanoparticles (AgNPs) and modified using PEG. Due to the PEG coating, the developed sensor exhibits a wide range of selectivity in ascorbic acid oxidation. It has also been noted that it showed a varied range of detection from (10 nm–100 μM) [20]. Interestingly, it has been well recorded that D2B antibody fragments of single-chain variable showed good affinity to prostate-specific membrane antigens (PSMA) in metastatic prostate cancer (CaP) [21]. The synthesized PEGylated scFvD2B-AuNPs were tested for their biocompatibility and immunogenicity in the human blood sample. Before blood incubation, the prepared complex's physicochemical properties were accessed with the help of various techniques. Interestingly, PEG chains grafting on AuNPs-scFvD2B disallowed the binding of proteins present in blood plasma and decreased the activation level of neutrophils compared with naked AuNPs-citrate [21]. It is likely due to a hydrated negative PEG cloud shielding the nanocomposites and rendering blood compatibility with less than 10% hemolysis. It has been well noted that AuNPs-scFvD2B-PEG is biocompatible and showed favorable features for the targeted therapy of CaP, with insignificant protein adsorption affinity, minimum immunorecognition, and very low hemolytic activity [21].

3.1.1 Citrate-stabilized particles

The predominant and practical approach to coating and functionalizing plasmonic nanoparticles with PEG is thiol-terminated derivatives (PEG-SH), which can be grafted onto the surfaces of nanoparticles via covalent bonds. In the context of citrate-stabilized nanoparticles, this can be accomplished by simply stirring the solution by adding PEG-SH with the preferred molecules to the nanoparticles. After a set period, citrate ligands gradually exchange with PEG-SH, causing the formation of colloidal solutions, and were found to be highly stable in solutions of high ionic strength as well as different biological fluids [22]. For example, Holmes and colleagues [22] observed the durability of the PEGylated-Au nanoparticles under set physiological conditions (0.157 M, NaCl) using UV—visible spectroscopy and recorded that the introduction of high salt concentration minimally impacted the colloidal stability of PEG-stabilized nanoparticles. Kim and co-workers have also presented it, nanoconjugates made up of AuNPs and photosensitizers (PSs) produced by conjugation of disulphide between Chlorin e6 (Ce6) and glutathione-coated-Au nanoparticles used extensively for such studies [23]. PEGylated-lactoferrin (Lf-PEG) was also amalgamated onto the surface of AuNP for oral absorption and glioblastoma multiforme (GBM) targeting of the nanoconjugate (symbolized as Ce6—AuNP-Lf). Furthermore, it has been found that Ce6—AuNP-Lf interacts with PEGylated-lactoferrin (Lf-PEG) at the blood—brain barrier and intestinal level and recorded that penetration efficiency through these barriers was very high. In glioblastoma multiforme (GBM) mice, the oral bioavailability of Ce6—AuNP-Lf was improved. Interestingly, it has been observed that photodynamic therapy followed by photothermal therapy was effective in the treatment because of the plasmonic effect produced by Au nanoparticles to increase the ability of reactive oxygen species (ROS) generation. Consequently, GBM-phototherapy after Ce6—AuNP-Lf administration through oral mode showed an excellent antitumor property owing to increased photoconversion efficiency and GBM targeting. It has also been noted that the obtained nanoconjugates enhanced the generation of ROS through plasmonic crossover between Ce6 and AuNPs. So, nanoconjugate Ce6—AuNP-Lf could be a strong GBM phototherapeutic agent [23].

Similarly, nanovesicles of Au have strong plasmonic coupling within the nearby nanoparticles in the vesicular shell, making them possible for ultrasensitive bioimaging and biosensing. The designed multifunctional plasmonic vesicle are arranged in such a way to obtain gold nanocrystals like gold nanorods and as gold nanoparticles of amphiphilic nature. The nanocrystals were coated with hydrophobic as well as hydrophilic polymer brushes or deblock co-polymer brushes of amphiphilic nature. To justify the various necessities of its applications in biomedical sciences, various polymers, which may be, biodegradable, photoactive, or responsive to different pHs, can be utilized to obtain brushes of hydrophobic nature. In contrast, PEG retained the hydrophilic nature of the compound. This prepared nanocomposite can be used in various biomedical sciences for diagnostics, like cancer of various origins [24].

3.2 PEG coating of magnetic NPs

Magnetic nanoparticles (MNPs) have been increasingly popular in recent years for a variety of biomedical uses. Their inherent magnetic characteristics have been studied for many applications such as cell labeling, cell separation, bioassay development, drug delivery, local hyperthermia induction using an external alternating magnetic field, and targeted death of cancer cells [25]. MNPs are utilized in clinical diagnostics as a contrast agent for magnetic resonance imaging (MRI) [26].

The uncoated magnetic nanoparticles are structurally unstable and prone to aggregation due to the interface and surface effect of the nanoparticles. Once it enters the human body, the proteins absorb the magnetic nanoparticles, leading to phagocytosis by the macrophages in the vascular endothelial system and rendered useless. However, it has been well noted that after the surface modification, it can be stabilized to show improved surface functionalization. For example, when there is the coating of active material by carboxyl and hydroxyl, the obtained nanoparticles would bind with the DNA fragments, proteins, as well as drugs and perform a function like transportation and target-based therapy. Currently, various compounds like PEG that cause surface modification are available. It has been well noted that modification of the surface can increase the biocompatibility, solubility in water as well as nanoparticles stability, and owing to such properties, they can be utilized as a vector for delivery of drugs, Magnetic resonance imaging (MRI), gene transfer as well as thermotherapy. Few compounds like PEG after the surface modification showed good water solubility for magnetic NPs. Owing to this feature, good application in MRI and other biomedical examinations and treatments has been recorded [27,28].

It has also been recorded that only limited numbers of polymers are suitable for in vivo injection; however, PEG has admirable water solubility, nontoxicity, and biocompatibility. Through end-group reactivity, the PEG can bind onto the surface of the nanoparticles, drugs, biological fragments, and DNA fragments and extend the blood circulation time [29,30]. In addition, by phagocytosis, the PEG-modified ferrite NPs can enter different cells and overwhelm the release of iron ions when it is broken down in the lysosome [31]. Interestingly, the magnetic NPs have special surface modifications that can bind with the targeted cells, therefore serving as a good nanoprobe for the early tumors diagnosis.

3.3 PEG coating of quantum dots (QD)

For the synthesis of the QDs generally, a hot injection organometallic route is followed, leading to the production of hydrophobic QDs that are not soluble in water [32]. Water soluble QDs production required intensive coating methodologies. Moreover, high toxicity can be produced by coating technologies, such as QDs coated with mercaptopropionic acid (MPA). Moreover, MPA is known to be toxic, and its use in coating to make them water-soluble is not fruitful for biological purposes. It has also been well known that the water-soluble coating of QDs might also lead to a reduction in its photostability, and as compared to the bare one, a decline in luminescent intensity was observed [33]. A diagnostic system like cancer needs specific sensitivity and targeting to utilize the available nanotools as a competent diagnostic tool.

Interestingly, hydrophilic surface coating of QDs is essential to obtain water-soluble QDs. PEG is an excellent biocompatible material that is extensively used to obtain a good nanotool [34]. The conjugation of lipids with PEG can effectively generate good biocompatible QDs without losing their fluorescence intensity. The liposomal formulations are known to have hydrophilic surfaces and are efficiently observed by the live cells without any hurdle or loss. It is also noted that, owing to highly reactive functional groups, PEG-Lipid conjugates are extensively used for biofunctionalization and surface modification, helping in the conjugation of different types of antibodies, peptides, and other useful molecules for targeting the cancer cells' specificity [35,36].

3.4 PEG interaction with proteins

In the exposure of nanoparticles to biofluids having proteins, such as the serum of humans, a dense protein layer is generally absorbed on the surface of the nanoparticles [37]. Protein corona greatly impacts the stability and behavior of the nanoparticles in biological fluids. In general, the protein corona plays an important role in deciding the fate of nanoparticles in blood circulation and macrophage uptake and functionalities [38]. Therefore, the main focus should be preventing or decreasing protein corona formation. Protein adsorption is primarily dependent on the PEG grafting density. The PEG grafting density and size of the nanoparticle reduce the adsorption of different proteins present in the serum to various levels [39]. The highest PEG density was tested (1.25 PEG/nm^2), and the adsorption of protein from the serum was reduced by 94%–99% compared with citrate-stabilized Au NPs. Furthermore, it was also recorded that the density of the PEG also determines the mechanism and efficacy of further macrophage uptake. It has been well reported that with PEG density below $\sim$0.16 PEG/nm^2, the macrophage uptake is mainly dependent on the presence of adsorbed serum protein, known as serum-dependent uptake, whereas, above $\sim$0.64 PEG/nm^2, adsorbed proteins do not have any effect on the macrophage uptake.

3.5 Zwitterionic ligands

3.5.1 Zwitterionic coating of QDs

Zwitterionic coating of QDs has a great impact on the biological system. The impact of various zwitterionic surface coatings on quantum dots (QDs) on their interaction with a serum-enhanced cell medium and their uptake by human cervical cancer (HeLa) cells has also been investigated. The adsorption of protein and human serum albumin (HSA) by Zwitterionic QDs was insignificant compared with similar types but negatively charged QDs. It has been recorded that the zwitterionic QDs incorporation by the HeLa cells was lower for negatively charged QDs. Interestingly the uptake yield was large for the positively charged QDs. Various studies have indicated that suppression of excessive protein adsorption was inhibited by zwitterionic QD surfaces [40].

Recent developments have also seen an increase in the production of unique surface coatings for semiconductor QDs based on heterobifunctional ligands that overwhelm the fluorescent probes for applications in the bioimaging process. It has been well noted that QDs capped with bidentate zwitterionic dihydrolipoic acid-sulfobetaine (DHLA–SB) ligands are a good substitute for PEG-coated based nanoparticles. Moreover, they lead to very little nonspecific protein adsorption, conserve good optical properties, offer outstanding stability within a specific period, and have a wider range of pH and salinity. QDs are functionalized with different biomolecules like streptavidin and biotin without much difficulty. The streptavidin-functionalized DHLA–SB QDs were utilized to know the intracellular recycling pathway of cannabinoid receptor 1 (CB1R) within live cells of different regions. It has also been observed that QDs can selectively reorganize the pool receptors through interactions of SA–biotin with insignificant nonspecific adsorption within different cell surfaces. In addition, the activity of the cell was seemingly unaffected by the used probe [41].

Interestingly, the multi-coordinating imidazole- and zwitterion-based ligands appropriate for surface modification and functionalization of QDs are prepared, and their effects are recorded. The obtained QDs capped with different new ligands reveal good long-lasting colloidal stability toward a wider pH range, surplus electrolytes, cell-growth media, and natural reducing agents like glutathione. Zwitterion-based QDs are resistant to oxidizing agents such as H_2O_2 and have a hydrophilic coating that allows for compact dimensions. These QDs are able to self-assemble with full-size proteins and can be tagged with a polyhistidine tag through metal-histidine coordination. Furthermore, the amalgamation of amine groups permits the covalent coupling of the QDs to Dopamine. The redox-active QD platforms can be obtained and utilized for tracking pH changes and concentrations of Fe ions and cysteine via charge-transfer interactions. It has also been observed that QDs cap-exchanged with folic acid functionalized ligands might efficiently target the various cancerous cells. This is also well reported that the folate-receptor-mediated endocytosis of QDs within the living cells was concentration- and time-dependent [42].

3.5.2 Zwitterionic coating of magnetic NPs

Magnetic nanoparticles after zwitterionic coating are known to have various biological applications. Nanoparticles obtained from different oxides were used extensively for such purposes. Recently, nanoparticles obtained from manganese oxide have attracted the attention of researchers as contrast agents for MRI. The ultrasmall MnO NPs (USMnO) synthesized by a one-pot synthetic method display a far enhanced ability of T1-weighted contrast enrichment for MRI ($r1 = 15.6 \pm 0.4\ \text{mM}^{-1}\ \text{s}^{-1}$ at 0.5 T). Furthermore, the coating of zwitterionic dopamine sulfonate molecules was done, preventing nonspecific binding of serum albumin protein and its biocompatibility. Remarkably, the obtained composite with zwitterionic coating can pass across the blood—brain barrier and produce clear image of brain structures. Thus, the USMnO coated with zwitterionic dopamine sulfonate can be used to accurately identify different brain diseases, including tumors. The USMnO coated with zwitterionic dopamine sulfonate molecules has improved biocompatibility and inhibits the nonspecific binding of serum albumins.

USMnO-ZDS can penetrate the blood—brain barrier, allowing for clear imaging of anatomical brain areas using T1-weighted contrast-enhanced MRI. Our USMnO ZDS has the potential to serve as a reliable MRI contrast agent for precise and flexible diagnosis of brain tumors and various other disorders [43]. Ultrasmall Fe_3O_4 nanoparticles have been prepared after coating with zwitterion L-cysteine for improved T1-weighted magnetic resonance imaging applications. The designed Fe_3O_4-PEG-Cys NPs have good antifouling properties, hemocompatibility, and cell compatibility and might be utilized as a contrast agent for increased blood pool and MRI of tumor and cancerous cells [44].

3.5.3 *Drawbacks of zwitterionic coatings*

Poly(dimethyl siloxane) (PDMS) is commonly utilized for various biomedical applications owing to its easy fabrication, low cost, good flexibility, high durability, permeability of oxygen, as well as promising self-healing properties. However, PDMS is known to possess some major drawbacks as well. It has been reported that PDMS causes excessively very high levels of aggregation of nonspecific protein whenever used with different biological samples due to its superhydrophobic features. Unfortunately, the methods like conventional surface modification do not work properly for PDMS. This is due to their low glass transition temperature [45].

3.6 Lipid bilayer

Lipid-coated noble metal nanoparticles merge the biomimetic surface characteristics of a self-assembled lipid membrane with the plasmonic features of a nanoparticle core. Various derivatives of cholesterol and other terpenoids were studied as synthetic platforms for functionalizing lipid nanoparticles. The authors incorporated side chains of varying lengths and polarities, each containing a terminal alkyne group serving as a Raman label, into cholesterol and Betulin structures. These labels can exist in two different conformations in the lipid layer of lipid nanoparticles, known as "head-out" and "head-in" orientations. This dimorphism in tag orientation allows for orthogonal functionalities in the nanoparticle surfaces, enabling selective targeting and Raman sensing for identifying and imaging cancer cells that overexpress the epidermal growth factor receptor [46].

Because of its rapid and often asymptomatic progression, high metastatic potential, and chemoresistance, pancreatic cancer has an incredibly dismal prognosis with an 85% fatality rate. One interesting finding in the field of pancreatic cancer treatment is the use of plasmonic hollow Au-nanoshells coated with PEGylated thermosensitive lipids to co-deliver the medications bortezomib and gemcitabine (GNS-L/GB). An ammonium sulfate-driven pH gradient technique was used to load Gemcitabine into the hydrophilic interior of the porous Au nanoshells, whereas Bortezomib was loaded within the lipid bilayers. Various biological and physicochemical experiments were conducted on GNS-L/GB. These included apoptosis, cellular uptake and cytotoxicity, and western blot analyses of pancreatic cancer cell lines. The nanoshells exhibited adjustable drug release upon near-infrared laser exposure for targeted administration. GNS-L/GB exhibited synergistic cytotoxic effects and enhanced internalization by cancer cells. A high-powered near-infrared continuous wave laser with a wavelength of 808 nm successfully destroyed cancer cells through the photothermal effect of GNS-L/GB, regardless of cell type. This method showed promise in combining chemotherapy and photothermal therapy synergistically, even in cases of resistant pancreatic cancer, depending on power density, time, and GNS dose [47].

4. Biocompatibility and toxicity of protein-based nanocomposites

Protein-based nanocomposites have been used in various biomedical applications (Fig. 2.3.). Biocompatibility is important for any nanoparticles inside the biological system. Biocompatibility ensures that the biological system-nanomaterial interaction does not cause any toxic effects such as oxidative stress, macromolecular damage, mutagenesis, or apoptosis [12]. Kim and colleagues [48] have prepared nanocomposites of gelatin-derived gelatin/hydroxyapatite (HA) for the purpose of a tissue engineering platform. Due to better cell viability and lack of antigenicity, clinicians use gelatin for wound dressing and adhesive. Moreover, hydroxyapatite is bioactive and osteoconductive and can be used in bone fillers and replacements. Combining these two components in nanocomposite form gives a well-developed porous scaffold to promote blood circulation and cell growth. Similarly, collagen-based scaffolds are gaining rapid attention in bone tissue engineering. Collagen is one of the essential components of the extracellular matrix in bone tissue and is suitable in tissue engineering because of low immunogenicity and high plasticity. The cross-linking of collagen nanocomposite and hydroxyapatite with recombinant human bone morphogenetic protein-2 molecules can be used in the grafting of bone defects in weight-bearing sites [49].

Similarly, chitosan silk sericin/hydroxyapatite nanocomposites showed cytocompatibility in osteoblast cells and are promising for bone tissue

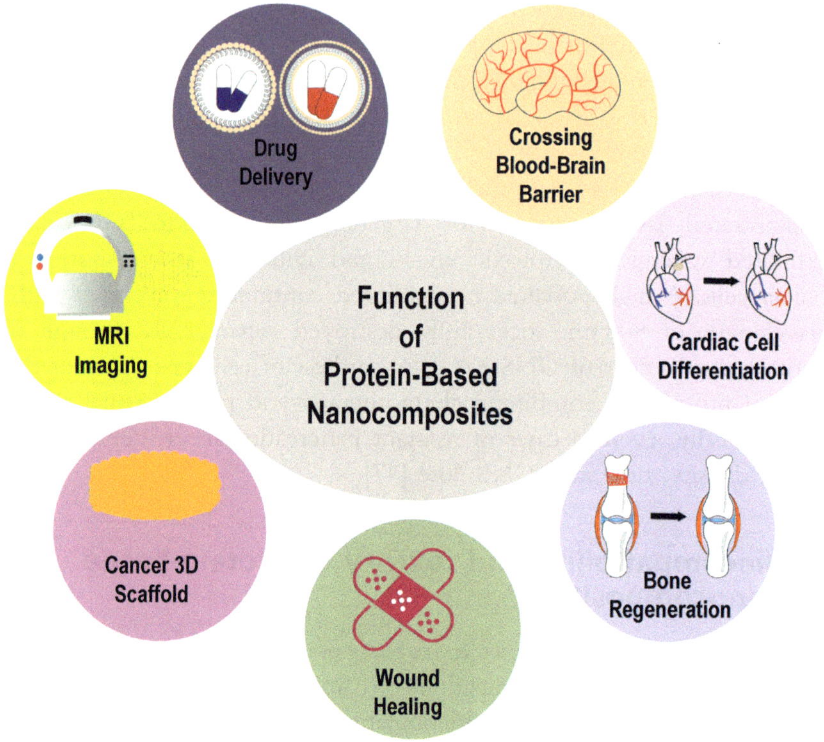

Figure 2.3 ***Different applications of protein-based nanocomposites in the biomedical field.*** The protein-based nanocomposites have found their application in drug delivery MRI, cancer, wound healing, brain blood barrier, and cardiac cell differentiation.

engineering. The chitosan-silk sericin/hydroxyapatite showed nontoxicity in the osteoblast cell lines and promoted cell growth [50]. Ahmed and co-workers [51] have reviewed the role of chitosan center scaffolds and their possible use in tissue engineering. Chitosan has three reactive functional groups that can be easily modified to create several chitosan-based derivatives and scaffolds. Carboxymethyl chitosan immobilized by alkaline phosphatase can be used to enhance the deposition of calcium by osteoblasts. Moreover, an increased cellular LAP activity was observed due to the incorporation of ALP-immobilized chitosan. In addition, chitosan-poly-L-arginine and chitosan PEG promote cell viability and prevent erythrocyte hemolysis.

Another study reported that the bio-nanocomposite scaffolds prepared by incorporating a varying percentage of zirconium in the chitosan-hydroxyapatite-wollastonite scaffold via freeze-drying method had shown zero cytotoxicity. Interestingly, the scaffold has hydrophilic components, so the scaffolds can readily absorb water. The high water absorption capacity and the nanocomposite structure give the scaffold a high degree of resemblance to the bone structure and porosity, which can be beneficial in bone tissue remodeling [52]. Mixing a small amount of graphene with silk protein to prepare a bio-nanocomposite has various benefits in biomedical applications. The biological system can easily handle a small amount of graphene and easily degrade it.

Moreover, the nanocomposite showed no change in the cellular morphology of mouse fibroblast cells even after 72 h. Moreover, graphene-silk nanocomposites showed a significant increase in cell density, supporting that a low amount of graphene mixed with silk protein helps increase cell viability. The nanocomposite can be used in various biomedical applications, including drug delivery and organ remodeling [53]. Artificial electronic skin or E-skin is lucrative tissue that can be used in various biomedical devices. Engineered silk protein hydrogel makes artificial electronic skin that resembles skin tissue and can be seamlessly interfaced with biological tissues. Moreover, piezo-electric energy-generating skin can sense biomechanical motions by harvesting biomechanical energy. Incorporating ZnO nanorods into silk protein hydrogels has piezo-electric properties, softness, deformability, and biocompatibility [54].

In another study, bacterial cellulose, a known biocompatible and natural polymer, was modified by incorporating keratin isolated from human hair to form a nanocomposite. The keratin-modified bacterial cellulose nanocomposites showed adhesion of skin fibroblasts on the bacterial cellulose surface. The protein/cellulose polymer-based nanocomposites can be a bio-artificial skin material [55]. Rad and co-workers [56] have prepared a novel composite scaffold using PCL/Zein/gum arabic, which has more than 77% porosity. The scaffold showed antibacterial properties and had a diameter suitable for biomedical applications. Moreover, the protein/polysaccharide polymers favored the proliferation of skin cells showing their good potential in artificial skin tissue engineering. The protein-based nanocomposites have enhanced biocompatibility, increased porosity, accurate hydrophobicity, and decreased toxicity.

Although in general organ engineering, it is important that nanocomposites are biocompatible and less toxic, in cancer therapy, it is acceptable for the nanocomposites to show cytotoxic properties. Nanocomposites help in precision medicine and create a tumor microenvironment to investigate the effect of drugs and drug delivery. Magnetic

Bio-metal-organic framework coated with folic acid-chitosan conjugate is a tumor-targeting nanocarrier that has shown few to zero toxicities on the biological system. Interestingly, nanocarrier loaded with drugs such as Curcumin and 5-Fluorouracil has shown selective uptake and higher toxicity in the cancer microenvironment [57]. Nanocomposites are also used in creating a bioengineered 3D cancer model. In an interesting research, Zhu and co-workers [58], integrated the 3D printer into cancer therapy. The authors created a unique 3D printer ink by suspending hydroxyapatite nanoparticles in the hydrogel. The ink helps create the bone-specific environment and investigate breast cancer bone metastasis. The 3D bone matrix was observed to mimic microenvironments of bone tumors, and breast cancer cells were allowed to grow in the 3D printed hydroxyapatite nanoparticles-based bone matrix, making it easy to understand the mechanism of breast cancer bone matrix. Hybrid self-assembling peptide (EFK8) carbon nanotube hydrogels are used to form in vitro 3D cancer spheroid and tissue engineering. The hybrid peptide hydrogels are used in studying the effect of tumor microenvironment stiffness.

Moreover, these hybrid peptides help investigate the cell-scaffold adhesion on cancer cell invasion by forming cancer cell spheroid [59]. Hydrophobic anticancer agents conjugated with solvent-based carriers are often used for many solid tumors. The development of novel delivery vehicles is crucial in addressing the dose-limiting toxicities of anticancer therapies and augmenting their antitumor efficacy. Nab-Paclitaxel is the first commercial protein nanoparticle made with 130 nm albumin-bound paclitaxel. Albumin is hydrophobic, forms noncovalent and reversible hydrophobic bonds with the substances, and can be easily transported inside the body. Phase I study of nab-Paclitaxel demonstrated that the nanocomposites do not show hypersensitivity or toxicity in the patient [60].

5. Conclusion

Tissue engineering is one of the growing interdisciplinary fields that require the inclusion of biology and technology to deliver the demand of the biomedical field. Organ failure, rejection of organ transplants by the human body, precision medicine, drug delivery, etc., requires the advancement of scaffolds that can help deliver the therapy as needed by the body. Nanotechnology has gained the interest of many researchers due to the difference in the compound's behavior and properties at the nano and bulk levels. The use of nanocomposites in tissue engineering has opened the pandora box of the biomedical fields. Researchers have begun to explore the use of protein-based nanocomposites in tissue engineering, as they have shown exceptional biomedical properties and are less toxic in biological systems. These properties make them a promising option for organ tissue engineering. In addition, protein-based nanocomposites have also been observed to serve as a carrier for cancer drugs, specifically delivering the drugs to the cancer microenvironment and helping to eliminate cancer cells. Researchers are actively developing new protein-based nanocomposites and optimizing their properties for specific applications. However, there are still challenges to be addressed before protein-based nanocomposites can be successfully clinically implemented and commercialized.

References

[1] Lanza R, Langer R, Vacanti JP, Atala A, editors. Principles of tissue engineering. Academic Press; 2020.

[2] Papalazarou V, Salmeron-Sanchez M, Machesky LM. Tissue engineering the cancer microenvironment—challenges and opportunities. Biophys Rev 2018;10(6):1695–711.

[3] Hasan A, Morshed M, Memic A, Hassan S, Webster TJ, Marei HE. Nanoparticles in tissue engineering: applications, challenges and prospects. Int J Nanomed 2018;24:5637–55.

[4] Hassan T, Salam A, Khan A, Khan SU, Khanzada H, Wasim M, et al. Functional nanocomposites and their potential applications: a review. J Polym Res 2021;28:1–22.

[5] Omanović-Mikličanin E, Badnjević A, Kazlagić A, Hajlovac M. Nanocomposites: a brief review. Health Technol 2020;10:51–9.

[6] Zhao R, Torley P, Halley PJ. Emerging biodegradable materials: starch- and protein-based bio-nanocomposites. J Mater Sci 2008;43:3058–71.

[7] Wang Z, Kang S, Cao S, Krecker M, Tsukruk VV, Singamaneni S. Protein-based functional nanocomposites. MRS Bull 2020;45(12):1017–26.

[8] Liu D, Tian H, Jia X, Zhang L. Effects of calcium carbonate polymorph on the structure and properties of soy protein-based nanocomposites. Macromol Biosci 2008;8(5):401–9.

[9] Liu H, Jian R, Chen H, Tian X, Sun C, Zhu J, et al. Application of biodegradable and biocompatible nanocomposites in electronics: current status and future directions. Nanomaterials 2019;9(7):950.

[10] Naskar A, Lee S, Ko D, Kim S, Kim KS. Bovine serum albumin-immobilized black phosphorus-based γ-Fe_2O_3 nanocomposites: a promising biocompatible nanoplatform. Biomedicines 2021;9(8):858.

[11] Liu S, Yu H, Huang K. Structural characteristics and biocompatibility of a casein-based nanocomposite for potential biomedical applications. J Mater Sci 2018;53(6):3959–71.

[12] Dara PK, Raghavankutty M, Balaraman G, Ashraf PM, Visnuvinayagam S, Tejpal CS, et al. Biocompatibility and histopathological evaluation of chitosan nanoparticles grafted fish gelatin bio-nanocomposite membranes in rats. Iran Polym J (Engl Ed) 2021;30(9):953–64.

[13] Sarkar S, Gulati K, Mishra A, Poluri KM. Protein nanocomposites: special inferences to lysozyme based nanomaterials. Int J Biol Macromol 2020;151:467–82.
[14] Kianfar E. Protein nanoparticles in drug delivery: animal protein, plant proteins and protein cages, albumin nanoparticles. J Nanobiotechnol 2021;19(1):159.
[15] Yasmin R, Shah M, Khan SA, Ali R. Gelatin nanoparticles: a potential candidate for medical applications. Nanotechnol Rev 2017;6(2):191–207.
[16] Liu H, Lin M, Liu X, Zhang Y, Luo Y, Pang Y, et al. Doping bioactive elements into a collagen scaffold based on synchronous self-assembly/mineralization for bone tissue engineering. Bioact Mater 2020;5(4):844–58.
[17] Nazari H, Heirani-Tabasi A, Hajiabbas M, Salimi Bani M, Nazari M, Pirhajati MV, et al. Incorporation of SPION-casein core-shells into silk-fibroin nanofibers for cardiac tissue engineering. J Cell Biochem 2020;121(4):2981–93.
[18] Hoffmann T, Peters D, Angioletti B, Bertoli S, Péres L, Reiter M, et al. Potentials nanocomposites in food packaging. Chem Eng Trans 2019;75.
[19] Singh D, Khan MA, Siddique HR. PLGA-based nanoparticles for the treatment of inflammatory diseases. In: Poly (lactic-co-glycolic acid)(PLGA) nanoparticles for drug delivery. Elsevier; 2023. p. 211–33.
[20] Agrawal N, Zhang B, Saha C, Kumar C, Kaushik BK, Kumar S. Development of dopamine sensor using silver nanoparticles and PEG-functionalized tapered optical fiber structure. IEEE Trans Biomed Eng 2019;67(6):1542–7.
[21] Mitri N, Rahme K, Fracasso G, Ghanem E. Human blood biocompatibility and immunogenicity of scFvD2B PEGylated gold nanoparticles. Nanotechnology 2022;33(31):315101.
[22] Rahme K, Nolan MT, Doody T, McGlacken GP, Morris MA, O'Driscoll C, et al. Highly stable PEGylated gold nanoparticles in water: applications in biology and catalysis. RSC Adv 2013;3(43):21016–24.
[23] Kim HS, Seo M, Park TE, Lee DY. A novel therapeutic strategy of multimodal nanoconjugates for state-of-the-art brain tumor phototherapy. J Nanobiotechnol 2022;20(1):14.
[24] Song J, Huang P, Chen X. Preparation of plasmonic vesicles from amphiphilic gold nanocrystals grafted with polymer brushes. Nat Protoc 2016;11(11):2287–99.
[25] Khan MA, Singh D, Ahmad A, Siddique HR. Revisiting inorganic nanoparticles as promising therapeutic agents: a paradigm shift in oncological theranostics. Eur J Pharm Sci 2021;164:105892.
[26] Sun H, Zhu X, Zhang L, Gu X, Wang J, Li J, et al. PDEA-coated magnetic nanoparticles for gene delivery to Hep G2 cells. Biotechnol Bioprocess Eng 2013;18:648–54.
[27] Corti M, Lascialfari A, Marinone M, Masotti A, Micotti E, Orsini F, et al. Magnetic and relaxometric properties of polyethylenimine-coated superparamagnetic MRI contrast agents. J Magn Magn Mater 2008;320(14):e316–9.
[28] Zhang Y, Zhang L, Song X, Gu X, Sun H, Fu C, et al. Synthesis of superparamagnetic iron oxide nanoparticles modified with MPEG-PEI via photochemistry as new MRI contrast agent. J Nanomater 2015;16(1):31.
[29] Gryparis EC, Hatziapostolou M, Papadimitriou E, Avgoustakis K. Anticancer activity of cisplatin-loaded PLGA-mPEG nanoparticles on LNCaP prostate cancer cells. Eur J Pharm Biopharm 2007;67(1):1–8.
[30] Tu Z, Zhang B, Yang G, Wang M, Zhao F, Sheng D, et al. Synthesis of poly (ethylene glycol) and poly (vinyl pyrrolidone) co-coated superparamagnetic iron oxide nanoparticle as a pH-sensitive release drug carrier. Colloids Surf A Physicochem Eng Asp 2013;436:854–61.

[31] Sui Y, Li Y, Li Y, Jin H, Zheng Y, Huang W, et al. Tumor-specific design of PEGylated gadolinium-based nanoscale particles: facile synthesis, characterization, and improved magnetic resonance imaging of metastasis lung cancer. J Photochem Photobiol B 2020;202:111669.

[32] Song EQ, Zhang ZL, Luo QY, Lu W, Shi YB, Pang DW. Tumor cell targeting using folate-conjugated fluorescent quantum dots and receptor-mediated endocytosis. Clin Chem 2009;55(5):955–63.

[33] Lee J, Ji K, Kim J, Park C, Lim KH, Yoon TH, et al. Acute toxicity of two CdSe/ZnSe quantum dots with different surface coating in Daphnia magna under various light conditions. Environ Toxicol 2010;25(6):593–600.

[34] Tong S, Hou S, Ren B, Zheng Z, Bao G. Self-assembly of phospholipid–PEG coating on nanoparticles through dual solvent exchange. Nano Lett 2011;11(9):3720–6.

[35] Al-Jamal WT, Al-Jamal KT, Tian B, Cakebread A, Halket JM, Kostarelos K. Tumor targeting of functionalized quantum dot– liposome hybrids by intravenous administration. Mol Pharm 2009;6(2):520–30.

[36] Chu M, Zhuo S, Xu J, Sheng Q, Hou S, Wang R. Liposome-coated quantum dots targeting the sentinel lymph node. J Nanopart Res 2010;12:187–97.

[37] Dobrovolskaia MA, Patri AK, Zheng J, Clogston JD, Ayub N, Aggarwal P, et al. Interaction of colloidal gold nanoparticles with human blood: effects on particle size and analysis of plasma protein binding profiles. Nanomedicine 2009;5(2):106–17.

[38] Carril M, Padro D, Del Pino P, Carrillo-Carrion C, Gallego M, Parak WJ. In situ detection of the protein corona in complex environments. Nat Commun 2017;8(1):1542.

[39] Unsworth LD, Sheardown H, Brash JL. Protein-resistant poly (ethylene oxide)-grafted surfaces: chain density-dependent multiple mechanisms of action. Langmuir 2008;24(5):1924–9.

[40] Ashraf S, Park J, Bichelberger MA, Kantner K, Hartmann R, Maffre P, et al. Zwitterionic surface coating of quantum dots reduces protein adsorption and cellular uptake. Nanoscale 2016;8(41):17794–800.

[41] Muro E, Pons T, Lequeux N, Fragola A, Sanson N, Lenkei Z, et al. Small and stable sulfobetaine zwitterionic quantum dots for functional live-cell imaging. J Am Chem Soc 2010;132(13):4556–7.

[42] Wang W, Ji X, Kapur A, Zhang C, Mattoussi H. A multifunctional polymer combining the imidazole and zwitterion motifs as a biocompatible compact coating for quantum dots. J Am Chem Soc 2015;137(44):14158–72.

[43] Wei R, Liu K, Zhang K, Fan Y, Lin H, Gao J. Zwitterion-coated ultrasmall MnO nanoparticles enable highly sensitive T 1-weighted contrast-enhanced brain imaging. ACS Appl Mater Interfaces 2022;14(3):3784–91.

[44] Ma D, Chen J, Luo Y, Wang H, Shi X. Zwitterion-coated ultrasmall iron oxide nanoparticles for enhanced T 1-weighted magnetic resonance imaging applications. J Mater Chem B 2017;5(35):7267–73.

[45] Keefe AJ, Brault ND, Jiang S. Suppressing surface reconstruction of superhydrophobic PDMS using a superhydrophilic zwitterionic polymer. Biomacromolecules 2012;13(5):1683–7.

[46] An X, Majumder A, McNeely J, Yang J, Puri T, He Z, et al. Interfacial hydration determines orientational and functional dimorphism of sterol-derived Raman tags in lipid-coated nanoparticles. Proc Natl Acad Sci U S A 2021;118(33). e2105913118.

[47] Poudel BK, Gupta B, Ramasamy T, Thapa RK, Pathak S, Oh KT, et al. PEGylated thermosensitive lipid-coated hollow gold nanoshells for effective combinational chemo-photothermal therapy of pancreatic cancer. Colloids Surf B Biointerfaces 2017;160:73–83.

[48] Kim HW, Kim HE, Salih V. Stimulation of osteoblast responses to biomimetic nanocomposites of gelatin–hydroxyapatite for tissue engineering scaffolds. Biomaterials 2005;26(25):5221–30.
[49] Itoh S, Kikuchi M, Koyama Y, Takakuda K, Shinomiya K, Tanaka J. Development of a hydroxyapatite/collagen nanocomposite as a medical device. Cell Transplant 2004;13(4):451–62.
[50] Chen L, Hu J, Ran J, Shen X, Tong H. A novel nanocomposite for bone tissue engineering based on chitosan–silk sericin/hydroxyapatite: biomimetic synthesis and its cytocompatibility. RSC Adv 2015;5(69):56410–22.
[51] Ahmed S, Ali A, Sheikh J. A review on chitosan centred scaffolds and their applications in tissue engineering. Int J Biol Macromol 2018;116:849–62.
[52] Maghsoudlou MA, Nassireslami E, Saber-Samandari S, Khandan A. Bone regeneration using bio-nanocomposite tissue reinforced with bioactive nanoparticles for femoral defect applications in medicine. Avicenna J Med Biotechnol (AJMB) 2020;12(2):68.
[53] Wang F, Aravind SJ, Wu H, Forys J, Venkataraman V, Ramanujachary K, et al. Tunable green graphene-silk biomaterials: mechanism of protein-based nanocomposites. Mater Sci Eng C Mater Biol Appl 2017;79:728–39.
[54] Gogurla N, Roy B, Kim S. Self-powered artificial skin made of engineered silk protein hydrogel. Nano Energy 2020;77:105242.
[55] Keskin Z, Urkmez AS, Hames EE. Novel keratin modified bacterial cellulose nanocomposite production and characterization for skin tissue engineering. Mater Sci Eng C Mater Biol Appl 2017;75:1144–53.
[56] Rad ZP, Mokhtari J, Abbasi M. Fabrication and characterization of PCL/zein/gum arabic electrospun nanocomposite scaffold for skin tissue engineering. Mater Sci Eng C Mater Biol Appl 2018;93:356–66.
[57] Nejadshafiee V, Naeimi H, Goliaei B, Bigdeli B, Sadighi A, Dehghani S, et al. Magnetic bio-metal–organic framework nanocomposites decorated with folic acid conjugated chitosan as a promising biocompatible targeted theranostic system for cancer treatment. Mater Sci Eng C Mater Biol Appl 2019;99:805–15.
[58] Zhu W, Holmes B, Glazer RI, Zhang LG. 3D printed nanocomposite matrix for the study of breast cancer bone metastasis. Nanomedicine 2016;12(1):69–79.
[59] Sheikholeslam M, Wheeler SD, Duke KG, Marsden M, Pritzker M, Chen P. Peptide and peptide-carbon nanotube hydrogels as scaffolds for tissue & 3D tumor engineering. Acta Biomater 2018;69:107–19.
[60] De Luca R, Profita G, Cicero G. Nab-paclitaxel in pretreated metastatic breast cancer: evaluation of activity, safety, and quality of life. OncoTargets Ther 2019;2:1621.

CHAPTER 3

Advantages and limitations/challenges of protein-based nanocomposite

Khalid Umar[1], Tabassum Parveen[2], Showkat Ahmad Bhawani[3], Jayanudin[4], Mohd Jameel[5] and M. Hazwan Hussin[1]

[1]School of Chemical Sciences, Universiti Sains Malaysia, Penang, Malaysia; [2]Department of Botany, Aligarh Muslim University, Aligarh, Uttar Pradesh, India; [3]Faculty of Resource Science and Technology, Universiti Malaysia Sarawak (UNIMAS), Kota Samarahan, Sarawak, Malaysia; [4]Department of Chemical Engineering, Universitas Sultan Ageng Tirtayasa, Banten, Indonesia; [5]Molecular Cancer Genetics & Translational Research Laboratory, Section of Genetics, Department of Zoology, Aligarh Muslim University, Aligarh, Uttar Pradesh, India

1. Introduction

Composites are made by combining different materials with different properties to create a new material with unique properties. The system consists of a matrix and reinforcement, each having its functions [1,2]. The matrix protects the reinforcement, while the reinforcement strengthens and rigidifies the composite. Pretreatment is needed to employ the nano-bridging technique in polymer composites since different reinforcement materials are used [2]. Composites can be classed as macro-, micro-, or nanocomposites based on reinforcing scale. The high surface-to-volume ratio of nanocomposites with reinforcing phases smaller than 100 nm makes them exceptional. These materials are used in engineering, plastics, rubber, coatings, adhesives, electronics, and optics. The increased use of nano-composites has raised environmental concerns about their slow decomposition. To solve these issues, nanocomposite components made from renewable materials such as vegetable oils, cellulose, starch, proteins, and more are being developed [2]. Composites with bio-renewable matrix and reinforcing are available. Biorenewable nanocomposites should be biocompatible, biodegradable, low-density, cost-effective, and adaptable [3]. However, they may demonstrate reduced thermal, mechanical, and chemical stability in comparison with petroleum-based alternatives, which

Protein-Based Nanocomposites for Tissue Engineering
ISBN 978-0-323-99357-9
https://doi.org/10.1016/B978-0-323-99357-9.00008-9

restricts their extensive utilization in industry [4,5]. Although they have limits, nanocomposites made from renewable resources (bio-nanocomposites) could offer a more ecologically sustainable option compared with composites manufactured from petroleum. It includes bio-nanocomposites based on protein such as dairy protein, soybean protein, and gelatin that serve essential functions from extending the food shelf life to enhancing food quality. This section will provide a comprehensive analysis of the chemistry, structure, benefits, and drawbacks of nano-composites derived from protein-based materials.

2. Protein-based nanocomposites: Fundamentals and preparation

2.1 Structural characteristics of protein for nanocomposites

The classification of proteins as biopolymers stems from their intricate primary and secondary structures, offering a broad spectrum of properties that render them ideal for developing innovative nanocomposites. These naturally occurring biopolymers are sourced from various outlets, including plants, microbes, and animals [6]. Their abundance and scalability make them promising for widespread and practical applications.

The amphiphilic nature and highly flexible chains of proteins contribute to their ability to undergo diverse modifications and establish specific interactions with synthetic materials. Recent advancements in material manufacturing techniques have enabled the precise manipulation of proteins' secondary and tertiary architectures. This control facilitates the arrangement of proteins into various configurations, enhancing their distinct characteristics and efficacy for use in nanocomposites. The resulting nanocomposites exhibit enhanced features, unique capabilities, and a reduced environmental impact [7]. To address the challenges posed by the low water solubility, weak physicochemical stability, and poor oral bioavailability of these bioactive ingredients, encapsulation technology utilizing diverse nanocarriers (Fig. 3.1) becomes crucial. This technology enhances the compatibility of these ingredients with the food matrix while improving their stability and bioavailability. Such challenges make it difficult to fortify bioactive ingredients into food products [9–11].

Protein structures comprise individual polypeptides, serving as the fundamental building blocks. These polypeptides consist of specific amino acids arranged in a manner crucial for diverse biological functions. Cellular processes, namely transcription and translation, generate macromolecules by

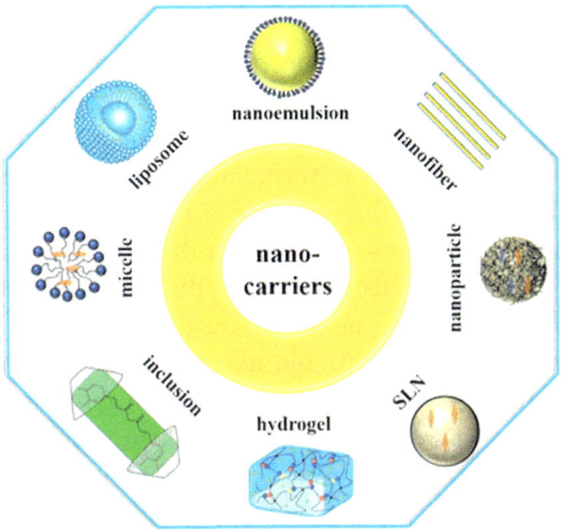

Figure 3.1 Nanocarriers suitable for food applications containing bioactive compounds [8].

forming lengthy chains linked through amide bonds. The hierarchical organization of these chains varies, ranging from large-scale to atomic structures, depending on the protein's origin. Proteins exhibit primary, secondary, tertiary, and quaternary structures determined by interactions such as hydrogen bonding, resulting in distinct structures like alpha-helices, beta-sheets, and beta-turns. Each structure plays a pivotal role in defining the protein's functionality and potential incorporation into nanocomposites.

The capability of proteins to enhance mechanical properties in nanocomposites stems from their structural flexibility and various inter- and intrachain interactions. For instance, protein fibers serve as reinforcement components, effectively transmitting loads and mediating stress to enhance mechanical characteristics. The presence of interfacial solid contacts between proteins and inorganic materials significantly amplifies reinforcing effects, leading to a substantial improvement in mechanical strength. Moreover, the structural flexibility of proteins facilitates the elongation and reorganization of polypeptide chains. This phenomenon enhances the energy absorption capacity, decelerates crack propagation, and prevents material failure [7]. The inherent characteristics and structural attributes of proteins, coupled with their ability to adopt various conformations and undergo shape modifications, make them highly suitable for fabricating nanocomposites with enhanced mechanical properties applicable across various domains.

2.2 Preparative methods and techniques

Bionanocomposites are formulations combining organic and inorganic elements, with the inorganic components referred to as nanofillers, typically featured in biorenewable nanocomposites. Nanofillers are categorized based on their dimensional structure, including one-dimensional linear, two-dimensional layered, and three-dimensional powder forms. Integrating nanofillers with a size below 100 nm into the polymer matrix allows for modifying composite material properties. Bionanocomposites comprise a polymer matrix, nanofillers, and an interaction zone [12], attracting significant attention from academia and industry. Adding a small quantity of nanofillers to polymer-based nanocomposites can result in improved mechanical properties, increased strength, and elastic stiffness. These nanocomposites may also exhibit exceptional attributes such as heightened electrical and optical resilience, enhanced durability, superior flame retardancy, and magnetic characteristics [13]. Manufacturing bionanocomposites primarily involves established procedures for processing plastics or composite materials. Various processing approaches aim to achieve a homogeneous and consistent dispersion of nanoparticles or nanofibers within the polymer matrix [14]. However, the challenge lies in achieving an accurate distribution of nanofillers within the polymer matrix, as they tend to aggregate and form clusters on a micron scale. This uneven dispersion of nanofillers within the polymer matrix decreases the properties of renewable nanocomposites. Extensive literature focuses on creating bionanocomposites, utilizing different combinations and processes specifically designed for each combination. One of the methods used is solution intercalation. As described by Zhao et al. (2008), solution intercalation operates within a solvent system where the bio-polymer or bio-prepolymer, like starch or protein, is soluble, and its inorganic nanofillers, commonly silicate platelets, are capable of expanding [15]. The layered silicate undergoes swelling in solvents such as water, chloroform, or toluen. Still, when the bio-polymer mixes with the solution of swollen nanoparticles, the polymer chains begin to intercalate, displacing the solvent from the interlayer spaces of the silicate. The resulting structure retains the intercalated arrangement after the removal of the solvent, leading to the formation of a bio-polymer/layered silicate bio-nanocomposite [16]. In situ, intercalative polymerization is also crucial for producing nanocomposites from biorenewable materials. This method entails the expansion of nanofillers into a liquid monomer or a monomer with low molecular weight. This results in the creation of a polymer within the interlayers of the nanofillers. Polymerization can be initiated by introducing an organic initiator or by inducing heat through cationic substitution within the layers prior to swelling with the monomer. In situ, intercalative polymerization is more effective than other procedures because it results in superior exfoliation.

Furthermore, it permits the integration of responsive and catalytically active organometallic entities into numerous strata of nanofillers. These species can interact with the monomer matrix, resulting in polymerization within the porous layers [16]. This approach was originally utilized for creating nylon-montmorillonite nanocomposites, but it has since been applied to produce a wide range of thermoplastics and thermoset nanocomposites. A flowchart showing an in situ intercalative polymerization is presented in Fig. 3.2.

Melt intercalation has gained recognition for its straightforwardness and efficiency, emerging as the established technique for producing polymer/ layered silicate bio-nanocomposites. This method entails heating a polymer to the requisite temperature, transforming it into a liquid state, and directly blending it with nanoparticles to ensure their even distribution within the polymer matrix. Typically conducted within an extruder, this process involves melting a high molecular weight polymer matrix at elevated temperatures and combining it with nanofillers to achieve a uniform composite structure [17]. The success of dispersion hinges on the compatibility between nanofillers and the polymer matrix, surface modifications of the

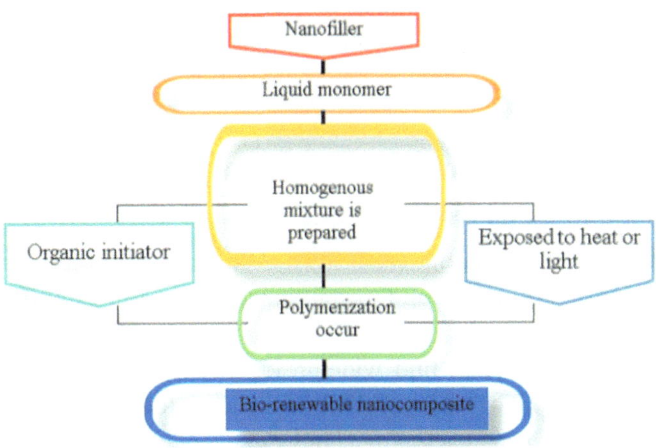

Figure 3.2 Flowchart of an in situ intercalative polymerization [16].

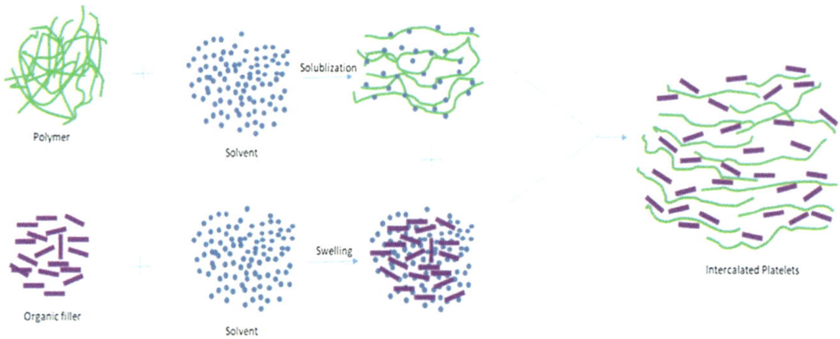

Figure 3.3 Melt-intercalation method [19].

nanofillers, and the specific processing conditions employed. In this operation, the molten polymer matrix infiltrates the nanofiller spaces, determining the formation of an intercalated or an exfoliated hybrid structure based on how effectively the polymer matrix disperses into the nanofillers [18]. Fig. 3.3 illustrates the melt-intercalation method.

The melt-mixing technique is exclusively applicable to thermoplastics, a requirement well-matched by proteins such as soy, wheat gluten, corn zein, caseinate, whey, and gelatin. Previously unsuitable polymers can now be used with the melt intercalation method, which was not feasible with in situ polymerization or the solution intercalation method. This method proves to be versatile and environmentally friendly as it does not depend on solvents for synthesizing nanocomposites. Its compatibility with various processes in the polymer industry, like extrusion, blending, and injection molding, renders it cost-effective and adaptable. Nonetheless, a notable drawback is its reliance on high temperatures, potentially leading to nanofiller surface modification degradation [19,20].

3. Nanomaterials incorporation in protein matrices

3.1 Metal and metal oxide nanoparticles

The advancement of various sectors has been driven by the unique functional properties of metal and metal oxide nanoparticles (NPs). Nanostructures like zinc oxide (ZnO-NPs), titanium dioxide (TiO_2-NPs), and copper oxide (CuO-NPs) find widespread applications, particularly in the food industry [21]. They are crucial in enhancing food quality, prolonging shelf life, and improving packaging. They can even function as gas sensors for toxin detection. These nanoparticles offer superior mechanical durability, antibacterial features, oxygen removal capacity, and enzyme fixation, extending storage duration and fortifying food resilience against external factors [22]. Various synthesis techniques are employed for these nanoparticles, including green synthesis, sol—gel processes, microwave radiation, and chemical reduction, among others, as outlined by Shkodenko et al. (2020). Zinc oxide nanoparticles (ZnO-NPs), recognized for their antimicrobial properties and low toxicity, are particularly valuable in the food industry due to their ability to exhibit UV-blocking characteristics at a reasonable cost [23]. Research by Petchwattana et al. (2016) indicates their effectiveness in inhibiting the growth of pathogens like Escherichia coli and *Staphylococcus aureus*. Consequently, integrating these nanoparticles into active materials enhances optical, thermal, mechanical, and physicochemical capabilities, although concerns exist regarding potential toxicological characteristics compared with bulk forms [24—26]. Incorporating these nanoparticles into protein-based applications significantly impacts attributes such as barrier functions, water resistance, antibacterial activity, mechanical strength, and thermal stability. Fig. 3.4 shows the synthesis of NP(Nanoparticles)/PU(Polyurethane) foam composites using ex situ-synthesized NPs.

3.2 Layered nonmetal nanomaterials

Layered nanomaterials, also known as two-dimensional nanomaterials (2DNMs), have garnered significant attention across various fields due to

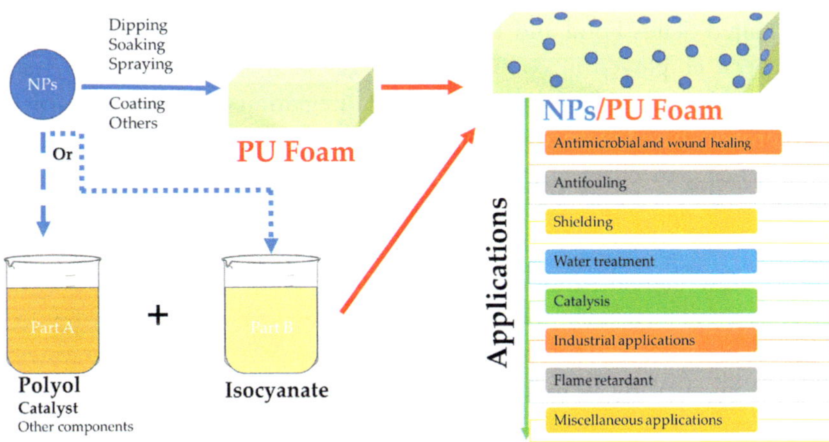

Figure 3.4 Illustrate the development of NP (Nanoparticles)/PU (Polyurethane) foam composites using ex situ-synthesized NPs and showcase their applications through a schematic representation [27].

their unique attributes, including high electron transfer rates, mechanical strength, biocompatibility, and light absorption [21]. In the food industry, nonmetal layered materials such as graphene, graphene oxide (GO), nanoclays like montmorillonite (MMT), graphitic carbon nitride (g-C_3N_4), silica nanoparticles (SiO_2-NPs), and black phosphorene (BP) are frequently utilized. These materials enhance antimicrobial activity, mechanical strength, barrier properties, and thermal stability in packaging films [25–31]. Despite having only a few thick atomic layers, 2DNMs offer substantial surface areas and advantageous contact points due to their interaction with proteins, enhancing physical and chemical characteristics [25,30]. A notable example is graphene, which possesses exceptional qualities such as specific surface area, mechanical stiffness, and electron mobility. Graphene becomes a valuable agent for improving thermal, mechanical, and barrier properties when coupled with biopolymers. Graphene oxide (GO), a derivative of graphene, has been successfully incorporated into various food packaging materials, including SPI [32], cellulose paper [33], chitosan [34], and gelatin [35]. Research indicates substantial enhancements in these composite films' durability, tensile strength, and barrier properties. Kumar et al. (2010) incorporated MMT into SPI, resulting in improved thermal stability and reduced water sensitivity, leading to more robust and durable films. Combining silicate clay like MMT with SPI/polyvinyl alcohol (PVA) forms composite films exhibiting enhanced tensile strength, improved thermal stability, and decreased water sensitivity [36]. Biocompatible and biodegradable SiO_2-NPs, recognized by the United States Food and Drug Administration (FDA) as cost-effective, have been employed in composite materials such as chitosan [28,37] and cellulose [38]. Overall, the utilization and integration of these nanoparticles into protein-based matrices of stacked nanomaterials show promising results in enhancing mechanical, barrier, and antibacterial characteristics.

3.3 Natural nanocomposites

Only a few natural nanomaterials exhibit biocompatibility and biological advantages in nanoscale materials. Due to their distinctive characteristics, Chitosan nanostructures and cellulose nanocrystals (CNCs) are extensively applied, particularly in food applications. When incorporated into various composite films, CNCs have shown promising outcomes. A study employing CNCs mixed with Zein/Catechin/β-Cyclodextrin revealed biodegradable films with reduced water vapor permeability (WVP), increased tensile strength, and elongation at break [21]. These composite films effectively prevented the oxidation of soybean oil and significantly reduced its moisture content [39]. Adding CNCs to SPI films significantly enhanced their tensile strength, surpassing unmodified SPI films. Notably, these films exhibited reduced water vapor permeability, indicating enhanced resistance to moisture infiltration. Vahedikia et al. (2019) discovered that incorporating cinnamon essential oil (CEO) and chitosan nanoparticles (CNPs) into zein-based biodegradable films enhanced their mechanical properties compared with films composed entirely of zein [40]. Although the films created by the CEO-CNPs did not exhibit antibacterial properties against specific microorganisms, they demonstrated reduced water vapor permeability, improved tensile strength, and lower elongation at the fracture point, suggesting uniform dispersion of CNPs across the films [40]. Adding functionalized nano-silica to nanocomposite biodegradable films made of SPI infused with CNFs enhanced tensile strength and decreased water vapor permeability compared with films without additives. Incorporating cellulose nanofibrils and nano-silica improved thermal degradation and reduced moisture content, as demonstrated by Qin et al. in 2019. In a distinct study, Zhao et al. (2021) documented the manufacturing process of SPI/cotton nanocrystalline cellulose (C-NCC) films. The addition of C-NCC significantly enhanced the films' gas barrier properties, water sensitivity, and mechanical properties, with the most significant benefits observed at a 7% C-NCC content [15]. These findings underscore the potential of natural nanomaterials like chitosan nanostructures, CNCs, CNFs, and cellulose-based nanomaterials to enhance the mechanical strength, barrier properties, and moisture resistance of biodegradable films used in food packaging. However, the efficacy of these materials often hinges on their concentration and interaction within the film matrix—the classification of natural nanocomposite, as shown in Fig. 3.5.

4. Properties of protein-based nanocomposites

4.1 Mechanical strength

Improving the mechanical properties of protein-based polymers is crucial, as they often exhibit less favorable characteristics compared with synthetic polymers. Key properties, including tensile strength, elongation at break, and Young's Modulus, need enhancement. These mechanical attributes are influenced by factors such as inherent polymer properties, production

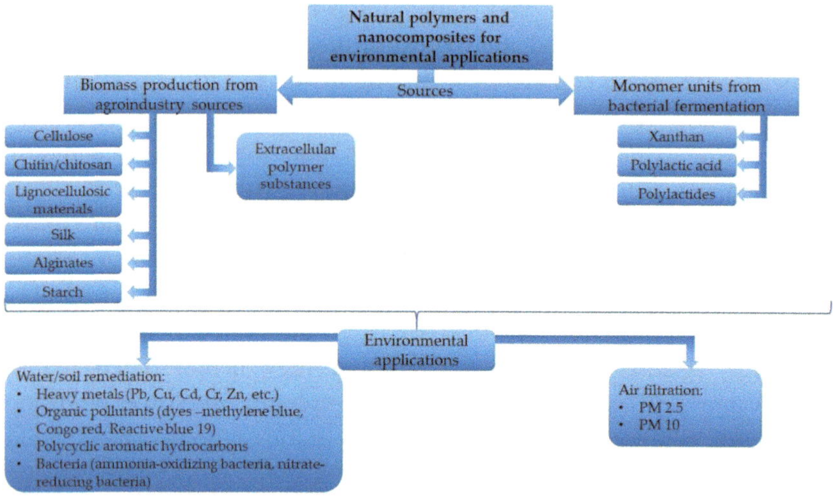

Figure 3.5 Leverage natural polymers and nanocomposites for environmental applications [41].

methods, and composition. Various protein polymers derived from plants (e.g., soy protein, zein maize, and wheat gluten) and animals (e.g., gelatin, casein, and whey protein) find widespread use, particularly in the production of edible films. Ideal polymers are achieved through the development of protein-based nanocomposites, wherein reinforcing nanomaterials like nanoparticles or nanofibers are incorporated into the protein matrix. This integration serves to enhance mechanical strength and durability, thereby influencing key properties such as tensile strength, modulus, and toughness. Inorganic nanomaterials, such as silicate layers or nanoclays like MMT, are frequently utilized to fortify protein-based nanocomposites. Metal oxide nanoparticles, including ZnO and TiO_2, have also been explored for their potential to enhance mechanical strength. Tang et al. (2019) demonstrated the efficacy of ZnO nanoparticles in strengthening films made from SPI [42]. In addition, cellulosic nanoparticles, as natural nanomaterials, play a vital role in reinforcing plant protein-based films. Innovative methods involve modifying the surface and enhancing functionality at the nanoparticle interface to improve mechanical characteristics further. Researchers continue to focus on integrating nanomaterials to advance the mechanical properties of protein-based polymers.

4.2 Barrier properties: Water vapor permeability

Various organic and inorganic nanomaterials have undergone testing to evaluate their impact on water vapor permeability (WVP) in protein-based applications. Nanomaterials such as cloisite Na^+ and MMT are commonly employed to enhance the water resistance of corrosive applications. These nanoclays create tight channels for air molecules, diminishing the passage of water vapor through coatings containing proteins [21]. Nevertheless, the influence of metal oxide nanoparticles on the water vapor permeability of plant protein-based films may differ. Higher concentrations of nanoparticles can lead to increased fragmentation and fluctuations in protein chains, consequently creating more pathways for water vapor transmission. For instance, studies indicate that cellulose nanocrystals (CNCs), as natural nanomaterials, significantly boost the water resistance of plant protein films, resulting in a reduction in WVP by over 60% [39]. Cellulosic nanoparticles have also been successfully incorporated into SPI and wheat gluten, both contributing to improved water resistance [43].

Furthermore, El-Wakil et al.'s (2015) research demonstrates that the incorporation of wheat gluten/nanocellulose/TiO_2 nanocomposites into active food packaging materials substantially enhances the barrier properties of the film for food packaging applications. Homogeneous nanomaterials have shown notable improvements in water resistance as well. For instance, with a CNC content of 12.5%, the WVP was reduced to 1.02×10^{-9} g (measured in meters per kilopascal per second). It highlights the influence of varying nanomaterial levels on water vapor permeability, underscoring the potential applications of bionanocomposites [44].

4.3 Antimicrobial and antioxidant properties

Active films, incorporating antimicrobials, are employed in the preservation of food during storage and transportation, particularly those based on plant proteins. Two categories of active nanocomposites exist. The first comprises nanostructured materials, such as metal oxide nanoparticles (NPs), which function as controlled drugs and antimicrobials [21]. Zinc oxide (ZnO), titanium dioxide (TiO_2), and silver (Ag) are frequently utilized in plant protein-based films due to their antibacterial properties. Research indicates that the incorporation of nanoparticles, such as ZnO-NPs, into films may hinder bacterial growth, the extent of which depends on the concentration [45,46]. For instance, Tang et al. (2019) observed that SPI films containing ZnO-NPs at specific concentrations significantly inhibited the development of *E. coli* and *S. aureus* bacteria [42]. While droplets of added carbon displayed antibacterial activity in the presence of microorganisms, no bactericidal effect was observed. According to research, two types of nanomaterials can be combined with proteins to produce different effects:

one type acts as an antibiotic, while the other serves as a reinforcing additive [47]. Xiao et al. (2020) successfully produced films with enhanced bactericidal activity against tested microorganisms by combining two different nanomaterials, CNCs and ZnO-NPs [43]. In addition, some films utilize chemical methods to activate antibacterial agents while employing nanoparticles to enhance their potency. In wheat gluten films containing titanium dioxide nanoparticles (TiO_2-NPs) and CNCs, exposure to UV light resulted in reduced bacteria presence, showcasing the collaborative effect of chemical additives and metal oxide nanoparticles [48].

The composition of bacterial cell walls influences the efficacy of these active nanocomposite films against gram-negative bacteria. Gram-positive bacteria exhibit increased resistance due to their larger, multilayered peptidoglycan cell walls, preventing nanoparticle entry. Plant protein-based nanocomposite films utilize nanoparticles to enhance strength and serve as controlled-release vehicles for antibacterial agents. Interactions between constituents provide potential strategies for regulating the release and effectiveness of antimicrobial agents in these films, influencing polymer chain motion and the dispersion of active compounds.

4.4 Thermal stability

Protein-based applications are typically evaluated for their thermal properties by utilizing methods like differential scanning calorimetry and thermogravimetric analysis. Cellulose nanostructures, specifically CNC and CN, have shown some significant improvements in the thermal properties of plant protein-based materials. Their addition increased the temperature at which disintegration happens. It altered the temperature at which the protein backbone degrades, indicating that there are improvements in resistance to heat by forming a more compact film structure [43]. The incorporation of MMT also yielded comparable results since the distributed MMT layers acted as insulating agents. Consequently, this resulted in an enhanced route for the spread of combustion gas, ultimately elevating the temperature at which the films began to deteriorate. Other studies have also demonstrated that by incorporating GO-NPs [49] and Chitosan NPs [50,51] into zein-based films, they are able to enhance their thermal resistance. This is because the nanoparticles are able to establish interactions with the zein molecules, thereby enhancing the overall stability of the films. However, with the addition of certain nanomaterials, such as lignin NPs and peanut protein NPs, it could be seen that it improved only the thermal stability of wheat gluten and SPI films, respectively. The study conducted by Tang et al. (2019) again discovered that zinc oxide nanoparticles (ZnO-NPs) and the research conducted by Han and Wang (2016) on silicon dioxide nanoparticles (SiO_2-NPs) have demonstrated the ability to improve the strength of films composed of SPI by establishing a stronger connection with the SPI matrix [34,42]. This diminishes the motion of protein chains and amplifies the film's resilience to high temperatures. Various categories of nanomaterials have generally exhibited favorable results in enhancing the thermal properties of proteins. The observed enhancements are attributed to increased interactions within the structure, reduced protein chain mobility, and improved bonding between the nanoparticles and the protein matrix.

5. Advantages of protein-based nanocomposites

5.1 Enhanced mechanical properties

Protein-based nanocomposites represent a promising field of research, capitalizing on the advantageous characteristics of both nanotechnology and proteins [52]. Lysozyme, a protein known for its multifunctional aspects, structural stability, and ease of production, has gained significant attention in biomedical applications [52]. Its versatility has led to the creation of nanocomposites either entirely composed of lysozyme or formed through their conjugation with other materials, underscoring its significance in biotechnological applications [52].

In the realm of tissue engineering, researchers have explored the synthesis of chitosan-sodium alginate (CS) nanocomposites incorporating zirconia nanoparticles [53]. These biomimetic nanocomposite scaffolds exhibited enhanced mechanical properties, with different weight percentages of zirconia nanoparticles influencing the physico-chemical and thermal behavior of the scaffolds [53]. The interaction between zirconia nanoparticles, chitosan, and sodium alginate resulted in a biocompatible scaffold suitable for tissue engineering applications [53].

Graphene oxide, renowned for its extensive surface area and interaction with proteins and peptides, has been incorporated into nanocomposites to optimize scaffold architectures in tissue engineering [54]. The review highlights the physiochemical and biological features of graphene oxide in protein-based nanocomposites, discussing its impact on protein conformation and structural stability [54]. Exploring nanocomposite bioconjugates reveals their positive effects on cell viability, proliferation, and the formation of new and functional tissue [54]. Inspired by the hierarchical architecture of nacre, a hybrid protein polymer incorporating graphene oxide and nanofibrillated cellulose demonstrated improved mechanical properties, acting as a spacer molecule to tune ion sorption and transport [54]. This protein-mediated binding of nanofibrillated cellulose and reduced graphene oxide reduced internal resistance, rendering it suitable for flexible electronic devices [55].

In the study investigating protein conformational changes on nanocomposites, Discosoma recombinant red fluorescent proteins adhered to silver nanoparticles exhibited distinct conformations identified through surface-enhanced Raman scattering (SERS) [56]. The study's originality lies in exploring dehydrated protein layers and achieving a strong electromagnetic field enhancement, enabling the detection of Raman signals from discontinuous protein layers [56]. The findings confirm the reversible and dynamic nature of the relationship between protein structure and function, highlighting the potential for mechanically modulating protein-based nanocomposites [56].

5.2 Biocompatibility and biofunctionality

Protein-based nanocomposites, situated at the intersection of nanotechnology and protein science, have gained significant attention, particularly for their distinctive merits in the realms of biocompatibility and biofunctionality [52]. The protein lysozyme, known for its multifaceted properties such as antibacterial, anti-inflammatory, anti-cancer, and analgesic attributes, emerges as a focal point in diverse biomedical applications, owing to its ease of production, modifiability, and structural stability [52]. This section explores key instances where the biocompatibility and biofunctionality of protein-based nanocomposites, with an emphasis on lysozyme, have been harnessed for various applications. In the domain of tissue engineering, the synthesis of chitosan-sodium alginate (CS) nanocomposites utilizing zirconia nanoparticles serves as an illustrative example of enhanced biocompatibility [53]. Through a comprehensive analysis of physicochemical and thermal behaviors, the interaction between zirconia nanoparticles and the chitosan-sodium alginate matrix is elucidated, resulting in biomimetic nanocomposite scaffolds with superior biocompatibility [53]. Moreover, the incorporation of zirconia nanoparticles at specific weight percentages enhances the bioactivity of the scaffolds, showcasing their potential for interactions with proteins in simulated body fluid and phosphate-buffered saline [53]. Addressing the urgent need for effective

COVID-19 diagnostics, a novel on-site testing method employing spike protein-conjugated quantum dot (QD) nanotags in a lateral flow immunoassay is proposed [57]. The advanced silica-core@dual QD-shell nanocomposites not only exhibit superior luminescence and stability but also underscore their biofunctionality in ensuring high sensitivity and reliability for detecting SARS-CoV-2-specific IgM and IgG in human serum [57]. This application highlights the critical role of nanocomposites in the rapid and accurate identification of infected individuals, emphasizing their potential in diagnostics and disease monitoring [57]. The integration of graphene oxide and proteins in nanocomposites has revolutionized the landscape of bioengineered tissues and organs [54]. Leveraging graphene oxide's substantial surface area and interaction with proteins, these nanocomposites exhibit enhanced biofunctionality, particularly in applications ranging from skin to cardiac tissue engineering [54]. The incorporation of protein-graphene oxide structures as nanocomposites or complexes demonstrates their positive impact on cell viability and proliferation, showcasing their potential functionality in the development of new and functional tissue [54]. Inspired by the hierarchical architecture of nacre, a hybrid protein polymer incorporating graphene oxide and nanofibrillated cellulose demonstrates remarkable biofunctionality [55]. Acting as a spacer molecule, this protein complex tunes ion sorption and transport, leading to improved supercapacitance suitable for flexible electronic devices [55]. This innovative molecular engineering approach offers a pathway to develop biomimetic composites with tailored biofunctionality for specific applications [55]. Exploring protein conformational changes on silver nanoparticle-based nanocomposites provides insights into the dynamic relationship between protein structure and function [56]. Utilizing surface-enhanced Raman scattering (SERS), the study delves into the reversible nature of conformational changes, highlighting the biofunctionality of proteins on nanocomposites [56]. These findings provide valuable insights into the potential applications of such materials in bioelectronics and related fields, underscoring their unique advantages in terms of biocompatibility and biofunctionality [56].

5.3 Sustainability and environmental impact

The imperative to address environmental concerns and promote sustainability has notably shaped the trends in protein-based nanocomposites. The increasing market preference for plant protein as a renewable resource reflects a substantial shift toward sustainability in recent years [58]. Plant protein production stands out for its robust sustainability factors and lower environmental impact compared with animal protein sources [58]. This recognition is crucial with the rising global demand for protein and the growing prominence of environmentally friendly alternatives. The utilization of plant protein-based carriers further supports sustainability efforts by improving the water solubility, stability, and bioavailability of bioactive substances through various delivery systems [58]. Renewable biomaterials, particularly green nanocomposites based on cellulose nanofibers (CNF), are emerging as lightweight, flexible, and sustainable materials for water purification [33]. Chemically modified CNFs with carboxylic surface functional groups achieved through TEMPO oxidation, play a key role in creating robust and highly efficient nanocomposites [33]. These green nanocomposites significantly contribute to the sustainability of water resources by providing a versatile material for various environmental applications, including water purification [33]. The functionalization of CNFs, influencing porosity and providing active functional groups, represents an environmentally conscious approach to composite film formation, showcasing the potential for sustainable water treatment solutions [33]. The application of nanotechnology in the synthesis of ZrO_2 nanoparticles and their nanocomposites offers a pathway to address major environmental issues, including pollution and diseases such as the COVID-19 pandemic [59]. The use of compounds from bacteria, fungi, microalgae, and plants in the synthesis process highlights the potential for green and sustainable practices [59]. The distinctive properties of green ZrO_2 nanoparticles, such as nanoscale size, diverse morphologies, high stability, and biocompatibility, make them suitable for biomedical and environmental applications, including water treatment and pollutant removal [59,60]. The emergence of green ZrO_2-based nanocomposites further expands their applications to catalytic reduction, nanoelectronic devices, and anti-biofilms, demonstrating their potential contributions to sustainable technologies [59,61,62]. In the context of food security and environmental impact, studies increasingly focus on extending the shelf life of food products using natural and environmentally friendly compounds, with whey protein (WP) playing a pivotal role [63]. The incorporation of natural bioactive compounds in WP films, facilitated by nanotechnology, enhances their antimicrobial and antioxidant properties, offering sustainable alternatives for food preservation [63]. The review highlights the potential applications of WP films in various food products. It discusses their impact on shelf life and chemical and microbiological quality indices, illustrating the intersection of nanotechnology, sustainability, and food security [63]. These findings underscore the pivotal role of nanotechnology in advancing sustainable solutions, showcasing the versatility of protein-based nanocomposites across diverse applications. As we progress toward a more sustainable future, these insights significantly contribute to the evolving landscape of materials science and biotechnology.

6. Limitations and challenges of protein-based nanocomposites

6.1 Limitations and challenges of protein-based nanocomposites

Protein-based nanocomposites, despite their considerable potential, face various limitations and challenges that demand thorough exploration to ensure their successful integration into diverse applications. One inherent limitation arises from the structural sensitivity of proteins within nanocomposites, rendering them prone to denaturation or degradation over time. These alterations, influenced by environmental factors like temperature and pH, present challenges to the stability and performance of nanocomposites, especially in applications requiring prolonged durability. In addition, navigating the intricate fabrication processes of protein-based nanocomposites poses challenges in terms of reproducibility and scalability. It is crucial to achieve consistent results on a large scale, as variations in processing conditions can impact the size, shape, and distribution of nanoparticles within the protein matrix. Developing standardized, scalable manufacturing techniques is imperative for the widespread adoption of these nanocomposites. Moreover, biodegradability, often considered an advantage, can transform into a limitation depending on the application. The rapid biodegradation of protein-based nanocomposites may compromise structural integrity, restricting their utility in environments requiring long-term stability. Striking a balance between structural robustness and controlled biodegradability becomes a significant challenge, necessitating optimization for specific applications. Lastly, the environmental implications of protein-based nanocomposites extend to safety, migrations, and toxicity concerns. A meticulous examination is required to evaluate potential ecological consequences, particularly regarding the release of nanoparticles into the environment during the life cycle of these materials. In biomedical applications, where interactions with biological systems occur, understanding the safety, toxicity, and migration aspects of protein-based nanocomposites is imperative for their successful utilization [7,64].

6.2 Processing challenges and scalability

The integration of proteins into nanocomposites for various applications brings forth promising opportunities, yet challenges in processing and scalability emerge as pivotal considerations. Examining notable examples from recent studies sheds light on the intricate nature of processing challenges associated with Protein-Based Nanocomposites. Lysozyme, known for its multifunctional attributes, stands as a prime example in protein nanocomposite research [52]. Despite its structural stability and ease of production, the fabrication of nanocomposites involving lysozyme encounters challenges in achieving uniformity and scalability. The versatility of lysozyme in different biomedical applications demands meticulous attention to processing techniques for widespread implementation [52]. A pioneering approach inspired by nacre involves the molecular engineering of proteins to create high-performance biomimetic composites [55]. The resilin-based hybrid protein polymer, designed with selective binding motifs for reduced graphene oxide (RGO) and nanofibrillated cellulose (NFC), exhibits superior mechanical properties. However, challenges arise in tuning ion sorption and transport across NFC/RGO interlayers based on specific processing conditions, demanding a nuanced understanding of the material's behavior during fabrication [65]. The exploration of protein conformational changes in Discosoma recombinant red fluorescent proteins (DsRed) adhered on silver nanoparticles (AgNPs)-based nanocomposites introduces challenges related to processing dynamics [56]. Achieving reproducible results requires a delicate balance during the dehydration of DsRed thin protein layers, a critical step in the interaction of proteins with solid surfaces. The reversible transitions between different conformations, as identified in this study, underscore the need for precise control over processing parameters to ensure consistency [56]. Plant protein-based nanocomposites, as renewable carriers for bioactive substances, face processing challenges linked to the diverse functions of plant proteins [58]. The intricate balance between acting as carriers for transportation systems, shells, or cores of a system demands careful consideration in processing to optimize these functions. Achieving scalability while improving water solubility, stability, and bioavailability necessitates innovative processing approaches for plant protein-based nanocomposites [58]. In conclusion, the processing challenges and scalability issues encountered in Protein-Based Nanocomposites, exemplified by the cases of lysozyme, biomimetic composites, protein conformational changes, and plant protein-based carriers, emphasize the importance of nuanced and tailored fabrication techniques. Addressing these challenges is paramount for harnessing the full potential of Protein-Based Nanocomposites in diverse applications, from biomedical technologies to sustainable food and nutrition fields.

6.3 Biodegradability concerns

In the context of developing protein-based nanocomposites, addressing biodegradability concerns is pivotal, considering the increasing environmental focus on sustainable materials. Nanostructured materials, exemplified by zirconia nanoparticles integrated into chitosan-sodium alginate (CS) nanocomposites, present unique properties for tissue engineering applications [53]. The study explores the biocompatibility of zirconia nanoparticles within CSZ scaffolds, emphasizing their potential in biomedical applications. The investigation underscores the importance of understanding how nanocomposite materials interact with biological systems, especially in the realm of tissue engineering [53]. Furthermore, the utilization of renewable biomaterials, such as cellulose nanofibers (CNFs), in green nanocomposites raises intriguing possibilities for sustainable water purification [66]. The modification of CNFs through TEMPO oxidation and their bonding with various metal components enhances the environmental efficiency of the resulting nanocomposites. This innovation not only contributes to the sustainability of water resources but also demonstrates the adaptability of nanocomposite materials for diverse environmental applications [66]. Expanding the scope to food packaging, an urgent need arises to counter the environmental impact of non-biodegradable materials. The development of polymer-based biodegradable materials and edible films, particularly biopolymer-based nanomaterials, emerges as a promising solution [66]. These nanocomposites exhibit multifunctional characteristics, including biodegradability, antimicrobial activity, and biocompatibility, offering a potential alternative to traditional non-biodegradable packaging materials. This aligns with the broader sustainability goals by reducing the environmental footprint of materials used in the food packaging industry [66]. In summary, the exploration of biodegradability concerns in protein-based nanocomposites spans various applications, from tissue engineering to water purification and food packaging. The integration of sustainable materials and the development of environmentally friendly nanocomposites underscore the importance of balancing technological advancements with ecological considerations.

6.4 Environmental implications, safety, migrations, and toxicity aspects

The advent of protein-based nanocomposites in various applications necessitates a meticulous examination of their environmental implications, safety profiles, potential migrations, and toxicity aspects. The integration of advanced nanotechnologies, as exemplified by the use of silica-core@dual QD-shell nanocomposites for SARS-CoV-2 detection [57], underscores the importance of evaluating the environmental impact of nanomaterials. While the application serves a critical function in healthcare, the use of quantum dots raises concerns about the potential long-term environmental consequences, necessitating comprehensive studies on their fate and impact postapplication [57]. In the domain of tissue engineering, the incorporation of graphene oxides into nanocomposites introduces a new dimension of materials with potential biomedical applications [54]. However, the environmental safety and toxicity of graphene oxides, particularly concerning their interactions with proteins, demand a thorough investigation. Balancing the benefits of enhanced physiochemical and biological features with potential environmental concerns is crucial for the responsible development and deployment of these nanocomposites [54]. Expanding the scope to the synthesis of ZrO_2 nanoparticles and their nanocomposites using compounds from bacteria, fungi, microalgae, and plants [63], the potential for environmental applications is vast. However, understanding the ecological impact of the synthesis process and the behavior of these nanoparticles postapplication is essential. The review emphasizes the need for a holistic approach that considers the broader implications of nanotechnological interventions, particularly in areas like water treatment and pollutant removal [63]. Similarly, in the context of using whey protein-based films enhanced by nanotechnology for food preservation, addressing the potential environmental consequences becomes paramount. While these nanocomposite films offer solutions for increasing the shelf life of food products, a comprehensive understanding of their impact on food quality and potential ecological effects is essential for responsible implementation [64]. In conclusion, the deployment of protein-based nanocomposites demands a nuanced evaluation of their environmental implications, safety, migrations, and toxicity aspects. This necessitates a multidisciplinary approach to ensure the responsible development and application of nanotechnological solutions in diverse fields.

7. Applications in various industries

7.1 Food packaging applications

The increasing environmental concerns associated with non-biodegradable and non-renewable materials used in daily food packaging applications have prompted a shift toward sustainable alternatives. A prominent avenue in this endeavor involves the development of bio-based materials, particularly biopolymer-based nanocomposites derived from natural sources such as polysaccharides and proteins. The concept of a bio-based economy gains traction as these materials offer a viable alternative to fossil resources, contributing to a more sustainable and eco-friendly approach [67]. One notable application lies in the realm of Poly(butylene succinate-co-butylene adipate) (PBSA)-based materials, acknowledged for their promising biodegradability in the packaging industry [68]. Despite their biodegradable nature, challenges related to poor gas barrier properties and low durability have impeded widespread adoption. To address these limitations, the incorporation of layered double hydroxide (LDH) fillers into PBSA has been explored. This innovative approach not only improves gas barrier properties and stabilizes PBSA against photoaging but also retains the biodegradability of the material, presenting a scalable solution for enhanced food packaging applications [68]. In a distinct approach, the utilization of microalgae protein biomass, such as spirulina (SP), has been explored to create thermoplastic blends and algal-based bioplastics for food packaging applications [69]. By incorporating SP into plasticized starch films, the resulting spirulina-starch-glycerol composite films exhibit a compelling combination of mechanical and chemical properties. These bio-composites, characterized through various analyses, showcase the potential for the development of environmentally friendly bio-nanocomposites for diverse applications in food packaging [48]. The multifaceted applications of nanotechnology in food packaging, encompassing natural nano-materials, biodegradable polymers, and innovative filler materials, underscore the versatility and potential of protein-based nanocomposites in addressing the environmental impact of packaging materials. The application of food packaging is shown in Fig. 3.6.

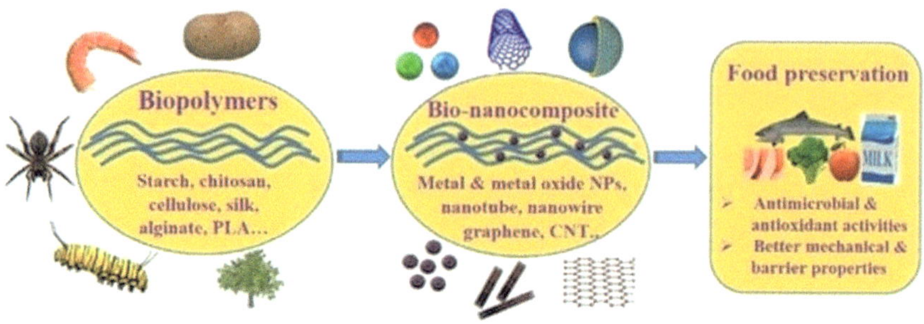

Figure 3.6 Process of food packaging [70].

7.2 Agricultural applications

Protein-based nanocomposites have become integral in various industries, and their impact on agricultural practices is particularly noteworthy. In this section, we explore how these nanocomposites contribute to sustainable solutions in agriculture. One promising avenue is the utilization of agri-food biomasses to produce biodegradable and edible plastics. Seeds used for oil extraction generate organic by-products, such as seed oil cakes (SOCs). A study on Argania spinosa (argan) SOC reveals its potential as a protein-rich resource for biodegradable films. Films produced with argan seed protein concentrate exhibit hydrophobicity, suitable mechanical properties, and antioxidant activity. These findings suggest the viability of using argan SOC in the cosmeceutical and food industries, aligning with the principles of a bio-based economy [71]. Another facet of agricultural applications lies in the realm of environmentally friendly packaging. Plant protein-based films, as alternatives to synthetic plastics, have gained attention for their biodegradability. Recent advancements involve the development of nanocomposite films, incorporating nanoparticles to enhance packaging properties. These nanocomposites exhibit improved functional performance, barrier properties, and antimicrobial effects. Applications extend to various food products, demonstrating increased shelf life during storage. This underscores the potential of nanocomposite plant protein-based materials in addressing consumer demands for sustainable packaging solutions [21]. Beyond packaging, protein-based biostimulants (PBBs) derived from plant and animal raw materials offer a sustainable approach to enhancing crop growth and yield. The hydrolysis of protein-rich by-products results in active ingredients influencing plant physiological processes. Two examples, hydrolyzed wheat gluten and potato protein, show significant stimulation of early sugar beet growth. The discussion extends to the potential development of PBBs into superabsorbent polymers (SAPs), emphasizing their role in sustainably supplying water and nutrients in agricultural systems. This highlights the multifaceted benefits of protein-based nanocomposites in promoting sustainable agriculture [72].

7.3 Industrial applications

Protein-based nanocomposites have become indispensable elements in a wide range of industrial applications, demonstrating their adaptability and influence across diverse sectors. In the dynamic field of tissue engineering, the integration of graphene oxide structures with proteins opens new horizons for bioengineered tissues and organs. Graphene oxides, with their expansive surface area and interaction capabilities with proteins and peptides, offer physiochemical and biological features crucial for optimizing scaffold architectures. A critical review focuses on the use of protein-graphene oxide structures, emphasizing their role as nanocomposites or biocomplexes. The analysis delves into their effects on protein conformation and structural stability, assessing applications in tissue engineering and regenerative medicine. Notably, recent applications demonstrate the biological activity of nanocomposite bioconjugates, underscoring their impact on cell viability, proliferation, and the formation of functional tissue. The review also explores novel strategies involving stem cell therapy and the integration of the extracellular matrix, paving the way for smart nanoplatforms in tissue engineering [54]. Shifting to industrial applications in environmentally friendly packaging, plant protein-based films stand out as sustainable alternatives to synthetic plastics. The incorporation of nanoparticles in nanocomposite films enhances their functional performance, barrier properties, and antimicrobial effects. This review explores recent findings on plant-based protein nanocomposites applicable to food packaging. The investigation extends to the characterization of these nanocomposite films and coatings, emphasizing their application on fruits, vegetables, meat, seafood, and other food products. The results indicate that the integration of nanomaterials extends the properties of plant protein-based materials, enhancing their functionality and contributing to increased shelf life for stored food products. This highlights the crucial role of protein-based nanocomposites in addressing consumer demands for sustainable and efficient packaging solutions in various industries [21]. Industrial application of the food packaging as shown in Fig. 3.7.

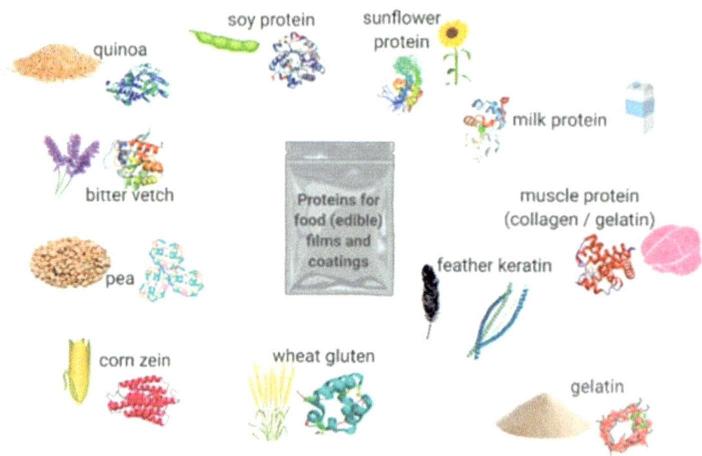

Figure 3.7 Protein-based (edible) films and coatings predominantly employ a variety of materials [73].

8. Comparison with other biopolymers and nanocomposites

8.1 Polymer-based nanocomposites

Polymer-based nanocomposites stand as an innovative class of materials created by integrating nanoscale fillers into a polymer matrix. These fillers, commonly nanoparticles or nanotubes, impart unique and improved properties to the resulting composite when compared with traditional polymers. The synergy between polymers and nanoscale materials combines the adaptability of polymers with the exceptional characteristics of nanoparticles [74]. The preparation of nanoparticle-based polymer nanocomposites typically involves three consecutive steps. Initially, nanoparticles and the polymer matrix undergo individual preparation. Subsequently, a synthesis step merges these raw materials through various physical and chemical processes. This chapter provides a comprehensive overview of these steps, highlighting the crucial role played by the physical modifications and functionalization of nanoparticles and matrix size in tailoring the nanocomposites for specific applications. The applications of polymer nanocomposites are intricately linked to the constituent materials, with both the matrix and filler materials significantly impacting the final properties and applications of the nanocomposites. From one perspective, the chapter delves into popular approaches employed for fabricating ceramic, metal, and polymer nanocomposites [65]. In addition, it explores the categorization of polymer nanocomposite coatings into conductive, biocompatible, and smart varieties, each serving distinct applications. A parallel investigation into nanocomposite adhesives reveals their classification into structural, biomimetic, pressure-sensitive, and conductive types based on performance characteristics.

8.2 Strengths and weaknesses compared with biopolymers from natural sources

The increasing demand for advanced materials has made the exploration of polymer nanocomposites and biopolymers derived from natural sources crucial. This section provides a review of the strengths and weaknesses of polymer nanocomposites concerning their applications, particularly in comparison with biopolymers. Polymer nanocomposites signify a revolutionary advancement in material science, finding utility across various domains like coatings, adhesives, biomedical fields, and energy storage. Their adaptability spans conductive to biocompatible coatings and smart nanocomposites, showcasing their versatility, fabrication methods, and nuanced applications that make them integral to modern-day technology. Notably, they play a vital role in corrosion protection and tissue healing [72,75]. On the contrary, biopolymers sourced from natural origins, especially those utilized in sustainable packaging, present a promising alternative. These materials are characterized by biodegradability, environmental friendliness, and a focus on mechanical properties, cost, and safety. The use of plant-based protein films as biodegradable materials, enhanced through nanocomposites, demonstrates their potential to extend the shelf life of food products while aligning with consumer demands for eco-friendly packaging [21,76]. A significant application of biopolymeric nanocomposites is their role in designing UV-protective sustainable packaging materials. By incorporating biocompatible nanomaterials, these materials ensure the protection of products from UV-induced changes during storage and transportation. The review underscores the importance of UV protection, discussing challenges and prospects in sustainable packaging and providing insights into the future of next-generation packaging technologies [76]. In the field of tissue engineering, biopolymers like protein-graphene oxide structures play a crucial role. Graphene oxide, with its physiochemical and biological features, contributes to optimizing scaffold architectures for tissue engineering. The review delves into recent applications, highlighting the biological activity of nanocomposite bioconjugates and their potential in regenerative medicine [54].

In conclusion, while polymer nanocomposites excel in versatile technological applications, biopolymers derived from natural sources, particularly in sustainable packaging and tissue engineering, offer unique strengths. The careful consideration of their respective strengths and weaknesses is essential for informed material selection and application in diverse fields.

9. Conclusion

In summary, the investigation into protein-based nanocomposites has provided a thorough understanding of their composition, manufacturing methods, properties, advantages, and limitations across various applications. The showcased adaptability in manufacturing methods complements the foundational understanding of composition and structure. The incorporation of diverse nanomaterials contributes to enhanced functionality, impacting mechanical strength, barrier characteristics, antimicrobial and antioxidant properties, and thermal stability. Noteworthy advantages of these nanocomposites include improved mechanical properties, biocompatibility, biofunctionality, sustainability, and a reduced environmental impact. However, it is crucial to acknowledge limitations and challenges such as stability concerns, processing difficulties, and biodegradability issues, emphasizing the need for careful consideration. Furthermore, a comparative analysis with other biopolymers and nanocomposites underscores the distinct features of protein-based nanocomposites. In essence, this comprehensive exploration highlights the promising attributes of protein-based nanocomposites while acknowledging the challenges that require further attention in their ongoing development and application as innovative materials [77–79].

Acknowledgments

The authors are thankful to Universiti Sains Malaysia for providing a financial support (short-term grant; 304/PKIMIA/6315580).

References

[1] Kim YH, Murakami RI, Park SJ. Advanced composites engineering and its nanobridging technology: applied research for polymer composites and nanocomposites. Singapore: World Scientific; 2020.

[2] Ates B, Koytepe S, Ulu A, Gurses C, Thakur VK. Chemistry, structures, and advanced applications of nanocomposites from biorenewable resources. Chem Rev 2020;120:9304–62.

[3] Ulu A, Noma SAA, Gurses C, Koytepe S, Ates B. Chitosan/polyvinylpyrrolidone/MCM-41 composite hydrogel films: structural, thermal. Surf Antibact Prop 2018;70:1700303.
[4] Rallini M, Kenny JM. Nanofillers in polymers. In: Modification of polymer properties; 2017. p. 47–86.
[5] Sinha Ray S, Bousmina M. Biodegradable polymer/layered silicate nanocomposites. In: Polymer nanocomposites; 2006.
[6] Zubair M, Ullah A. Recent advances in protein-derived bionanocomposites for food packaging applications. Crit Rev Food Sci Nutr 2019;60(3):406–34.
[7] Wang Z, Kang S, Cao S, Krecker M, Tsukruk VV, Singamaneni S. Protein-based functional nanocomposites. MRS Bull 2020;45(12):1017–26.
[8] Zhang R, Han Y, Xie W, Liu F, Chen S. Advances in protein-based nanocarriers of bioactive compounds: from microscopic molecular principles to macroscopical structural and functional attributes. J Agric Food Chem 2022;70(21):6354–67.
[9] McClements DJ, Li F, Xiao H. The nutraceutical bioavailability classification scheme: classifying nutraceuticals according to factors limiting their oral bioavailability. Annu Rev Food Sci Technol 2015;6:299–327.
[10] de Souza Simões L, Madalena DA, Pinheiro AC, Teixeira JA, Vicente AA, Ramos ÓL. Micro- and nano bio-based delivery systems for food applications: in vitro behavior. Adv Colloid Interface Sci 2017;243:23–45.
[11] Benshitrit RC, Levi CS, Tal SL, Shimoni E, Lesmes U. Development of oral food-grade delivery systems: current knowledge and future challenges. Food Funct 2012;3(1):10–21.
[12] Das PP, Chaudhary V, Ahmad F, Manral A. Effect of nanotoxicity and enhancement in performance of polymer composites using nanofillers: a state-of-the-art review. Polym Compos 2021;42(5):2152–70.
[13] Nayak RK, Mahato KK, Ray BC. Processing of polymer-based nanocomposites. Reinforc Polym Compos Process Character Post Life Cycle Assessm 2019;21:55–75.
[14] Tanahashi M. Development of fabrication methods of filler/polymer nanocomposites: with focus on simple melt-compounding-based approach without surface modification of nanofillers. Materials 2010;3(3):1593–619.
[15] Zhao R, Torley P, Halley PJ. Emerging biodegradable materials: starch- and protein-based bio-nanocomposites. J Mater Sci 2008;43:3058–71.
[16] Thakur M, Chandel M, Rani A, Sharma A. Introduction to biorenewable nanocomposite materials: methods of preparation, current developments, and future perspectives. In: Biorenewable nanocomposite materials, Vol. 2: Desalination and wastewater remediation. American Chemical Society; 2022. p. 1–24.
[17] Dlamini DS, Li J, Mamba BB. Critical review of montmorillonite/polymer mixed-matrix filtration membranes: possibilities and challenges. Appl Clay Sci 2019;168:21–30.
[18] Mittal V. Polymer layered silicate nanocomposites: a review. Materials 2009;2:992–1057.
[19] Jali S, Mohan TP, Mwangi FM, Kanny K. A review on barrier properties of cellulose/clay nanocomposite polymers for packaging applications. Polymers 2024;16(1):51.
[20] Khan MA, Ahmad A, Umar K, Nabi SA. Synthesis, characterization, and biological applications of nanocomposites for the removal of heavy metals and dyes. Ind Eng Chem Res 2015;54(1):76–82.
[21] Jafarzadeh S, Forough M, Amjadi S, Kouzegaran VJ, Almasi H, Garavand F, Zargar M. Plant protein-based nanocomposite films: a review on the used nanomaterials, characteristics, and food packaging applications. Crit Rev Food Sci Nutr 2023;63(29):9667–93.

[22] Galstyan V, Bhandari MP, Sberveglieri V, Sberveglieri G, Comini E. Metal oxide nanostructures in food applications: quality control and packaging. Chemosensors 2018;6(2):16.

[23] Shkodenko L, Kassirov I, Koshel E. Metal oxide nanoparticles against bacterial biofilms: perspectives and limitations. Microorganisms 2020;8(10):1545.

[24] Petchwattana N, Covavisaruch S, Wibooranawong S, Naknaen P. Antimicrobial food packaging prepared from poly(butylene succinate) and zinc oxide. Measurement 2016;93:442–8.

[25] Yu Y, Zheng J, Li J, Lu L, Yan J, Zhang L, Wang L. Applications of two-dimensional materials in food packaging. Trends Food Sci Technol 2021;110:443–57.

[26] Afridi SK, Umar K, Parveen T, Razali MR. Nanocomposites in the degradation of organic pollutants. In: Nanocomposites-advanced materials for energy and environmental aspects. Woodhead Publishing; 2023. p. 321–47.

[27] Fierascu RC, Lungulescu EM, Fierascu I, Stan MS, Voinea IC, Dumitrescu SI. Metal and metal oxide nanoparticle incorporation in polyurethane foams: a solution for future antimicrobial materials? Polymers 2023;15(23):4570.

[28] Yu M, Zhao S, Yang L, Ji N, Wang Y, Xiong L, Sun Q. Preparation of a superhydrophilic SiO_2 nanoparticles coated chitosan-sodium phytate film by a simple ethanol soaking process. Carbohydr Polym 2021;271:118422.

[29] Cai W, Wang BB, Wang X, Zhu YL, Li ZX, Xu ZM, Song L, Hu WZ, Hu Y. Recent progress in two-dimensional nanomaterials following graphene for improving fire safety of polymer (nano)composites. Chin J Polym Sci 2021;39(8):935–56.

[30] Zhou Y, Yin H, Ai S. Applications of two-dimensional layered nanomaterials in photoelectrochemical sensors: a comprehensive review. Coord Chem Rev 2021;447:214156.

[31] Haseen U, Umar K, Ahmad H, Parveen T, Mohamad Ibrahim MN. Graphene and its composites: applications in environmental remediation. Modern Age Waste Water Probl Solut Using Appl Nanotechnol 2020:85–91.

[32] Sun L, Du T, Hu C, Chen J, Lu J, Lu Z, Han H. Antibacterial activity of graphene oxide/g-C_3N_4 composite through photocatalytic disinfection under visible light. ACS Sustain Chem Eng 2017;5(10):8693–701.

[33] Li J, Jiang S, Wei Y, Li X, Shi SQ, Zhang W, Li J. Facile fabrication of tough, strong, and biodegradable soy protein-based composite films with excellent UV-blocking performance. Compos B Eng 2021;211:108645.

[34] Han Y, Wang L. Improved water barrier and mechanical properties of soy protein isolate films by incorporation of SiO_2 nanoparticles. RSC Adv 2016;6(113):112317–24.

[35] Nor AA, Hean CG, Nur Hanani ZA. Incorporation of graphene oxide to enhance fish gelatin as bio-packaging material. Food Packag Shelf Life 2021;28:100679.

[36] Kumar P, Sandeep KP, Alavi S, Truong VD, Gorga RE. Preparation and characterization of bio-nanocomposite films based on soy protein isolate and montmorillonite using melt extrusion. J Food Eng 2010;100(3):480–9.

[37] Tian B, Xu D, Cheng J, Liu Y. Chitosan-silica with hops β-acids added films as prospective food packaging materials: preparation, characterization, and properties. Carbohydr Polym 2021;272:118457.

[38] Rukmanikrishnan B, Ramalingam S, Kim SS, Lee J. Rheological and anti-microbial study of silica and silver nanoparticles-reinforced k-carrageenan/hydroxyethyl cellulose composites for food packaging applications. Cellulose 2021;28(9):5577–90.

[39] Jiang L, Han Y, Meng X, Xiao Y, Zhang H. Cellulose nanocrystals reinforced Zein/Catechin/β-cyclodextrin inclusion complex nanoparticles nanocomposite film for active food packaging. Polymers 2021;13(16):2759.

[40] Tang S, Wang Z, Li W, Li M, Deng Q, Wang Y, Li C, Chu PK. Ecofriendly and biodegradable soybean protein isolate films incorporated with ZnO nanoparticles for food packaging. ACS Appl Bio Mater 2019;2(5):2202−7.
[41] Matei E, Predescu AM, Râpă M, Țurcanu AA, Mateş I, Constantin N, Predescu C. Natural polymers and their nanocomposites used for environmental applications. Nanomaterials 2022;12(10):1707.
[42] Xiao Y, Liu Y, Kang S, Wang K, Xu H. Development and evaluation of soy protein isolate-based antibacterial nanocomposite films containing cellulose nanocrystals and zinc oxide nanoparticles. Food Hydrocolloids 2020:105898.
[43] Fortunati E, Luzi F, Jiménez A, Gopakumar DA, Puglia D, Thomas S, Kenny JM, Chiralt A, Torre L. Revalorization of sunflower stalks as novel sources of cellulose nanofibrils and nanocrystals and their effect on wheat gluten bionanocomposite properties. Carbohydr Polym 2016;149:357−68.
[44] El-Wakil NA, Hassan EA, Abou-Zeid RE, Dufresne A. Development of wheat gluten/nanocellulose/titanium dioxide nanocomposites for active food packaging. Carbohydr Polym 2015;124:337−46.
[45] Rani S, Kumar KD, Mandal S, Kumar R. Functionalized carbon dot nanoparticles reinforced soy protein isolate biopolymeric film. J Polym Res 2020;27(10):1−10.
[46] Abdullah A, Abdullah AZ, Ahmed M, Khan J, Shahadat M, Umar K, Alim MA. A review on recent developments and progress in sustainable acrolein production through catalytic dehydration of bio-renewable glycerol. J Clean Prod 2022;341:130876.
[47] Luecha J, Sozer N, Kokini JL. Synthesis and properties of corn zein/montmorillonite nanocomposite films. J Mater Sci 2010;45(13):3529−37.
[48] Schmitz F, de Albuquerque MBS, Alberton MD, Riegel-Vidotti IC, Zimmermann LM. Zein films with ZnO and ZnO: Mg quantum dots as functional nanofillers: new nanocomposites for food package with UV-blocker and antimicrobial properties. Polym Test 2020;91:106709.
[49] Rouf TB, Schmidt G, Cakmak M, Kokini JL. Design and mechanistic understanding of graphene oxide reinforced zein nanocomposites with improved mechanical, barrier and thermal properties. J Mater Sci 2019;54(19):12533−52.
[50] Cui H, Surendhiran D, Li C, Lin L. Biodegradable zein active film containing chitosan nanoparticle encapsulated with pomegranate peel extract for food packaging. Food Packag Shelf Life 2020;24:100511.
[51] Safian MT, Umar K, Ibrahim MN. Synthesis and scalability of graphene and its derivatives: a journey towards sustainable and commercial material. J Clean Prod 2021;318:128603.
[52] Sarkar S, Gulati K, Mishra A, Poluri KM. Protein nanocomposites: special inferences to lysozyme based nanomaterials. Int J Biol Macromol 2021;151:467−82.
[53] Shanmugam B, et al. Biomimetic development of chitosan and sodium alginate-based nanocomposites contains zirconia for tissue engineering applications. J Biomed Mater Res B Appl Biomater 2022.
[54] Biru EI, Necolau MI, Zainea A, Iovu H. Graphene oxide−protein-based scaffolds for tissue engineering: recent advances and applications. Polymers 2022;14(5):1032.
[55] Dhar P, Josphat P, Szilvay GR, Westerholm-Parvinen A, Maloney T, Laaksonen P. Genetically engineered protein based nacre-like nanocomposites with superior mechanical and electrochemical performance. J Mater Chem A Mater Energy Sustain 2020;8(2):656−69.

[56] Scarangella A, Marvine S, Mlayah A, Bonafos C, Monje M, Roques C, et al. Detection of the conformational changes of Discosoma red fluorescent proteins adhered on silver nanoparticles-based nanocomposites via surface-enhanced Raman scattering. Nanotechnology 2019;30(16):165101.
[57] Wang C, et al. Development of spike protein-based fluorescence lateral flow assay for the simultaneous detection of SARS-CoV-2 specific IgM and IgG. Anal R Soc Chem (RSC) 2021.
[58] Guan T, Zhang Z, Li X, Cui S, McClements DJ, Wu X, et al. Preparation, characteristics, and advantages of plant protein-based bioactive molecule delivery systems. Foods 2022;11(11):1562.
[59] Tran TV, et al. Green synthesis of ZrO_2 nanoparticles and nanocomposites for biomedical and environmental applications: a review. Environmental chemistry letters. Springer Science and Business Media LLC; 2022.
[60] Zhao G, Zhou C, Fan F. Preparation and properties of soy protein isolate/cotton-nanocrystalline cellulose films. Int J Polym Sci 2021:5518136.
[61] Vahedikia N, et al. Biodegradable zein film composites reinforced with chitosan nanoparticles and cinnamon essential oil: physical, mechanical, structural and antimicrobial attributes. Colloids Surf B Biointerfaces 2019;177:25–32.
[62] Wei N, et al. High-performance soy protein-based films from cellulose nanofibers and graphene oxide constructed synergistically via hydrogen and chemical bonding. RSC Adv 2021;11(37):22812–9.
[63] Marashi SM, Hashemi M, Berizi E, Raeisi M, Noori SM. Elaboration of whey protein-based films in food products: emphasis on the addition of natural edible bio-nanocomposites with antioxidant and antimicrobial activity. Jundishapur J Nat Pharm Prod 2022;17(2).
[64] Suresh S, Pushparaj C, Subramani R. Recent development in preparation of food packaging films using biopolymers. Food Res Rynnye Lyan Resour 2021.
[65] Subbir Parvej M, Khan I, Forhad Hossain M. Preparation of nanoparticle-based polymer composites. Elsevier eBooks; 2022. p. 55–94.
[66] Jin S, Kuang L, Li J. Nature-inspired green procedure for improving performance of protein-based nanocomposites via introduction of nanofibrillated cellulose-stablized graphene/carbon nanotubes hybrid. Polymers 2018;10(3):270.
[67] Fahmy HM, Salah Eldin RE, Abu Serea ES, Gomaa NM, AboElmagd GM, Salem SA, et al. Advances in nanotechnology and antibacterial properties of biodegradable food packaging materials. RSC Adv 2020;10(35):20467–84.
[68] Delorme AE, Radusin T, Myllytie P, Verney V, Askanian H. Enhancement of gas barrier properties and durability of poly(butylene succinate-co-butylene adipate)-based nanocomposites for food packaging applications. Nanomaterials 2022;12(6):978.
[69] Soma DOM, Abdel-Hakim A. Characterization of biodegradable composite based on microalgae modified glycerol-plasticized-starch films. Polym Eng Sci 2023.
[70] Basavegowda N, Baek KH. Advances in functional biopolymer-based nanocomposites for active food packaging applications. Polymers 2021;13(23):4198.
[71] Fatemeh Mirpoor S, Mariniello CVL, D'Agostino A, Cristina d'Agostino M, Cammarota M, et al. Argan (*Argania spinosa* L.) seed oil cake as a potential source of protein-based film matrix for Pharmaco-Cosmetic applications. Int J Mol Sci 2022;23(15):8478.
[72] Okanlawon LJ, Ali HM, Ekblad T, Fredlund KM, Olsson M, Johansson E. Protein-based biostimulants to enhance plant growth—state-of-the-art and future direction with sugar beet as an example. Agronomy 2022;12(12):3211.
[73] Mihalca V, Kerezsi AD, Weber A, Gruber-Traub C, Schmucker J, Vodnar DC, Dulf FV, Socaci SA, Fărcaş A, Mureşan CI, Suharoschi R. Protein-based films and coatings for food industry applications. Polymers 2021;13(5):769.

[74] Liang S, Zhang M, Biesold GM, Choi W, He Y, Li Z, et al. Recent advances in synthesis, properties, and applications of metal halide perovskite nanocrystals. Polym Nanocompos 2021;33(50):2005888.
[75] Faiza Amin K, Mazdi Nahin A, Enamul Hoque Md. Polymer nanocomposites for adhesives and coatings. Elsevier eBooks; 2022. p. 235–65.
[76] Gore AH, Prajapat AL. Biopolymer nanocomposites for sustainable UV protective packaging. Front Mater 2022;9.
[77] Umar K. Water contamination by organic-pollutants: TiO_2 photocatalysis. Mod Age Environ Probl Remed 2018:95–109.
[78] Han LF, Tan CP, Zawawi RM, Nur Hanani ZA. Enhancing the mechanical and barrier properties of chitosan/graphene oxide composite films using trisodium citrate and sodium tripolyphosphate crosslinkers. J Appl Polym Sci 2021;138(26):50618.
[79] Silva NHCS, et al. Protein-based materials: from sources to innovative sustainable materials for biomedical applications. J Mater Chem B 2014;2:3715.

CHAPTER 4

Recent advances in design and development of protein nanocomposite

Sakshi Kapoor[1] **and Hilal Ahmad**[2]
[1]Nanoscale Research Facility, Indian Institute of Technology Delhi, New Delhi, India; [2]Interdisciplinary Research Center for Membranes and Water Security, King Fahd University of Petroleum & Minerals (KFUPM), Dhahran, Saudi Arabia

1. Introduction

Proteins may be designed to interact with synthetic materials because of the many functional moieties, amphiphilic nature, and flexibility of lengthy chains. Protein materials are appealing in biological applications and in reducing the adverse effects of human activities on the environment and diverse ecosystems due to their biocompatibility and biodegradability. Through covalent and noncovalent interactions including hydrogen bonding, hydrophobic contacts, and electrostatic interactions, protein materials' extensive chemical activity permits their simple integration with abiotic materials. Protein-based nanocomposites are optimized in their structural design to obtain improved performance [1].

The current tendency is to create eco-friendly nanocomposites to lower carbon emissions and promote material recycling. Because of their outstanding functionality and biodegradability, biomacromolecules (BMMs), which are essential for in vivo life and include proteins, polypeptides, enzymes, DNA, RNA, lipids, and polysaccharides, are employed in in vitro applications [2,3]. As large as 100 nm in one dimension can be employed with nanoparticles that are specifically used as medication or therapeutic chemical carriers. They are constructed from a variety of substances, including lipids, metals, and natural or manufactured polymers. Due to their speedier and more effective biological absorption than bigger macromolecules, nanoparticles are great materials for delivery systems. Numerous applications are possible when combined with nanomaterials

Protein-Based Nanocomposites for Tissue Engineering
ISBN 978-0-323-99357-9
https://doi.org/10.1016/B978-0-323-99357-9.00001-6

that have the appropriate photoelectric and thermal characteristics, including biosensors, artificial tissue, information storage, and medication delivery [4–7].

For instance, protein fibers which are frequently used as reinforcement components result in composite materials with superior mechanical characteristics due to their effective load transmission and stress mediation. Protein and inorganic materials have strong interfacial interactions that expand the molecular interfacial zones, greatly enhancing reinforcing effects and resulting in a synergistic improvement of mechanical traits [8]. In addition, polypeptide chains may be stretched and reoriented thanks to the structural flexibility of proteins, which is accompanied by a variety of intra- and interchain connections and multilayer secondary structures. The reduced fracture propagation and postponed eventual failure of the material are the results of the improved energy absorption. These nanocomposites are also made biocompatible with protein materials, which makes them appealing for biomedical uses such as drug delivery, tissue engineering scaffolds, and wearable biophysical and biochemical sensors [9–11].

The increasing prevalence of antimicrobial food additive-resistant bacterium types has had a significant influence on human mortality and healthcare. Finding substitute antimicrobial food additives that may mimic innate immune systems is therefore urgently needed [12]. In addition, multipurpose electronic gadgets carry out essential tasks due to their enormous potential in real-world Internet of Things applications. For human health detection, soft robot technologies, wearable electronics, energy storing and providing, etc., several flexible electronic devices have been created recently. Future electronic gadgets are expected to include flexible sensors that are portable, safe, extremely sensitive, and friendly to the environment. Multifunctional flexible sensors constructed of eco-friendly materials including silk, cellulose, natural rubber, gelatine, and polyvinyl alcohol have received a lot of attention up to this point. In addition, sensors that combine pressure, temperature, humidity, stress reactions, and other factors are acquired [13,14].

Artificial electronic skins (E-skins) that are bioinspired are appealing for a variety of uses, including soft robotics, implantable biomedical devices, healthcare monitoring, and artificial intelligence systems. For smooth interface and stand-alone functioning of E-skins, efficient energy generators that are compatible with biological tissues in both a mechanical and biological sense are necessary [15]. Because most tissues are naturally soft and in motion, piezoelectric (PZ, based on mechanical stress) and triboelectric

(TB, based on electrostatic induction) devices are appropriate for this usage. PZ devices in particular make it possible to create new electromechanical interfaces with human skin or tissue for the development of ultrasonic transducers and actuators as well as for monitoring and harvesting biomechanical movements [16,17].

We shall review current developments (year: 2020–23) in the creation of protein-based nanocomposites in this article. We will concentrate on how synthetic and naturally occurring proteins interact, go through several methods for creating hybrid nanostructures, and talk about how components' functions and properties relate to one another as well as the final nanocomposites.

2. Physicochemical properties

2.1 Structural features

- *Scanning electron microscope (SEM)*: A common biopolymer that has gained a lot of attention is soy protein isolate (SPI); plentiful, affordable, and sustainable. Therefore, it is necessary to create high-performance SPI-based materials. A bio-influenced heterostructure was created by inserting graphene oxide (GO) nanosheets into the SPI-glycerin (Gly) matrix using a vacuum evaporation self-assembly technique. Fig. 4.1C and D displays digitized images of the created SPI-Gly-GO and SPI-Gly-rGO nanocomposites. The front and side SEM images of the SPI-Gly-rGO nanocomposite are depicted in Fig. 4.1E and F demonstrating the withdrawal of rGO nanosheets from the SPI-Gly matrix and the usual hierarchical micro-/nanoscale structures [18].
- *Atomic force microscopy (AFM)*: Fig. 4.1A and B show that SPI-Gly-GO nanosheets had a thickness of around ~10 nm; significantly more than the thickness of a single GO nanosheet (~1.5 nm). This illustrates that the GO nanosheets had been effectively incorporated into the SPI chains and diffused throughout the SPI-Gly matrix. Eventually, the superfluous oxygen-comprising batch on the plane of GO nanosheets was eliminated to produce the SPI-Gly-rGO nanocomposite using hydroiodic acid (HI) reduction [18].
- *X-ray diffraction (XRD)*: The intact crystal structure of the alkali-treated SPI is shown by the α-helix and β-sheet diffraction peaks of SPI, situated at $2\theta = 8.6$ degree and $2\theta = 20.1$ degree, respectively (Fig. 4.1G); demonstrating that both structures had not been damaged even after the chemical reduction [18]. Furthermore, the SPI-Gly-GO nanocomposite

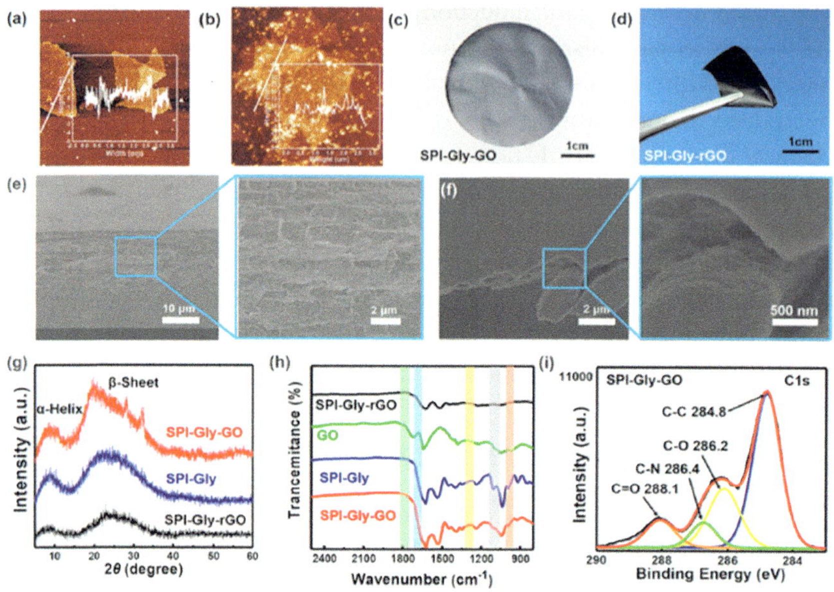

Figure 4.1 (A,B) An AFM picture of GO nanosheets and GO nanosheets coated with SPI-Gly. (C,D) Digital images of the nanocomposites made of SPI-Gly-GO and SPI-rGO-Gly. (E,F) multilayer structure of the SPI-Gly-rGO nanocomposites is visible in the SEM side- and front-view images. (G) XRD images of the SPI-Gly film and the nanocomposite SPI-Gly-GO, SPI-Gly-rGO. (I) XPS spectrum of the SPI-Gly-GO nanocomposite. (H) FTIR spectrum of the SPI-Gly film, GO nanosheets, and SPIs-Gly-GO and SPI-Gly-rGO nanocomposites. *(Reproduced with copyright permission from Ref. [18].)*

showed the signal of SPI chains without the characteristic GO nanosheet diffraction peak ($2\theta = 10$ degree), indicating that no agglomeration occurred for the SPI-Gly-GO system at low SPI concentrations.

- *Fourier transform infrared (FTIR)*: Fig. 4.1H depicts the covalent cross-linking in SPI-Gly-GO nanocomposites between SPI chains and nanosheets. The large peak of GO nanosheets at 1720 cm^{-1} is due to the vibrational symmetry-stretching of carboxyl groups (-C=O stretching). Amidol I of the SPI polypeptide chain (C=O stretching vibration), amide II (N—H bending), and amide III (C—H and N—H stretching), respectively, correspond to the distinctive peaks of SPI chains and SPI-Gly film at 1645, 1539, and 1239 cm^{-1}. At 1024 and 920 cm^{-1} of the SPI-Gly film, respectively, the typical peaks of —OH groups and -C-N groups developed, indicating the interaction of Gly plasticizers with SPI polypeptide chains [18]. The peak intensity of -N-H in the SPI-Gly-GO nanocomposite was noticeably higher than that of the SPI-Gly composites, indicating that an amidation reaction took place between the carboxyl groups of the GO nanosheets and the main amino groups on the SPI peptide chains. In addition, the SPI-Gly-GO nanocomposite's peak C—N intensity at 1042 cm^{-1} exhibits a negative trend, demonstrating that SPI chains and GO nanosheets underwent a cross-linking process that reduced the hydrogen connection between SPI chains and Gly plasticizers. In contrast, to GO nanosheets, SPI-Gly-GO nanocomposites showed evidence of the epoxide ring-opening process by the removal of C—O characteristic peaks at 1222 cm^{-1} and the stretching vibration of C—O—C characteristic peaks that formed at 1100 and 1250 cm^{-1}.

- *X-ray photoelectron spectra (XPS)*: Three peaks at 284.8, 286.1, and 288.1 eV, corresponding to the C—C, C—O, and C=O groups, respectively, divide the C1s regions of the SPI-Gly matrix. The intercalation of GO nanosheets into the SPI-Gly matrix was effective as evidenced by the enhanced C—O intensity in the SPI-Gly-GO nanocomposite (Fig. 4.14I). The covalent cross-linking between SPI chains and GO nanosheets was further demonstrated when a stronger C—N signal formed at 286.7 eV. The peak intensities of C=O and C—O in the SPI-Gly-rGO nanocomposite were much lower after chemical reduction, indicating redundant oxygen-comprising groups of the GO nanosheets were eliminated [18].

2.2 Mechanical strength

- One of the most important agricultural commodities in the world is soybeans, primarily used to produce soy oils and provide food for both people and animals. In fact, as a sustainable agricultural product, soybeans have the potential to replace a significant amount of nonrenewable petroleum oils, coals, and other minerals. This is in the production of environmentally friendly, carbon-neutral, and biodegradable goods that can support and enhance our quality of life while remarkably lowering greenhouse gas emissions and the degradation of water, soils, and the atmosphere [19].
- Soy protein isolates (SPIs), which were employed as the optimal material model for creating SPI-oxidized sugar (OS) nanocomposite films, were cross-linked using a green synthesis technique and soy-based sugars (glucose and sucrose) in aqueous solutions. SPIs were mass ratio to glucose or sucrose at 1:0.25, 1:0.50, and 1:0.75, respectively. The

identical SPI-OS mass ratios were used to construct the nanocomposite films reinforced with clay nanoparticles (CNPs) [20]. Both uncured (with limited SPI cross-linking) and cured (with maximum cross-linking) nanocomposite film samples were utilized for mechanical testing to conduct comparative research [19].

- The ultimate tensile strength and Young's modulus for either SPI-oxidized glucose or SPI-oxidized sucrose film specimens dropped sharply with increasing sugar mass fraction in the case of both uncured and cured film samples. Average ultimate tensile strengths for uncured SPI-oxidized glucose films without CNP reinforcement are 15.46, 3.61, and 0.68 MPa, respectively, and correspond to the films' SPI/glucose mass ratios of 1:0.25, 1:0.50, and 1:0.75. The average ultimate tensile strength of these films, however, increased after curing to 17.58, 7.13, and 3.80 MPa, respectively. For uncured SPI-oxidized glucose films with SPI/glucose mass ratios of 1:0.25, 1:0.50, and 1:0.75, respectively, the average Young's moduli are 574.29, 169.32, and 24.46 MPa. These average moduli went up to 872.09, 247.31, and 124.88 MPa after curing. Such findings suggest that, given an SPI/glucose mass ratio, curing increased both the ultimate tensile strength and Young's modulus of the resulting SPI oxidized glucose films. However, the modulus improvement was significantly more noticeable, increasing by up to 400% in the case of the SPI/glucose mass ratio of 1:0.75 compared with 1:0.25 and 1:0.50. In addition, the mechanical characteristics of the SPI-oxidized sucrose films tended to behave similarly to those of the SPI-oxidized glucose films. This improvement in the mechanical characteristics of the resultant SPI-OS films was brought about by the cross-linking degree that was increased during curing. It was discovered that the addition of CNPs roughly halved both the ultimate tensile strength and Young's modulus for uncured and cured SPI oxidized glucose films with SPI/glucose mass ratios of 1:0.25 and 1:0.50, while significantly increasing the strains at the break of these films, indicating CNP-induced softening. The impact of the CNPs on the mechanical characteristics of the resultant films was reversed in the case of the SPI/glucose mass ratio of 1:0.75. Thus, it was inferred that a small quantity of CNPs can change SPIs that are cross-linked, which in turn affects the resultant SPI-OS films' mechanical characteristics [19].

2.3 Thermal analysis

- Natural protein gelatin (GL) is manufactured and reinforced with poly 4-hydroxyphenyl methacrylate-carbon nano-onions (PHPMA-CNOs = f-CNOs) to create GL/f-CNOs composite hydrogels using the sonochemical approach [21].
- Fig. 4.2A shows the results of DSC study performed to determine the melting temperature and crystallinity of composite hydrogels. The degree of crystallinity (DOC) of pure GL hydrogel was 35.02 ± 0.17, whereas the DOC of GL/f-CNOs composite hydrogel with 1 mg/mL of f-CNOs was 46.19 ± 0.37. The results of the GL/f-CNOs composite hydrogel, on the contrary, showed 51.12 ± 0.13. In addition, the melting temperatures of all the hydrogels ranged from 95 to 155°C (Fig. 4.2A). Overall, DSC research showed that the addition of f-CNOs considerably improved the composite hydrogels' crystallinity and melting temperature [21].
- Fig. 4.2B shows the TGA plot for freeze-dried hydrogels. The TGA data revealed the relationship between the concentration of f-CNOs and the thermal stability of composite hydrogels. With increasing the f-CNOs content, a progressive improvement in the thermal stability of composite hydrogels was seen. Around 12%–14% of weight loss was seen, especially at 112°C caused by the release of water contained inside hydrogel samples. The hydrogels showed signs of heat breakdown between 295 and 425°C. In particular, the beginning temperature of degradation ($T_{0.1}$) for pure GL hydrogel was 298°C, while the halfway temperature ($T_{0.5}$)

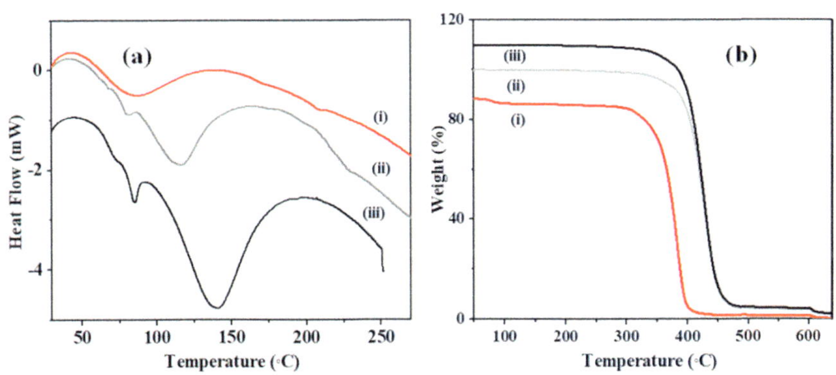

Figure 4.2 (A) DSC and (B) TGA graphs of (i) pristine GL, (ii) GL/f-CNOs (1 mg/mL), and GL/f-CNOs (2 mg/mL) composite hydrogels, respectively. *(Reproduced with copyright permission from Ref. [21].)*

was 345°C. With 1 mg/mL of f-CNOs, the GL/f-CNOs composite hydrogel displayed $T_{0.1}$ at about 345°C and $T_{0.5}$ at 420°C. As opposed to this, the GL/f-CNOs composite hydrogel showed $T_{0.1}$ at 347°C and $T_{0.5}$ at 424°C. TGA data showed that the high conductivity of CNOs as well as the Van der Waals or noncovalent electrostatic interaction between f-CNOs and GL chains significantly reduced the onset temperature of the GL/f-CNOs composite hydrogels [21].

2.4 Biocompatibility assay

- It is stated that employing bacterial cellulose nanofibrils (BCN) and protein zein nanoparticles (ZN) as natural building blocks makes it easy, quick, and ecologically friendly to manufacture a mechanically strong and multifunctional nanocomposite. A well-known, scalable papermaking technique successfully incorporates the nanoparticles ZN into the BCN networks to create a homogenous nanopaper composite [22].
- Further tests were conducted on the mouse L929 fibroblast cells to determine the biocompatibility of the BCN-ZN nanocomposites. The findings of the L929 fibroblast cells' adherence and growth on the nanocomposite surfaces are depicted in Fig. 4.3. Fig. 4.3A illustrates that none of the samples are harmful to the L929 fibroblast cells, indicating that nanocomposites are generally biocompatible. After 24 and 48 h of growth, the BCN-ZN nanocomposites exhibit considerably larger fibroblast quantities than pure BC, and these numbers modestly

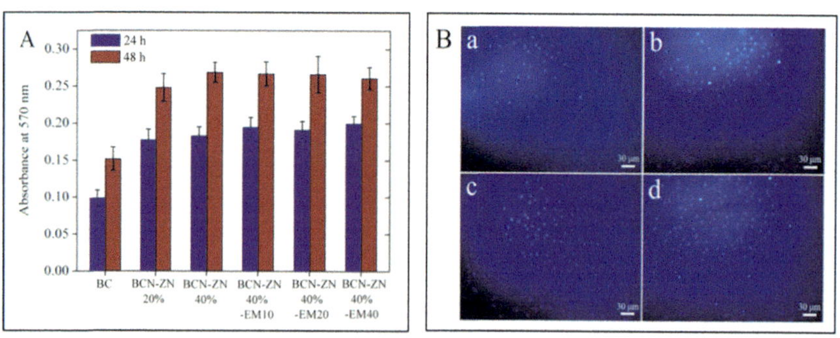

Figure 4.3 (A) MTT tests of L929 fibroblast cells after 24 and 48 h of growth on membranes made of pure BC, BCN-ZN nanocomposites, and BCN-ZN nanocomposites loaded with EM. (B) After 48 h of culture, fluorescent pictures of L929 fibroblast cells were taken on (a) pure BC, (b) BCN-ZN 20%, (c) BCN-ZN 40%, and (d) BCN-ZN 40%-EM40 nanocomposites. For fluorescence imaging, Hoechst stains were applied to all membranes. *(Reproduced with copyright permission from Ref. [22].)*

rise with increasing ZN concentration. Fig. 4.3B shows the fluorescence pictures of cells on the surfaces of nanocomposites after 48 h of incubation. The BCN-ZN nanocomposites exhibit larger cell densities than pure BC, which is in excellent accord with the outcome of MTT experiments (Fig. 4.3A). These findings suggest that ZN and BCN may be combined to efficiently enhance cell development and proliferation on BCN-ZN nanocomposites, increasing the biocompatibility of BC-based materials as a whole [22].

2.5 Electrochemical performance

- A viable option for creating "green" flexible electronics is thought to be soy protein isolate (SPI), which has a lot of potential for use in flexible wearable electronics. Several SPI-based nanocomposite films are created by incorporating $BaTiO_3$ (HBT), an inorganic filler with a high dielectric constant, as interleaved nanoparticles into a biodegradable SPI substrate [23]. Specifically, the manufactured film, SPI HBT0.5GL0.5, which contains 0.5 wt% HBT and glycerin (GL). The high specific capacitance and low charge transfer resistance of the fully biocompatible nanocomposites may present a viable path toward the creation of an environmentally benign electrode material for energy storage applications [24].
- The conductivity of all SPI-HBT films improved steadily as the HBT content rose (Fig. 4.4A), especially that of SPI-HBT0.5GL0.5, which reached a maximum conductivity of 0.24 S/m and is seven orders of magnitude higher than that of SPI-GL2.5 (3.74 10^{-8} S/m), demonstrating that the addition of HBT produced a remarkable increase in conductivity [23].
- This specific SPIHBT0.5GL0.5 film demonstrated equivalent (even greater) conductivity when compared to 10 different types of synthetic composite polymers in earlier investigations, reaching 0.912 S/m under conditions of low conductive filler loading (0.5 wt%) and high moisture content (48.2%) (Fig. 4.4B). At a 10% loading of supramolecular polymer functionalized graphene (SPFG), the conductivity of the poly (L-lactic acid) (PLLA) polymer (sample five in Fig. 4.4B) was as high as 0.96 S/m; however, when the loading was 1% (sample four in Fig. 4.4B), the conductivity decreased to 5.62 105 S/m, which was significantly lower than the conductivity of the SPIHBT0.5GL0.5 film [23].

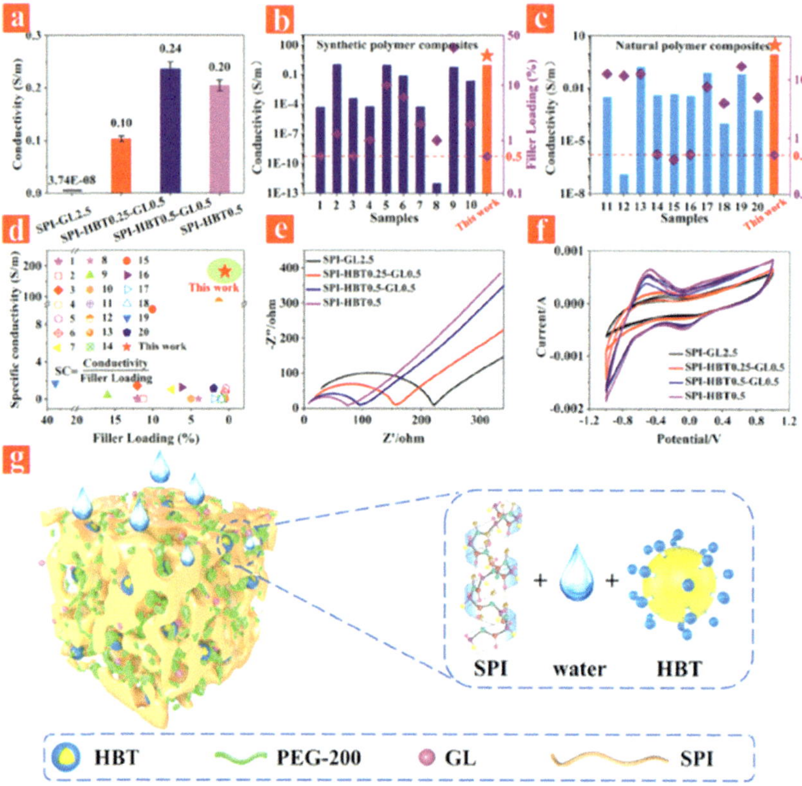

Figure 4.4 The SPI-HBT-GL0.5 film's conductivity and electrical conduction schematic. (A) A conductivity comparison of various SPI-based films. (B) A comparison of the synthetic polymer composites' conductivity with the SPI-HBT-GL film (C) SPIHBT0.5GL0.5 comparison of the conductivity of natural polymer composites. (D) A comparison of the specific conductivity of natural and synthetic polymer composites using the SPI-HBT0.5-GL0.5 film. (E) A schematic of impedance Nyquist for SPI-based films. (F) Curves of the SPI-based films' cyclic voltammetry. (G) The conductivity of the SPI-HBT-GL-0.5 film. *(Reproduced with copyright permission from Ref. [23].)*

- The SPIHBT0.5GL0.5 film's conductivity was also much greater than that of several bio-based and SPI-based conductive composites, including silk, electrical protein NWs, cellulose, starch, and bio-oil (Fig. 4.4C).
- The conflict between flexibility and conductivity would be a long-term design issue for flexible wearable devices. For instance, the high filler loading made the ionic conductive silk/laponite composite film prone to agglomerate, which made the film brittle and susceptible

to cracking when stretched by external pressures (sample 13). Intriguingly, the addition of only 0.5 weight percent (wt%) HBT to the SPI-based films successfully assisted in achieving a noticeably high specific conductivity [SC, = conductivity/filler loading (%)] (Fig. 4.4D); meanwhile, the relatively low content of the HBT filler was capable of evenly dispersing in the SPI substrate for good flexibility, pointing to its potential application in niche markets, such as wearable flexible electronics [23].

- It was hypothesized that the following can account for the SPI-HBT0.5-GL0.5 film's higher conductivity: First, the dielectric constant increases with increasing BT content because BT has a higher dielectric constant. Second, the grafted OH layer was strongly linked to the protein chains' COOH groups, which enhanced the dispersion of the HBT nanoparticles and encouraged the development of a consistent electric field in the composites that resulted. A greater effective conductivity was attained because ions and water molecules were able to more readily influence the polar hydroxyl groups. Third, the SPI substrate's development of a three-dimensional hydrogen bond network architecture provided a useful conductive channel (Fig. 4.4G).
- Impedance of the AC Films with various HBT contents had remarkably varied Nyquist diagrams. In particular, as the HBT content gradually increased, the high-frequency semicircle's diameter rapidly shrank until it was reduced by three times (i.e., Fig. 4.4E, from a black to a purple trace), most likely as a result of the increased quantity of conductive particles in the film brought on by the higher HBT content. In summary, the improvement in the films' electrical properties would mostly be attributed to the substrates' hydrogen bond cross-linking and the addition of HBT [23].
- The cyclic voltammogram curves of the SPI-based films are shown in Fig. 4.4F. SPIHBT0.5GL0.5 has a substantially bigger closed hysteresis loop area than SPIGL2.5. The primary cause was the strong dielectric property of the HBT nanoparticle, which significantly increased the conductivity of the films. However, the geometry of the filler, its dispersion, the local electric field distribution, and the interface polarization between various phases are all important factors that affect the electrochemical performance of the composite film. The formation of an interconnected filler network in the SPI substrate was aided by hydroxylated surface shell layers, and the −OH absorbent is more helpful in producing composite materials with high conductivity [23].

3. Industrial applications

3.1 Ischemic diseases treatment

(a) *Bio-Sketch*: The leading cause of mortality in the world is ischemic heart disease (IHD), and therapeutic angiogenesis is its potent method for treatment. Due to its high bioactive qualities, sericin (S), a natural silk protein, is frequently employed in regenerative medicine. Graphene oxide (GO), a derivative of graphene, is more readily manufactured and has the same desirable features as graphene. In addition, GO is more soluble in polar solvents and is easily functionalized due to an abundance of oxygen-containing groups on both its basal and edge planes. These characteristics support its broad applicability, particularly in nanocomposites with improved mechanical, electrical, and physicochemical properties. Due to their amphiphilic character and capacity to bear high mechanical stresses, proteins, and protein-like materials have been employed as matrix materials in GO-based composites instead of poisonous and harmful organic polymers or solvents. The primary goal is to create sericin-functionalized graphene oxide (SGO) nanocomposites for the treatment of illnesses characterized by inadequate angiogenesis [25].

(b) Synthesis:

- Graphite in solution was used to create modified Hummers' technique graphene oxide (GO) nanosheets.
- The high-temperature, high-pressure process was modified to carry out the degumming of sericin (S) from the silk cocoon. After being broken up into pieces, the silk cocoon was submerged in distilled water. The mixture was centrifuged after being held at 121°C and the supernatant was collected after membrane dialyze and storage at −20°C [25].
- In phosphate-buffered saline solution, GO was mixed continuously with 1-Ethyl-3-(3-dimethylaminopropyl) Carbodiimide (EDC) and N-hydroxysuccinimide (NHS) and sericin was added dropwise. The mixture was centrifuged and finally, SGO nanocomposite pellet was lyophilized. EDC's function is to activate the carboxyl groups on GO's surface.

(c) Application:

- *Hemolytic assay*: The hemocompatibility of SGO nanocomposites on human erythrocytes was evaluated using a hemolytic test. The centrifuged pellet from healthy human blood samples was washed in phosphate-buffered saline (PBS). The erythrocytes were diluted in phosphate-buffered saline and used for the assay. In general, any foreign particle that comes into touch with erythrocytes may cause cell membrane disruption and cause hemoglobin to leak out [25]. Therefore, it is crucial to research the produced nanocomposites' hemocompatibility. According to the American Standard for Testing Materials, a substance is regarded as nonhemolytic if the percentage of hemolysis is less than 2. The greatest concentration employed in the analysis for the current study revealed a percentage of hemolysis of 1.25, illuminating the hemocompatible nature of SGO nanocomposites (Fig. 4.5A).

- *Chick embryo angiogenesis (CEA) assay*: The CEA test was used to examine angiogenesis or vascular sprouting in the presence of SGO nanocomposites. It is the accepted test that uses egg yolk to look at the development of new blood vessels. The shells of the 2–3-day-old fertilized chicken eggs were cleaned with ethanol before being incubated. Furthermore, S, GO, and SGO nanocomposites were used to nurture chick embryos [25]. When compared to controls, the data obtained show that SGO-treated chick embryos generate more blood vessels, demonstrating their angiogenic ability (Fig. 4.5B).

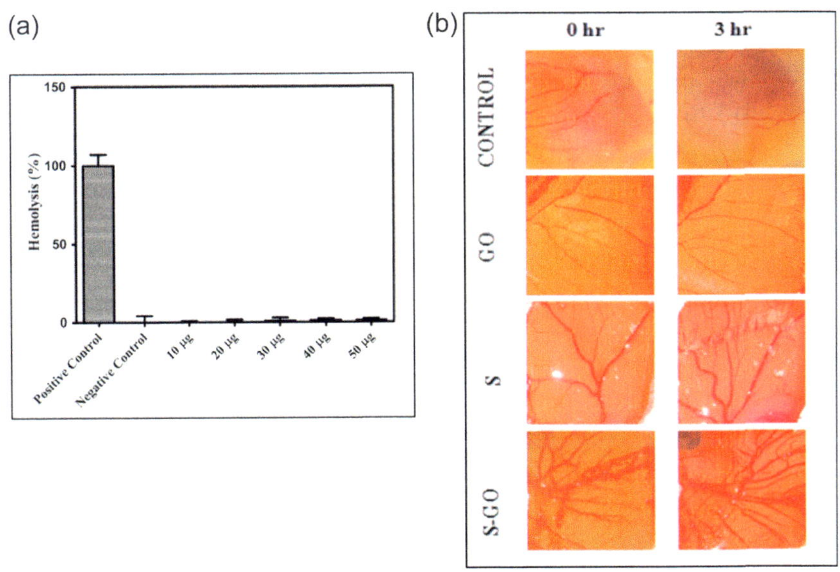

Figure 4.5 (A) Hemocompatibility testing for S-GO nanocomposites at various concentrations. The negative and positive controls were PBS and water, respectively. (B) In vivo CEA test for the untreated control, GO, S, and S-GO groups. *(Reproduced with copyright permission from Ref. [25].)*

3.2 Antimicrobial activity

(a) *Bio-Sketch*: A possible approach to suppress harmful bacteria is the use of nanomaterials, either alone or in composites with proteins [26,27]. To determine the antibacterial effectiveness of these nanocomposites, silver nanoparticles (AgNPs) were combined with either fenugreek or mung bean seed proteins (FNP or MNP, respectively). Fenugreek seed protein has a good amino acid profile and is rich in legumes, making it a possible source of bioactive agents. When digested, certain bioactive peptides are released that can suppress bacterial infections. The peptides that make up the mung bean protein hydrolyzate can serve as ACE inhibitors, antioxidants, and anticancer agents. In recent years, silver nanoparticles (AgNPs), which have antibacterial properties against bacteria plus fungi may combat multidrug-resistant bacterial strains and have emerged as one of the most researched and examined nanostructures created from nanotechnology. AgNPs can disrupt bacterial membranes and kill cells, resulting in severe disruptions of cell structure, function, and death [28].

(b) Synthesis:

- After being pulverized in a grinder, the mung bean, and fenugreek seeds were continuously stirred in n-hexane at room temperature (RT) before being filtered through cheesecloth. The defatted seeds were utilized for protein isolation after drying. The defatted slurry was mixed with distilled water, pH-adjusted to 9.0 at RT using 0.1 N NaOH; agitated, and centrifuged. To precipitate the protein, the extracts were mixed and the pH was raised to 4.5 using 1 N HCL. Centrifugation was used to separate the proteins, and the supernatant was then decanted out. Crude protein was dialyzed against distilled water, rinsed, dispersed in distilled water at pH 7.5, and then lyophilized. The isolated proteins from fenugreek and mung beans that were employed as source materials had purity levels above 98.5% and 99.8%, respectively. Sodium Dodecyl Sulfate-Polyacrylamide Gel Electrophoresis was used to further fractionate them (SDS−PAGE).
- Trisodium citrate (TSC) was used as a reducing and capping agent to produce silver nanoparticles using the coprecipitation technique. Before adding TSC, the $AgNO_3$ solution was first mixed in deionized water, brought to a boil, and heated until the mixture's color turned pale yellow. The mixture was then brought to RT while remaining black to protect against light [28].

- In a beaker of silver nitrate solution, mung bean or fenugreek dispersion in deionized distilled water was added, and the mixture was heated until boiling. Trisodium citrate was then added drop by drop while being stirred until the yellow hue was visible. The silver-fenugreek nanocomposite (Ag-FNP) or silver-mung-bean nanocomposite has now undergone synthetic synthesis (Ag-MNP).

(c) *Application*: Researchers investigated the antibacterial effects of protein nanocomposites (Ag-FNP, Ag-MNP), solo proteins (FNP and MNP), and AgNPs against Gram-positive and Gram-negative harmful bacteria (Table 4.1). Tube dilution was used to evaluate the Minimum inhibitory concentrations (MIC) of various compounds against various bacteria. After being serially diluted in bacterial growth media, the test substance was introduced to the test organisms, and they were then incubated [28]. All of the antimicrobial drugs that were put to the test demonstrated antibacterial activity with substantially different values ($P < .05$) at the MIC. Ag-FNP and Ag-MP both demonstrated wider antibacterial activity than either AgNPs or proteins did (FNP and MNP). The most susceptible organisms were found to be Gram-positive *S. aureus* and Gram-negative *S. typhimurium* (Table 4.1).

3.3 Ultrasensitive medical pressure sensor

- *Bio-Sketch*: Due to the advantages of high sensitivity to force-induced changes, quick response, reliable stability, low manufacturing cost, and relatively low energy consumption, pressure sensors—piezoresistive devices—have been considered as qualified candidates for next-generation pressure sensors [29]. Silk fibroin (SF) based on-skin electronics have drawn a lot of interest for use in creating electronic skins because of their inherent biodegradability, high porosity, superior biocompatibility, environmental sustainability, and ease of manufacture. MXene, a newly discovered two-dimensional (2D) transition-metal carbide and carbonitride with distinctive structural characteristics and excellent electrical properties, has been used in a variety of applications, including energy storage, gas detection, water purification, and electromagnetic interference shielding [13].
- *Synthesis*: By electrospinning the regenerated silk film, which could be acquired from the silkworm cocoons by degumming and dialyzing, the Silk Fibroin (SF) nanofiber membranes with a porous structure and dependable flexibility were created. By etching the Ti_3AlC_2

Table 4.1 Antibacterial activity of (at 1 MIC) AgNPs, FNP, MNP, Ag-FNP, and Ag-MNP, where 1 MIC expressed as 1 μg/mL.

Treatment/	Inhibition zone diameter (mm)				
Pathogenic bacteria	**AgNPs**	**FNP**	**MNP**	**Ag-FNP**	**Ag-MNP**
			Gram-negative bacteria		
K. pneumonia	$10.3 \pm 0.3^{j\text{-}o}$	$13.67 \pm 0.6^{h\text{-}l}$	$10.0 \pm 0.7^{j\text{-}o}$	$53.0 \pm 0.4^{b,c}$	43.0 ± 0.5^{d}
S. typhiurium	$12.0 \pm 0.6^{i\text{-}n}$	$15.3 \pm 0.5^{h\text{-}j}$	21.0 ± 0.2^{g}	$53.0 \pm 0.1^{b,c}$	$53.0 \pm 0.5^{b,c}$
E. coli	$14.0 \pm 0.4^{h\text{-}l}$	5.67 ± 0.6^{op}	$9.0 \pm 0.3^{k\text{-}p}$	43.0 ± 0.1^{d}	50.0 ± 0.8^{c}
P. aerugenosa	$14.67 \pm 0.5^{h\text{-}k}$	$9.0 \pm 0.3^{k\text{-}p}$	$6.3 \pm 0.8^{n\text{-}p}$	$40.0 \pm 0.3^{d,e}$	31.0 ± 0.1^{f}
P. mirabilis	$11.67 \pm 0.2^{i\text{-}n}$	4.3 ± 0.7^{p}	$6.3 \pm 0.1.1^{n\text{-}p}$	$52.0 \pm 0.3^{b,c}$	$53.0 \pm 0.6^{b,c}$
			Gram-positive bacteria		
S. pyogenes	$16.3 \pm 0.3^{g\text{-}i}$	$7.3 \pm 0.6^{m\text{-}p}$	$11.67 \pm 1.5^{i\text{-}n}$	31.0 ± 0.4^{f}	31.0 ± 0.3^{f}
S. aureus	$13.0 \pm 0.6^{i\text{-}m}$	$10.3 \pm 0.1^{j\text{-}o}$	$12.0 \pm 0.8^{i\text{-}n}$	66.0 ± 0.2^{a}	68.0 ± 1.0^{a}
L. monocytogenes	$18.67 \pm 0.5^{g,h}$	$11.3 \pm 0.4^{i\text{-}o}$	$8.67 \pm 1.2^{l\text{-}p}$	$35.3 \pm 1.3^{e,f}$	31.0 ± 0.5^{f}

Ag-FNP, silver fenugreek protein nanocomposite; *Ag-MNP*, silver mung bean protein nanocomposite; *AgNPs*, silver nanoparticles; *FNP*, fenugreek seed proteins; *MNP*, mung bean protein. Every value is the average of three replicates ± SE. Letters (a–p) in same column refer to significantly different values ($P < .05$).

Reproduced with copyright permission from Ref. [28].

MAX phase with a LiF/HCl solution, MXene ($Ti_3C_2T_x$) was created. Through a supramolecular interaction, the MXene nanosheets were dip-coated onto the SF nanofiber membrane to create the MXene-SF membrane. By screen-printing the MXene ink onto the SF nanofiber membrane, the MXene ink-SF interdigitated electrode was created. The biodegradable MXene-SF membrane and the MXene ink-SF interdigitated electrode, which could function as the sensing layer and the electrode layer, respectively, were assembled face to face to create the pressure sensor [13].

(d) Application:

- With high sensitivity (up to 298.4 kPa^{-1}), a broad operating range (up to 39.28 kPa), a quick response/recovery time (7/16 ms), acceptable breathability, great cycle stability, and ecologically benign degradability, the resulting sensor demonstrated outstanding sensing performance. It, therefore, has considerable promise for medical diagnosis and therapy since it might be used to detect finger motions, blood pressure, muscle, and throat movements [13].
- As seen in Fig. 4.6A, the sensor could detect finger bending when it was attached to a human finger, and the current response could further rise as the bending angles increased. In addition, the sensor might be used to measure the various pressures that the finger push produces. The sensory response increased in step with the steadily rising pressure (Fig. 4.6B).
- In the meantime, it was also possible to realize the physical signals of elbow bending (Fig. 4.6C), which is much more significant for the identification of physical rehabilitation training and healing muscle damage [13].
- The human wrist pulse is a crucial indicator of a person's heart rate and artery health, hence the pressure sensor's ability to detect a pulse is highly significant for potential medical diagnosis. Fig. 4.6D illustrates how the sensor was securely fastened to the wrist artery to measure the physical force produced by the heartbeats in real time. The sensor displayed regular pulse waveforms at a rate of about 90 beats per minute (bpm) for a man. To capture the detailed pulse wave, including the distinctive systolic peak (P1) and diastolic peak, high sensitivity is required (P2). In addition, the radial augmentation index (P2/P1), which is used to detect issues with arterial stiffness and vascular aging, is acknowledged as a crucial parameter. The value was determined to be 0.54, which is a typical value and in good agreement with the literature reference for a 27-year-old healthy adult volunteer (height of 175 cm)., using a series of waveforms obtained

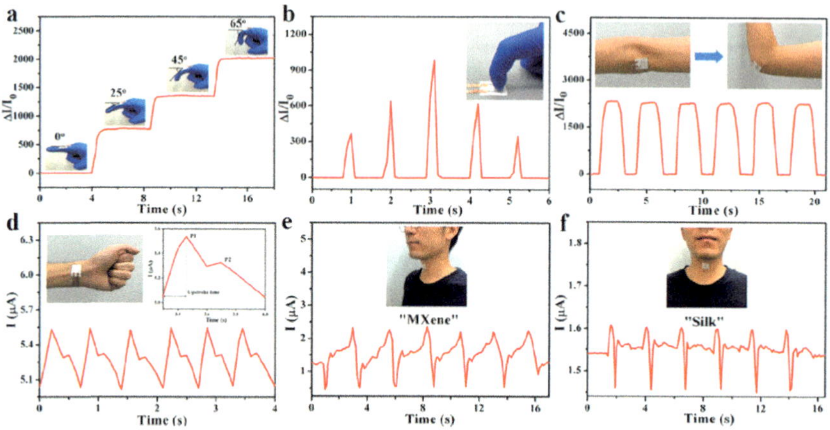

Figure 4.6 Applications of the protein/MXene-based pressure sensor in the detection of both small-scale and widespread human activities. (A) The sensor's reaction when the finger is bent. Images of the sensors mounted on a finger at various bending degrees are shown in the inset. (B) The sensor's ability to detect various pressures produced by finger tapping. Optical pictures of the sensor being touched by fingertips are included. (C) The sensor's ability to detect muscle movements. Optical pictures of the sensor mounted on an elbow are shown in the inset. (D) Monitoring the sensor's reaction to a wrist pulse. Magnified pulse waveforms and an optical picture of the sensor mounted on a wrist are shown in the inset (including P1, P2, and the upstroke time). (E and F) The sensor's response when it senses throat motions made while uttering certain phrases, such as "MXene" and "silk." Optical pictures of the sensors mounted on a throat are shown inset. *(Reproduced with copyright permission from Ref. [13].)*

with the MXene/protein-based sensor. On the contrary, the upstroke time, which stands for the systolic stage's rising time, is a crucial factor to consider while analyzing an artery. For a healthy individual, the upstroke time is often less than 180 ms. The male volunteer's average upstroke time from the radial pulse waves was 150 ms, indicating that his cardiovascular system was in good shape. The pressure sensor may therefore be used to diagnose issues with cardiovascular aging and stiffness in addition to heart rate, by measuring the upstroke duration and radial augmentation index in the pulse waveforms [13].

- The pressure sensor might also be utilized to discern between different neck motions while saying "MXene" and "silk" (Fig. 4.6E and F). When uttering various sentences, various distinctive peaks produced by minuscule vibration pressures might be precisely measured [13].

3.4 Ammonia detection and flame-retardant properties

(a) *Bio-Sketch*: Phytic acid (PA) a nontoxic organic acid generated from plants, serves as a green dopant for polyaniline (PANI) and provides abundant phosphorus, giving fabric nanocomposites excellent conductivity and fire resistance. The electronic textiles (E-textiles) also incorporated strain response with quick ammonia monitoring and high strain sensitivity, making use of the doping-de-doping process of creating a conductive PANI network. A revolutionary method for creating multifunctional flexible electronic devices with many qualities, including sensing, flame retardance, electromagnetic shielding, and energy storage, is provided by this easy and environmentally benign method [14,30].

(b) *Synthesis*: The E-textiles were created by homogeneous dispersions of PA-doped PANI@CNTs being dipped coated. Since CNTs and aniline molecules have strong $\pi-\pi$ conjugated contacts, they can act as templates for in situ polymerization of aniline with ammonium persulfate as the initiator. After that, PA was presented as doped acid while the oxidation structure of PANI is lowered by the addition of nitrogen atoms and protons, and the cationic radicals produced during the doping process give PANI electrical conductivity [14]. Next, the elastic, durable, and skin-friendly milk protein fabric is assembled layer by layer with conductive suspensions to create an efficient microfiber conductive network (MPF).

(c) Application:

- *Ammonia Detection*: The concept and procedure of ammonia detection are shown in Fig. 4.7A and B When exposed to ammonia, E-textile exhibits the exact conductivity and resistance. This may be attributed to the fact that NH_3 catches hydrogen ions in the PANI−NH−group and some PA-doped PANI is converted to a de-doping state. The resistance increases when polyaniline is lowered more; as a result, the current steps down in the same fashion (Fig. 4.7C). The PANI returns to a doped condition once the ammonia volatilizes, and the E-textile regains its initial resistance. The E-textile appears to respond to ammonia at considerably varying rates depending on the concentration (Fig. 4.7D), suggesting both its great sensitivity and stability in ammonia detection. Importantly, the multipurpose E-textile can respond to an ammonia decrease in 1.3 s and maintain a constant current signal for 10 s (Fig. 4.7B and E); making it useful for alarm systems that can detect and warn against severe ammonia leaks [14].

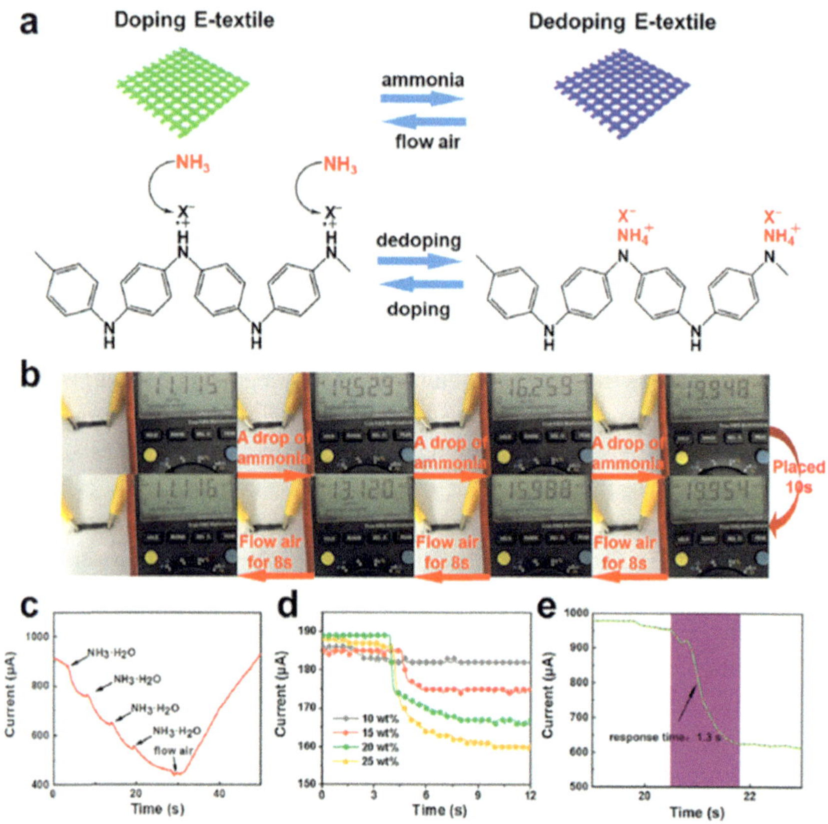

Figure 4.7 (A) Schematic representation of the great sensitivity to ammonium's operating system. (B) Images of resistance variations during ammonia-dropping and air-drying of a PANI@ CNTs/milk protein fabric sample. (C) The PANI@CNTs/milk protein fabric nanohybrids' responsiveness changed after four consecutive drops in ammonia and drying in moving air. (D) Ammonia response current at various concentrations. (E) The PANI@CNTs/milk protein fabric ammonia sensor's reaction time is 1.3 s. *(Reproduced with copyright permission from Ref. [14].)*

- *Flame-Retardant*: Our multifunctional E-textile has superior flame-retardant properties over neat MPF textile because of the phosphorus-rich groups in the PA-doped PANI@ CNTs composites. Here, lighting the samples in the air evaluated the flame retardance of the neat MPF textile and the E-textile, respectively. The resistance to the flame of E-textile results from phosphorus-based flame retardant-PA; thermally decomposing into phosphoric acid to facilitate the formation of the carbonized layer, while the

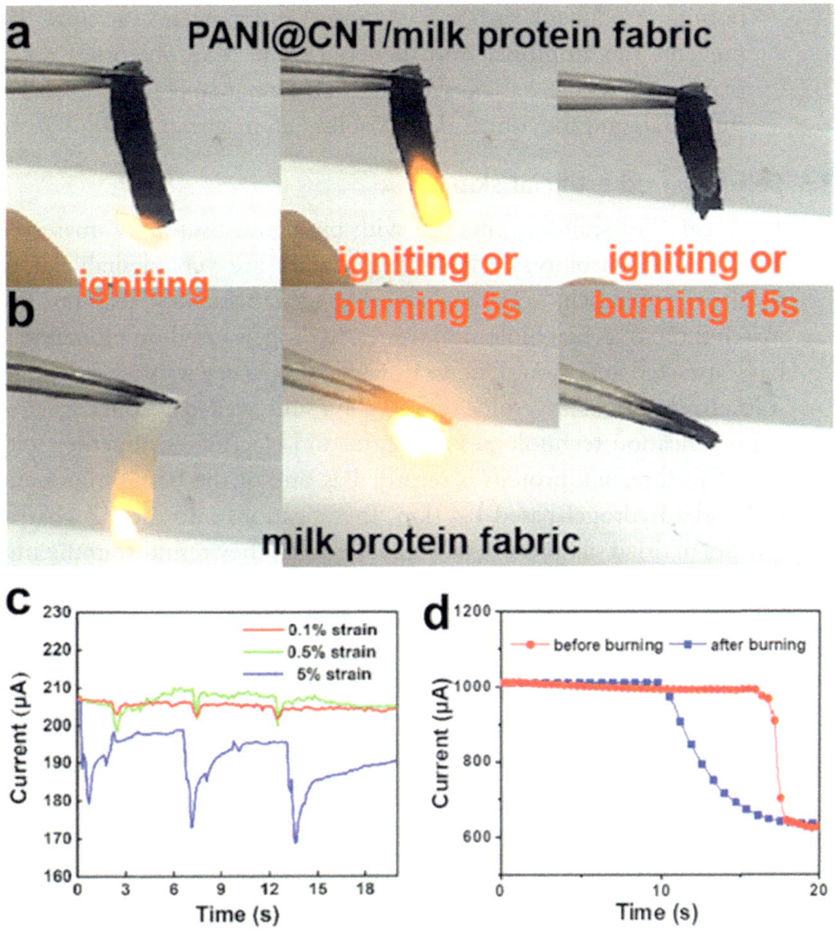

Figure 4.8 (A) Digital photographs of PANI@CNTs/milk protein fabric composites and (B) milk protein fabric after igniting 5 and 15 s, respectively. (C) Repeatedly compressing tests of a PANI@CNTs/milk protein fabric sensor at small strain after burning. (D) Ammonia-responsive sensitivity of the E-textile before and after burning. *(Reproduced with copyright permission from Ref. [14].)*

flammability of MPF can be attributed to abundant carbon and hydrogen elements (Fig. 4.8A and B). Importantly, following the fire treatment, repeating signal patterns were obtained under various strains as seen in Fig. 4.8C. High sensitivity can also be used for ammonia detection (Fig. 4.8D) through E-textile and can detect ammonia sensitively even after burning as seen by almost the same change in current. Response times are slower because burning produces a carbon layer with a micro–nano structure that prevents the ammonia from penetrating it. The outcomes reveal that the E-textile has outstanding flame retardance, and excellent structural, and functional dependability after ignition [14].

3.5 Self-powered artificial skin

(a) *Bio-Sketch*: For seamless interface with biological tissues, PZ materials' softness, deformability, and biocompatibility are very desirable. Due to their water-rich, soft-mechanical, and bio-friendly features that match those of actual biological tissues, hydrogels based on biomaterials have attracted attention. Due to its fascinating characteristics, including softness, deformability, biocompatibility, and well-developed micro/nanofabrication technologies for optics and electronics, together with its PZ feature, silk protein is regarded as one of the best components to build a hydrogel-based PZ skin. Investigations into the PZ characteristics of dried silk protein have revealed that they result from the mechanically stressed, broken symmetries of secondary molecular structures, and crystalline orientations [16].

(b) *Synthesis*: To completely remove the sericin protein, *Bombyx mori* cocoons were ripped apart and cooked in a Na_2CO_3 solution for 30 min. The fibroin fibers were repeatedly washed with distilled water before being dried in air at RT. The silk fibers were dissolved in a $CaCl_2$/glycerol/formic acid solution to create the silk hydrogel solution. ZnONRs, or zinc oxide nanorods, were created using a straightforward hydrothermal technique. Aqueous silver nanowire (AgNW) solution was applied to the PET substrate and dried on a hot plate to create the silver nanowires (AgNWs) embedded in a silk-ZnONR membrane. Then, by combining ZnONR in the silk hydrogel solution at ratios of 0, 1.6, 3.2, 4.8, and 6.4 wt%, silk-ZnONR nanocomposite solutions were created. The nanocomposite mixture was then cast onto the prepared AgNW electrodes and allowed to dry. After drying, the silk-ZnONRs nanocomposite membrane with the buried AgNW electrode was cut to the required shapes and peeled off the PET substrate. Two membranes were bonded together after being kept at 55% relative humidity (RH) for an hour to absorb water from the environment and complete the device's manufacturing. The two thin ZnONRs-silk/AgNW membranes were then put together to create a PZ EG-skin device with a thickness of around 0.81 mm. The buried AgNW electrodes were connected to thin copper wires for electrical measurements. A silk hydrogel solution was applied to the PET substrate for encapsulation and allowed to dry. The silk membranes were removed from the substrate after drying [16]. Then, to create a fully enclosed device, the as-prepared nanocomposite device with a buried AgNW electrode was sandwiched between two silk membranes and kept at 55% RH.

(b) Application:

- Two EG-skin devices were used to power an oximeter using charging capacitors and rectifier circuits at a mechanical frequency of 15 Hz for biomedical applications, as shown in Fig. 4.9A. The oximeter was attached to the charged capacitors, which were then discharged to activate it. Indicating that the EG-skin was

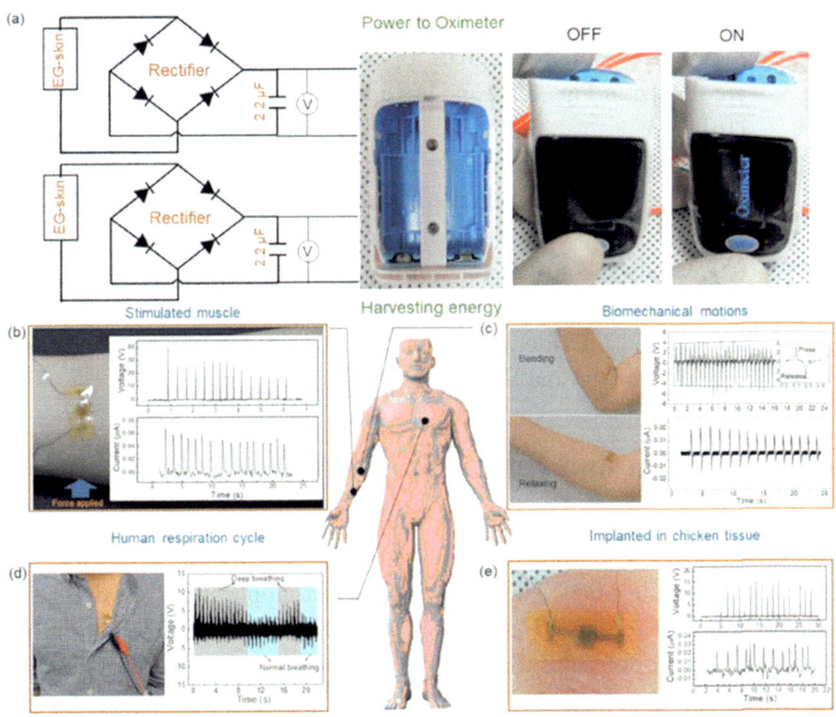

Figure 4.9 Applications of encapsulated EG-skins for activating commercial biodevices (oximeters) and capturing biomechanical energy from various human activities. (A) The circuit diagram for activating the oximeter by charging and discharging the capacitors. Energy production from the EG-skin connected to the (B) forearm by tapping the hand to stimulate the muscle, (C) elbow by bending and releasing, (D) chest to monitor breathing cycles, and (E) inserted in chicken breast tissue. *(Reproduced with copyright permission from Ref. [16].)*

suitable as a power source for low-power consumption biomedical devices; the power provided by the EG-skin was adequate to turn on the oximeter to monitor human health parameters [16].

- As shown in Fig. 4.9B, the EG-skin was fastened to a human hand (forearm) and used to measure the amount of muscle tension that occurred when a deforming force was applied to the hand's bottom side (by tapping it). The gadget might experience tension by stimulating the muscle and producing a stronger electrical signal and power of about 6.2 W/cm^2.
- In addition, a device was attached to the elbow to capture energy from biomechanical hand movements. Electrical power was produced upon elbow bending and releasing, with an output value of 0.2 W/cm^2 (Fig. 4.9C).
- The EG-skin was also placed on the chest to track breathing activities. The respiration signals for regular and deep breathing modes are shown in Fig. 4.9D and are adequate for monitoring respiration [16].
- The implantable electronic device was placed within a portion of biological tissue (chicken) and observed in response to light finger pressure from the outside (Fig. 4.9E). With a power of 0.9 W/cm^2, considerable results for the real-time voltage and current were obtained. As a result, the protein-based artificial EG skin would provide a flexible and biocompatible substrate for soft robotics and wearable/implantable bioelectronics [5].

4. Conclusion and future prospects

This chapter covered the interactions between artificial and naturally occurring proteins, various techniques for building hybrid nanostructures, and their characteristics. The various industrial applications of diversified nanohybrids are discussed in detail as reported in recent publications. Proteins are biopolymers that inspire the design and development of innovative nanocomposites. They make excellent structural and functional components because of their highly developed main and secondary structures, diverse characteristics, and functionalities. In combination, proteins' bio-physicochemical characteristics, ease of processing, and scalability make them desirable options for creating new materials. Therefore, these bio nanocomposites are encouraged to fabricate and can be used for several products.

References

[1] Wang Z, Kang S, Cao S, Krecker M, Tsukruk VV, Singamaneni S. Protein-based functional nanocomposites. MRS Bull December 2020;45(12):1017–26.
[2] Kim E. McKelvey school of engineering department of energy, environmental and chemical engineering (Doctoral dissertation, Washington University.
[3] Floriano R, Edalati K, Pereira KD, Luchessi AD. Titanium-protein nanocomposites as new biomaterials produced by high-pressure torsion. Sci Rep January 10, 2023;13(1):470.
[4] Pirsa S, Aghbolagh Sharifi K. A review of the applications of bioproteins in the preparation of biodegradable films and polymers. J Chem Letters July 1, 2020;1(2):47–58.
[5] Deshmukh RK, Kumar P, Tanwar R, Gaikwad KK. Pectin-polyvinylpyrrolidone based antimicrobial and antioxidant nanocomposite film impregnated with titania nanoparticles and bael shell extract. Food Bioprocess Technol December 2022;15(12):2839–53.
[6] Akbar MU, Athar MM, Bhatti IA, Bhatti HN, Khosa MK, Zia KM, et al. Biomedical applications of bionanocomposites. Bionanocomposites. vol 1. Elsevier; January 2020. p. 457–83.
[7] Sani IK, Alizadeh M. Isolated mung bean protein-pectin nanocomposite film containing true cardamom extract microencapsulation/CeO2 nanoparticles/graphite carbon quantum dots: investigating fluorescence, photocatalytic and antimicrobial properties. Food Packag Shelf Life September 1, 2022;33:100912.
[8] Du C, Du T, Zhou JT, Zhu Y, Jia X, Cheng Y. Enhanced stability and mechanical properties of a graphene–protein nanocomposite film by a facile non-covalent self-assembly approach. Nanomaterials April 1, 2022;12(7):1181.
[9] Asdagh A, Karimi Sani I, Pirsa S, Amiri S, Shariatifar N, Eghbaljoo–Gharehgheshlaghi H, et al. Production and characterization of nanocomposite film based on whey protein isolated/copper oxide nanoparticles containing coconut essential oil and paprika extract. J Polym Environ January 2021;29:335–49.
[10] Meydanju N, Pirsa S, Farzi J. Biodegradable film based on lemon peel powder containing xanthan gum and TiO2–Ag nanoparticles: investigation of physicochemical and antibacterial properties. Polym Test February 1, 2022;106:107445.
[11] Sharifi KA, Pirsa S. Biodegradable film of black mulberry pulp pectin/chlorophyll of black mulberry leaf encapsulated with carboxymethylcellulose/silica nanoparticles: investigation of physicochemical and antimicrobial properties. Mater Chem Phys July 15, 2021;267:124580.
[12] Hadidi M, Jafarzadeh S, Forough M, Garavand F, Alizadeh S, Salehabadi A, et al. Plant protein-based food packaging films; recent advances in fabrication, characterization, and applications. Trends Food Sci Technol February 1, 2022;120:154–73.
[13] Chao M, He L, Gong M, Li N, Li X, Peng L, et al. Breathable Ti3C2Tx MXene/protein nanocomposites for ultrasensitive medical pressure sensor with degradability in solvents. ACS Nano June 3, 2021;15(6):9746–58.
[14] Wang Y, Zhang X, Cao J, Huang X, Zhang X. Multifunctional E-textiles based on biological phytic acid-doped polyaniline/protein fabric nanocomposites. Adv Mater Technol June 2021;6(6):2100003.
[15] He Y, Zhang Z, Wang Y, Liu M, Liao C, Yuan J, et al. Synergistic effects of bioprotein decoration and WS2@ Ti3C2 nanohybrids on the interfacial and tribological performance of PPS/PTFE fabric composites. Tribol Int August 1, 2023;186:108587.
[16] Gogurla N, Roy B, Kim S. Self-powered artificial skin made of engineered silk protein hydrogel. Nano Energy November 1, 2020;77:105242.

[17] Manna S, Manna M, Jana S. Interpenetrating polymer network in microparticulate systems: drug delivery and biomedical application. Interpenet Polymer Network Biomed Appl 2020:1–23.
[18] Liu T, Liu Z, Zhang J, Shi SQ, Gong S, Li J. An ultrastrong bioinspired soy protein isolate-based nanocomposite with graphene oxide intercalation. Compos B Eng May 1, 2022;236:109805.
[19] Bukartyk M, Zholobko O, Wu XF. Green synthesis of soy protein nanocomposites: effects of cross-linking and clay nanoparticles on the mechanical performance. ACS Omega February 11, 2022;7(7):5883–93.
[20] Guan QF, Ling ZC, Han ZM, Yang HB, Yu SH. Ultra-strong, ultra-tough, transparent, and sustainable nanocomposite films for plastic substitute. Matter October 7, 2020;3(4):1308–17.
[21] Mamidi N, Castrejón JV, González-Ortiz A. Rational design and engineering of carbon nano-onions reinforced natural protein nanocomposite hydrogels for biomedical applications. J Mech Behav Biomed Mater April 1, 2020;104:103696.
[22] Li Q, Gao R, Wang L, Xu M, Yuan Y, Ma L, et al. Nanocomposites of bacterial cellulose nanofibrils and zein nanoparticles for food packaging. ACS Appl Nano Mater March 10, 2020;3(3):2899–910.
[23] Wei Y, Jiang S, Li X, Li J, Dong Y, Shi SQ, et al. "Green" flexible electronics: biodegradable and mechanically strong soy protein-based nanocomposite films for human motion monitoring. ACS Appl Mater Interfaces July 27, 2021;13(31):37617–27.
[24] Alam RB, Ahmad MH, Islam MR. Improved electrochemical performance of multi-walled carbon nanotube reinforced gelatin biopolymer for transient energy storage applications. PLoS One November 9, 2023;18(11):e0288113.
[25] Vedakumari SW, Jancy SJ, Pravin YR, Bhoopathy J, Iyswariya K, Thomas S, et al. Facile synthesis of sericin modified graphene oxide nanocomposites for treating ischemic diseases. Environ Res June 1, 2022;209:112925.
[26] Hosseini SN, Pirsa S, Farzi J. Biodegradable nano composite film based on modified starch-albumin/MgO; antibacterial, antioxidant and structural properties. Polym Test May 1, 2021;97:107182.
[27] Dhanalakshmi A, Natarajan B, Ragavan D, Palanimurugan A. Bio-protein fuctionalization of ZnO nanoparticles using chicken egg albumin and bovin serum albumin for enrichment bioactivity. Mater Today Proc January 1, 2022;68:506–14.
[28] Sitohy M, Al-Mohammadi AR, Osman A, Abdel-Shafi S, El-Gazzar N, Hamdi S, et al. Silver-protein nanocomposites as antimicrobial agents. Nanomaterials November 9, 2021;11(11):3006.
[29] Yang H, Wu B, Gao J, Zhang B, Zhao N, Qi F, et al. Composite nanofillers with a locust-like cushioned half-moon structure to improve the impact resistance of polyurethane. J Mater Res Technol November 1, 2023;27:2737–50.
[30] Peng H, Wang D, Fu S. Biomimetic construction of highly durable nacre-like MoS2 bio-nanocomposite coatings on polyacrylonitrile textile for intumescent flame retardation and sustainable solar-thermal-electricity conversion. Compos B Eng June 15, 2021;215:108742.

CHAPTER 5

Biomedical applications of protein-based nanocomposites

Hayfa Alajilani Abraheem Jamjoum[1,2], Khalid Umar[1], Rohana Adnan[1], Tabassum Parveen[3], Jayanudin[4] and H. Fadlullah[5]

[1]School of Chemical Sciences, Universiti Sains Malaysia, Penang, Malaysia; [2]Department of Chemistry, Faculty of Science, University of Sabratha, Sabratah, Libya; [3]Department of Botany, Aligarh Muslim University, Aligarh, Uttar Pradesh, India; [4]Department of Chemical Engineering, Universitas Sultan Ageng Tirtayasa, Banten, Indonesia; [5]Chemistry Education Department, Universitas Sultan Ageng Tirtayasa, Banten, Indonesia

1. Introduction

Proteins are gaining significant attention in various fields and research studies due to their rich chemical functionality, biocompatibility, biodegradability, and favorable mechanical properties [1]. Proteins are polyamides made up of hundreds of amino acids that are fundamental macromolecules in biological systems. In general, protein structure can be organized into four levels. The primary structure is the amino acid sequence, the secondary is the conformation, the tertiary is the overall folding of the polypeptide chain, and the quaternary structure is the specific association of multiple polypeptide chains. The multilevel structures of protein (secondary, tertiary, and quaternary) lead to the interactions and adhesions between different types of amino acids at various positions and different energies [2]. Proteins have been used in dietary or as green materials mainly to prepare biodegradable food packaging and are currently being actively investigated for medical applications. Proteins hold great potential to be applied in various biomedical applications like drug delivery, biosensors, and skin and bone tissue engineering. Proteins are produced by animal, plant, and some microbial agents. Some examples of protein obtained from animals and plants are stated in Table 5.1. The table also listed microbial agents producing protein by bacteria and fungus. The properties of these proteins differ depending on their sources and method of synthesis.

Protein-Based Nanocomposites for Tissue Engineering
ISBN 978-0-323-99357-9
https://doi.org/10.1016/B978-0-323-99357-9.00002-8

Table 5.1 Protein from different sources.

Animal-based protein	Plant-based protein	Microbial agent-producing protein
Whey protein	*Wheat gluten*	*Bacillus coagulans*
Casein	*Corn Zein*	*Cupriavidus necator*
Albumin	*Soy protein*	*Candida utilis*
Keratin	*Kafirin*	*Geotrichum candidum*
Collagen	*Peanut protein*	
Gelatin	*Gliadin*	
Silk	*Lectin*	
Elastin		

Various chemical and physical treatments and substances can alter the structure of proteins to improve their properties [3]. Besides, the integration of protein with organic and inorganic nanomaterials to produce nanocomposites results in synergetic properties improvement in comparison with the individual components [1]. This creates a motivation behind the continuous research and development of protein-based nanocomposites. This chapter highlighted the use of protein nanocomposites for biomedical applications. The discussion is categorized based on the protein sources. Initially, a study on animal-based protein is described, followed by plant-based protein and some examples of synthesis of microbial protein. Finally, the summary and future perspective of protein-based nanocomposites are presented.

2. Biomedical applications of protein nanocomposites derived from animals

This section explores the use of animal-based protein nanocomposites in biomedical applications. It focuses on various proteins such as whey protein, casein, albumin, keratin, collagen, gelatin, and silk. The discussion includes specific examples of each protein type.

2.1 Whey protein

Whey is a protein-rich, biocompatible, and biodegradable material available abundantly as a by-product of the dairy industry [4]. Whey protein is commercially occurring in three forms: whey protein concentrate (WPC), whey protein hydrolyzate (WPH), and whey protein isolate (WPI). Whey protein is made up of β-lactoglobulin, α-lactalbumin, immunoglobulin, glycomacropeptide, bovine serum albumin, and other constituents [5]. Given its high nutritional values, whey protein is widely used as a food supplement and is being actively investigated for its potential in food packaging and biomedical applications. In addition, it has been investigated for antimicrobial, antiviral, and anticarcinogenic properties [6]. A study was conducted to investigate the potential of whey protein isolate (WPI) incorporated with zinc oxide (ZnO) bio-nanocomposites as antibacterial films for wound dressing. The whey protein films were prepared using the solvent casting technique, while the nanostructured ZnO was synthesized through a modified wet chemical precipitation route. The synthesized ZnO exhibited an average size of 30 nm and a specific surface area of 49.5 m^2/g. Subsequently, the nanocomposites were prepared by mixing the WPI films with a different weight percentage of ZnO at 2% (WPI–ZnO-2), 4% (WPI–ZnO-4), and 6% (WPI–ZnO-6), respectively. The films were reported to be flexible, with an average thickness of approximately 60 μm. The appearance of the nanocomposites is depicted in Fig. 5.1. The pure WPI film showed a transparent characteristic. Upon the addition of ZnO, the films turned opaque, and a white film was obtained, which is a common finding for polymer-ZnO composites. The antibacterial activity of the nanocomposites was evaluated against *S. epidermidis* and *E. coli*, and their physicochemical characteristics were determined. ATR-FTIR and XRD analyses revealed that only weak physical interaction existed between the whey protein and ZnO filler. This study shows that the swelling ratio of the nanocomposite films increased at basic pH, which is an attractive property in terms of chronic wound exudate absorption. Meanwhile, the ZnO concentration affected the antibacterial properties of the nanocomposite films, at which a small amount of ZnO could inhibit the growth of *S. epidermidis*. In contrast, higher ZnO concentrations were needed to generate a weak response in *E. coli* [7].

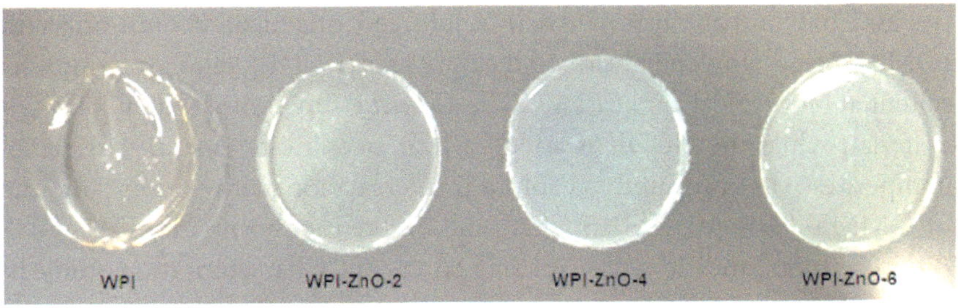

Figure 5.1 The appearance of whey protein isolate nanocomposites at different ZnO loading. *(Reproduced from Ref. [7] with MDPI permission.)*

In another study conducted by Slota et al. hydrogels based on WPI and nano-hydroxyapatite (HAp) were prepared for applications in bone regeneration, and their properties were investigated. HAp is known to have a high chemical and crystallographic similarity to the inorganic phase of bone; therefore, it has the potential to be used for bone regeneration studies. Despite this, it has some limitations, including brittleness, low tensile strength, and low fracture toughness. Therefore, this study proposed the use of hydrogel composites based on WPI and HAp to tackle the problem. Two types of HAp were prepared using the wet precipitation method, having slightly different physicochemical properties. Three different concentrations of HAp were used to prepare the hydrogels varying from 0, 5, 10, and 15 wt%. In vitro analysis of the hydrogels was conducted in four types of liquid, which are distilled water, Ringer's fluid, artificial saliva, and simulated body fluid. The incubation finding shows a successful formation of new layers of apatite, and the composite with 15 wt% of HAp showed the best bioactivity based on the formation of apatite. Besides, the microbiological analysis confirmed the safety of the composite with the absence of biomaterial-mediated cytotoxicity activity. This supports the WPI/HAp composite hydrogels as potential materials for novel bone substitutes [8].

2.2 Casein

Casein is a low-cost, nontoxic, highly stable, and readily accessible protein obtained from dairy manufacturing similar to whey. Casein is the major component of protein in milk that accounts for around 80% of the total protein [9], depending on the source of the milk. Casein is known to be an efficient transport for essential nutrients and minerals like calcium and phosphate. Due to this nature, casein has been used in drug delivery systems of modern medicine [10]. Casein exists in the form of αs1-casein, αs2-casein β-casein, and κ-casein. Liu et al. studied the structural characteristics and biocompatibility of casein-reinforced organized montmorillonite (OMMT) and ethylene glycol diglycidyl ether (EGDE) nanocomposites for potential biomedical applications. The OMMT functions as the reinforcing material, while the EGDE is added as the crosslinking agent. The nanocomposites were prepared via solution intercalation with various amounts of OMMT (0, 5, 10, and 15 wt.%) and different concentrations of EGDE (0, 10, 20, 30, and 40 wt.%) relative to casein. Characterization study by FTIR shows that EGDE reacted with casein to form a network structure, whereas increasing the amount of OMMT resulted in the change in

OMMT structure from exfoliated to intercalated, as proven by XRD and TEM. Furthermore, with SEM analysis, they observed a transition of the film surface from smooth to porous with the incorporation of OMMT. The nanocomposites with OMMT and EGDE have enhanced physical properties in terms of thermal stability, water resistance, mechanical properties, and biodegradation resistance compared with neat casein. Based on the cell culture studied, the addition of OMMT significantly improves the biocompatibility of the casein nanocomposites owing to the presence of Si element and higher surface area that can promote cell attachment. Overall, the prepared nanocomposites are suitable for cell adhesion and proliferation, and they can be used as substrates for cell growth in wound healing and tissue engineering applications [11]. Dumitrescu et al. conducted a study on hydrogels consisting of casein-loaded poly(2-hydroxyethyl methacrylate)-polyethylene glycol diacrylate (PHEMA-PEGDA) for potential applications in bone repair and regeneration. Although PHEMA hydrogel has been widely employed in tissue repair, it does not effectively promote mineralization. Therefore, it serves as a suitable matrix for evaluating the mineralization capability of casein. The objective of this study was to explore the impact of phosphoprotein on enhancing mineral deposition within the hydrogel.

The hydrogels were prepared through free radical bulk polymerization at room temperature, with varying casein loading. The PHEMA-PEGDA amount was maintained at a fixed 1:1 weight ratio, while the casein content ranged from 0% to 100% relative to PHEMA-PEGDA. Fig. 5.2 illustrates the representation of the samples. The results obtained from calcium/

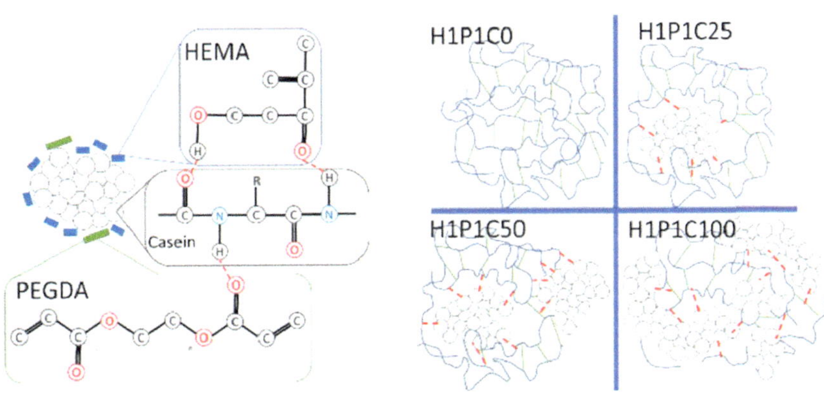

Figure 5.2 Representative of casein-loaded phema-PEGDA at 0, 25, 50, and 100 wt.% of casein. *(Reproduced from Ref. [12] with MDPI permission.)*

phosphate alternate incubation indicate that an increase in casein content contributes to enhanced mineralization. SEM analysis confirmed the formation of a nanoapatite phase in the protein areas. This characteristic is crucial for the hydrogel's suitability in applications related to bone repair and regeneration [12].

2.3 Albumin

Albumin is another type of protein that exists in different types, including ovalbumin, human serum albumin (HSA), and bovine serum albumin (BSA), depending on their origin. Albumin is usually used for drug delivery, carrier, and other uses in the pharmaceutical industry. Serum albumin is the most abundant plasma protein and is frequently used as a carrier [13]. Zewde et al. prepared hydrogel nanocomposites containing BSA-conjugated silver nanoparticles (BSA/Ag) to study the interaction between the hydrogel and the nanoparticle. The hydrogel was prepared by using tetrazine-modified polyethylene glycol and norbornene-modified hyaluronic acid, while the BSA-silver nanoparticle was encapsulated by using in situ reaction in the matrix. Based on the XPS analysis, they found out that there is a rearrangement of the hydrogel molecule at which the polyethylene glycol part is pointing up toward the surface, and the hyaluronic acid interacts with the bovine serum albumin through hydrogen bonding. Apart from that, another important finding from these nanocomposites is their antimicrobial properties. The neat hydrogel showed poor antimicrobial activity performance against *E. coli*, *L. monocytogenes*, and *S. sonnei*. In contrast, the addition of BAS/Ag nanoparticles to the hydrogel resulted in excellent bacterial activity against these three bacteria. This is a crucial criterion for the hydrogel nanocomposites to be used in wound dressing applications [14]. Another study on BSA was reported previously on BSA-stabilized manganese-based nanocomposites with sensitive tumor microenvironment response produced an efficient drug delivery system [15]. This study on human serum albumin nanocomposites has been conducted by Akbal et al. In this study, they synthesize a new saponin-loaded montmorillonite-human serum albumin (SAP-loaded Mt-HSA) as a drug delivery system for colorectal cancer therapy. HSA acts as the carrier due to its high binding affinity, high biocompatibility, and ability to form spherical nanoparticles. The Mt possesses excellent mucoadhesive properties that can help the nanocomposites to pass through the gastrointestinal barrier. Meanwhile, saponin is known to have antimicrobial, antifungal, antiinflammatory, and hypocholesterolemic effects. All these combined characteristics are useful for drug delivery systems. The SAP-loaded Mt-HSA nanocomposites were prepared by desolvation technique using precipitating and crosslinking agents, and their performance was evaluated. The nanocomposites were tested by colorectal cancer cell line (DLD-1) and L9292 fibroblast cells as a healthy cell model. Interestingly, the nanocomposites were found to be effective in destroying cancer cells with minimal or no toxicity toward healthy cells [16]. Aside from this, Elgohary et al. conducted a study on boronic acid decorated HSA nanocomposites for combined chemo/herbal therapy targeting sialic acid residues in lung cancer [17].

2.4 Keratin

Keratin is another type of natural protein usually found in hair, horns, wool, hooves, and nails. Keratin contains cell-binding groups such as leucine-aspartate-valine, glutamate-aspartate-serine, and arginine-glycine-aspartate that benefit proliferation and cell attachment [18]. A study on keratin-chitosan/ZnO (KCZnO) nanocomposites hydrogel was investigated by Zhai et al. for antimicrobial treatment of burn wound healing. Keratin powder used in this study was extracted from human hair. The hydrogel nanocomposites were prepared via the lyophilization technique and used as bandages. The addition of ZnO provides good antibacterial properties and tensile strength and sustains swelling. The KCZnO bandage has high porosity that is beneficial for the augmentation of fibroblast cells. Based on the in vivo assessments in SD rats, the bandage also showed increased wound curing with faster skin cell construction and collagen development. These findings support KCZnO nanocomposite bandages for burn wound healing [19]. A recent study by Das et al. reported on guar gum ester combined with chicken feather keratin interact films scaffold for tissue engineering. The guar gum was cross-linked with hydrolyzed keratin, and the films were prepared using different ratios of the polymer. The protein-polysaccharide combination produced films with enhanced physic-chemical properties, including mechanical properties and porosity. The films also give excellent antimicrobial properties against *E. coli* and *S. aureus* [20]. Furthermore, there is another study on keratin-modified bacterial cellulose (BC) nanocomposites for skin tissue engineering was reported. The keratin was isolated from human hair. It was added to the BC to enhance dermal fibroblast cells' attachment. This was proven by the cell culture studies in which dermal fibroblast demonstrated a good attachment profile, and keratinocytes maintained the original morphology of the surface of the nanocomposites [21].

2.5 Collagen

Collagen has been widely used for different types of medical applications. Collagen is known for its unique features, including biocompatibility, biodegradability, remarkable safety profile, and low antigenicity, and it can be found abundantly in vertebrate organisms [22]. One study examined the stability and biocompatibility of nanocomposite films from PLA/collagen/silver nanoparticles (AgNP). Hydrolyzed collagen obtained from the acid treatment of bovine tendon collagen was used in this work. The films were prepared by using melt blending and compression molding techniques with different amounts of AgNP (0.5, 1.0, and 1.5 wt.%) added, and the collagen was fixed at 5 wt.% for every ratio. It was revealed that, addition of AgNP improved the stability of the nanocomposites due to the blocking of the oxidation of PLA free radicals. They conducted in vitro biocompatibility analysis on the mouse fibroblast cell line NCTC, clone L929, using quantitative 3-(4,5-dimethylthiazol-2-yl)-2,5-diphenyltetrazolium bromide (MTT) and lactate dehydrogenase (LDH) assays. The MTT results revealed high values of cell viability of more than 80% with the presence of the nanocomposites for 48 h, while the LDH released were reduced to less than 15%. The lower LDH value indicates no damage to the cell membranes. The nanocomposites did not affect cell proliferation and maintained the normal cell growth rate, as proven by the cell cycle analysis [23]. Marin et al. conducted a study on collagen/clay/gentamicin nanocomposites aiming to be used for skin regeneration's purpose. There are four different kinds of commercial clays: Cloisite 20A, Cloisite 15A, Cloisite 93A, and Cloisite 30B, were used to investigate the effect of clay type on the release of gentamicin and overall properties of the nanocomposites. Alkaline-treated bovine cartilage-derived type II collagen gel was chosen in the interim. Clay layers are distributed uniformly throughout the collagen matrix, as shown by the XRD study. They found out from the in vitro kinetic profile test that the burst release of gentamicin from the nanocomposites retarded depending on the clay type compared with collagen-gentamicin. All the prepared nanocomposites displayed favorable antimicrobial activities against *E. coli* and *S. aureus*, as shown in Fig. 5.3. Based on the result obtained, the clay type of Cloisite 93A and Cloisite 30B presented the best performance for further use and investigation [24].

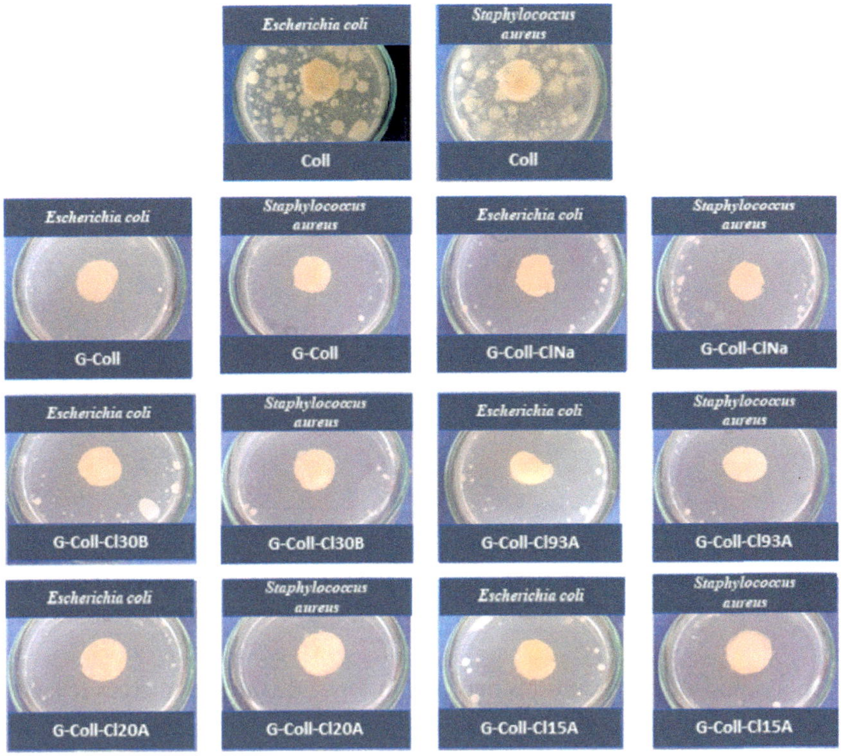

Figure 5.3 Photographic images of antimicrobial activity of collagen/clay/gentamicin nanocomposites. *(Reproduced from Ref. [24] with MDPI permission.)*

2.6 Gelatin

Gelatin is a heterogeneous mixture of high molecular mass proteins and high water solubility that can be derived from collagen of bones, tendons, skin, and ligaments via acidic or basic hydrolysis. Gelatin is tasteless and colorless with adequate transparency; it exists in flakes, sheets, or coarse powder forms [25]. Recently, Samadian et al. fabricated 3D scaffold nanocomposites based on poly (L-lactic acid)/polycaprolactone (PLLA/PCL) containing gelatin nanofibers (GNF) and gold nanoparticle (AuNP) for bone tissue engineering. In this study, GNF was prepared through electrospinning methods and was used as an extracellular matrix structure. The 3D scaffold was prepared using thermal-induced phase separation and subsequently undergoes characterization. The overview of the scaffold

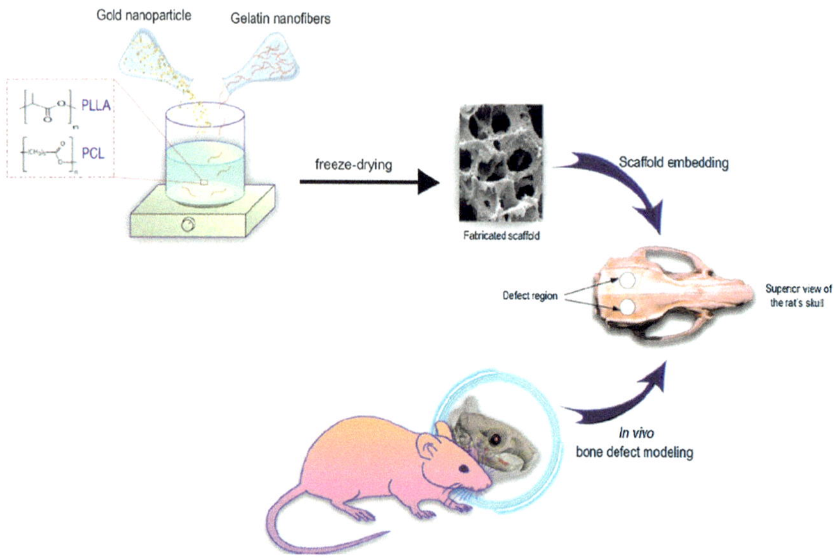

Figure 5.4 Overview of the scaffold nanocomposites preparation and application. *(Reproduced from Ref. [26] with Springer Nature permission.)*

nanocomposite preparation is depicted in Fig. 5.4. In vitro analysis revealed that the composite with 80 ppm AuNP exhibited the highest cell proliferation. In addition, PLLA/PCL/Gelatin/80 ppm AuNP give the highest neo-bone formation, osteocyte in lacuna woven formation, and angiogenesis in the defect site [26].

A study on gelatin-gallic acid/ZnO nanocomposites as bioadhesives for wound dressing applications has been conducted. In this work, silane was used as the crosslinker to promote gelatin-ZnO interactions. The nanocomposite films showed antimicrobial activity against *S. aureus* and *E. coli*, and bacterial proliferation was inhibited at lower ZnO contents of 1%. More importantly, a higher adhesion level was achieved for the sample containing gallic acid compared with the commercial cyanoacrylate adhesive [27]. Furthermore, Rakhshaei et al. reported a study on chitosan-gelatin/zinc oxide (CS-Gel/nZnO) nanocomposites hydrogel scaffold that possesses both drug delivery and antibacterial properties for skin tissue engineering. From the delivery studies, the CS-Gel/nZnO scaffold exhibited prolonged drug release. The scaffold nanocomposites also showed antimicrobial activity against *E. coli* and *S. aureus* [28]. Many researchers have explored gelatin-based nanocomposite for medical applications. Other examples of studies on gelatin reported previously were on chitosan/

gelatin/fluorohydroxyapatite cartilage scaffold [29], boron nitride nanosheets/gelatin nanocomposites for use as artificial nacre [30], gelatin/ciprofloxacin/polymyxin B sulfate for wound dressing [31], and cellulose acetate/gelatin/hydroxyapatite nanocomposites mats for wound dressing [32].

2.7 Silk

Silk is made up of two major types of protein, which are fibroin, a fibrous protein, and sericin, a sticky protein. Both types have been used for many tissue engineering researches. Sericin and fibroin-enriched nanocomposites hydrogel based on 3-hydroxyethyl methacrylate/2-acrylamido-2-methylpropane sulfonic acid/montmorillonite (HEMA/AMPSA/MMT) were investigated for soft tissue regeneration in the context of regenerative medicine. This study found that all the materials are biocompatible, and the cells' adipogenic differentiation was boosted by the addition of sericin and fibroin protein [33]. One study on nanocomposites made up of pectin-cellulose hydrogel/silk fibroin/magnesium hydroxide, $Mg(OH)_2$ was reported. The study revealed the enhancement of anti-biofilm activity with the presence of fibroin and $Mg(OH)_2$ by inhibiting *P. aeruginosa* film formation [34]. Moving forward, Mehrabani et al. prepared chitin/silk fibroin/TiO_2 nanocomposite with strong microbial activity for use as wound dressing bandage. The produced nanocomposites showed good biocompatibility, blood clotting capability, biodegradability, and water uptake. Chitin/silk fibroin had the best antibacterial and antifungal activities against *S. aureus* and *C. albicans* compared with neat chitin and silk fibroin [35]. Furthermore, fabrication of nanocomposites from gold nanorods reinforced silk fibroin has been conducted for peripheral nerve tissue engineering applications. The prepared nanocomposites are biocompatible, and they improve cellular attachments, cell connection, and proliferation; thus, they are suitable to be used as scaffolds for neural tissue engineering [36].

2.8 Elastin

Elastin stands as the main protein in the artery walls' extracellular matrix. It is essential for giving arteries their elastic and flexible characteristics, especially in response to changes in blood pressure. In addition, elastin is a key component in various tissues throughout the body, including the skin, lungs, and ligaments [37,38]. The components of elastin first come together

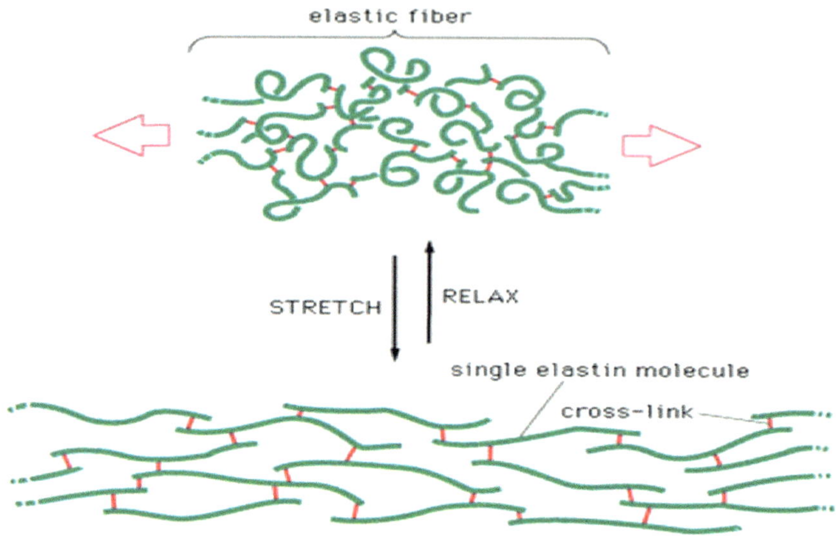

Figure 5.5 Elastin fiber and tissue exhibit elastic properties and flexibility by altering the arrangement of elastin molecule links [39].

in the natural environment to generate tropoelastin, a water-soluble precursor molecule. Subsequently, these precursor molecules unite, forming elastin fibers through the establishment of covalent cross-links, as illustrated in Fig. 5.5. Advancements in genetic engineering techniques have facilitated the creation of elastin-like polymers (ELPs) [40]. The basic structure of these proteins is similar to the repeating patterns found in natural elastin. But, using techniques from genetic engineering, specific sequences can be incorporated, allowing researchers to tailor the properties of these polymers according to their preferences [41]. Notably, because of how closely they resemble the body's natural elastin, these engineered proteins evade immune system responses, offering a unique advantage [42]. The ability to design and genetic engineering offers a number of benefits for the production of elastin-like proteins and their nanoparticles. These include the ability to produce monodisperse polymers (uniform size), precise control over molecular weight, and the ability to achieve the required pharmacokinetic parameters, the capacity to bind many drug molecules together as well as the attachment of nanoparticle targeting agents to particular bodily tissues or areas [39,43–45]. Moreover, various polymers designed using these methods can rapidly undergo phase changes in response to temperature fluctuations, as illustrated in Fig. 5.6.

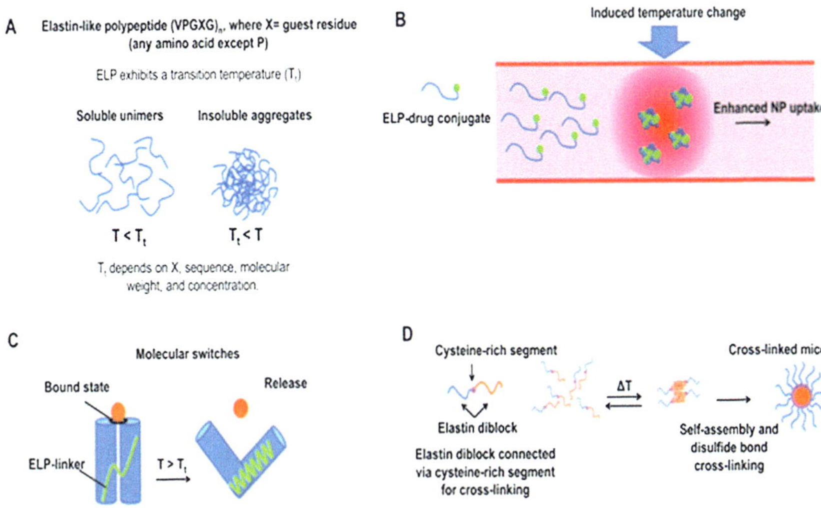

Figure 5.6 Temperature-responsive ELP nanoparticles result from the unique properties of ELP [45].

3. Plant-based protein nanocomposites for biomedical applications

This section highlights various types of plant-based protein nanocomposites, with a specific focus on wheat gluten, corn zein, soy protein, and kafirin. The discussion includes recent studies reporting on these nanocomposites and provides examples of their applications.

3.1 Wheat gluten

Wheat gluten is a type of protein produced as a by-product of the bioethanol and starch industry. It is cheap, environmentally friendly and has excellent physicochemical properties [46]. Wheat gluten is made up of two major components, which are glutenin and gliadin, and it found application in both food and nonfood industry [47]. Wheat gluten can produce polymers that are transparent, flexible, biodegradable, and suitable for medical applications [48]. Despite this, limited study has reported on wheat gluten nanocomposites for medical application. In one study, wheat gluten was incorporated into a hydroxyapatite-gelatin composite scaffold. This work aimed to investigate the effect of wheat gluten on thermal cross-linking and osteogenesis of the scaffold. Different ratios of gelatin to wheat gluten were used to prepare the composites. They found out that the ratio greatly influences the performance of the scaffold at which medium gluten concentration produced the optimum scaffold properties. They also observed that a high gluten amount produced a brittle scaffold, whereas, at a low gluten amount, the scaffold easily degraded during the in vitro test. Overall, the hydroxyapatite-gelatin/gluten supported new bone formation in critical-sized rat calvarial defect, supported by osteoconductive and osteointegrative nature [49].

3.2 Corn zein

Zein is a vegetal protein rich in prolamin extracted from corn. Zein is an alcohol-soluble protein with biodegradable and biocompatible characteristics. Zein can be classified into α-zein, β-zein, γ-zein, and δ-zein depending on their solubility and sequence homology [50]. Sodium citrate was applied topically to treat diabetic ulcers using corn zein as an efficient medication delivery vehicle. Two types of composites were prepared, which are in fiber and film form. In contrast to the film type, the interaction between sodium citrate and maize zein revealed a slower and more regulated release of sodium citrate from the fibers [51]. Delivery of curcumin using zein-xanthan gum nanocomposites was reported by Zhang et al. Initially, the zein-xanthan gum nanoparticle was prepared by antisolvent precipitation, and then curcumin was encapsulated in the composite. Xanthan gum acts as a stabilizer to improve the stability of zein, and it also considerably improves the encapsulation and efficacy loading capacity of nanocomposites with high loading of curcumin. This helps assist in the slow and sustained release of curcumin in simulated intestinal fluid [52].

Amjadi et al. studied the potential of carvone-loaded zein/pullulan nanofibers for medical applications. The zein/pullulan nanofibers were prepared at different ratios by the electrospinning method. They found out that the addition of carvone provides scavenging activity and inhibits the growth of *S. aureus* and *E. coli*. The cytotoxicity assay proves the biocompatibility of the nanofibers [53]. Meanwhile, Fereydouni et al. prepared nanofibers containing zein and nano-curcumin. The loading of oil in water (O/W) curcumin emulsion was varied at 5, 10, and 15 wt.%. The representation of the nanofiber's preparation is displayed in Fig. 5.7. Based on the viability and antioxidant studies, the best condition for cell proliferation was obtained for zein containing 10 wt.% curcumin nanofibers [54]. Another study reported nanofibrous zein was on PCL/zein/gum Arabic [55], calendula officinalis extract/PCL/Zein/Gum arabic [56] and Clay-corn-caprolactone [57], targeted for application in skin and bone tissue engineering.

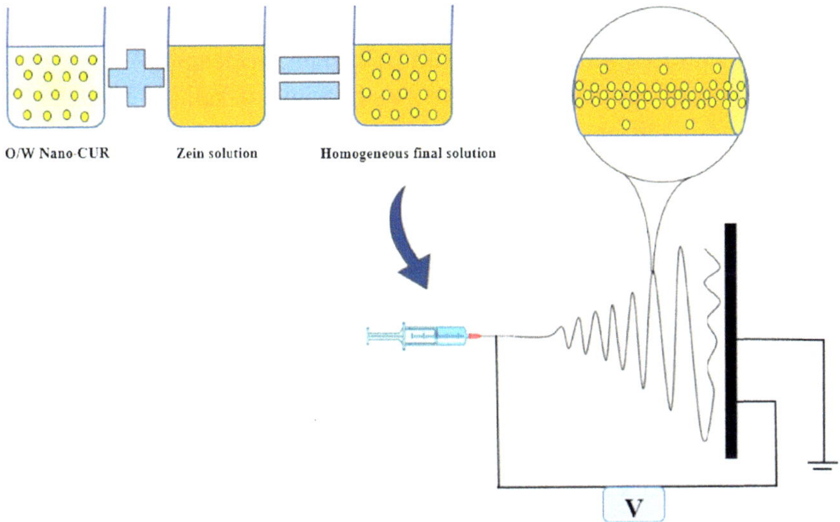

Figure 5.7 The preparation steps of zein/curcumin nanofibers. *(Reproduced from Ref. [54] with Springer Nature permission.)*

3.3 Soy protein

Soy protein can be obtained from the processing of natural soybeans. Soy protein can exist in different derivatives based on the method of extraction. They contain different amounts of protein. For example, soy protein concentrate contains 70% protein; soy protein isolate (SPI) has more than 90% protein, whereas defatted soy flour has around 50% protein. Soy protein film loaded with analgesic drug bupivacaine was investigated for wound healing application. This study was able to produce films with good biocompatibility, favorable mechanical properties, and excellent release profiles [58]. Besides this, a study on cinnamon essential oil-laden 45S5 bioactive glass/soy protein composite scaffolds for bone infection treatment has been carried out. The prepared scaffold showed antibacterial activity against *S. aureus* and *E. coli* [59]. Research on SPI reported previously include polyvinyl alcohol/SPI nanofibrous patches for wound healing [60], SPI/waterborne polyurethane composite sponge for implantable tissue engineering [61], hydroxyethyl cellulose/SPI scaffolds for bone regeneration [62], poly (ethylene terephthalate)/SPI hydrogel for wound dressing. SPI-modified hydroxypropyl chitosan film for skin wound healing [63].

3.4 Kafirin

Kafirin is a protein extracted from sorghum grain, made up of 70%–80% of total endosperm proteins. It can be classified into α-kafirin, β-kafirin, γ-kafirin, and δ-kafirin. It can be used in packaging materials, food coating, antimicrobial agents, and carrier in drug delivery [64]. One study reported on the effect of LAPONITE addition on the properties of biodegradable kafirin nanocomposite films. LAPONITE is a type of synthetic clay and is used as a rheology modifier. In this work, kafirin was plasticized with equal amounts of glycerol, lactic acid, and polyethylene glycol and incorporated with 1, 3, 5, and 10 wt.% of LAPONITE. The addition of LAPONITE did not create significant changes in the film, but it made the film less ductile and stiffer due to the interaction between the clay and amine group of kafirin [65]. In the same year, Li et al. developed hollow and solid kafirin-based nanoparticles as a delivery vehicle for curcumin. The nanoparticles were prepared by electrostatic layer-by-layer (LbL) deposition of dextran sulfate/chitosan. The hollow nanoparticle showed less release of curcumin compared with the solid type [66].

3.5 Peanut protein

One study has reported on the use of peanut protein isolate (PPI) with PLLA nanofibers for potential application in the biomedical field. PPI is obtained as a by-product from the peanut flour industry. It contains a variety of amino acids and is particularly rich in lysine. In this study, PLLA/PPI nanofibers were prepared by electrospinning method with different concentrations of PLLA to PPI. They found out that PLLA/PPI nanofibers exhibit better thermal stability compared with pure PPI, and the contact angle analysis revealed that the hydrophobicity of the nanofibers was significantly improved. Further studies are still needed to test the efficacy of these materials in medical applications.

3.6 Gliadin

Proteins called gliadin and glutenin make up the majority of wheat gluten, a complex mixture of carbohydrates and proteins, with the former being alcohol-insoluble and having a molecular weight of 106 kDa. Gliadin, a set of proteins separated from alcohol by 70% of gluten, exhibits a molecular weight ranging from 25 to 100 kDa. Interestingly, these proteins have a significant concentration of the amino acid glutamine, making up approximately 40% [67,68]. Gliadin demonstrates limited solubility in aqueous solutions [69–71]. Because of their structural similarity to creatine and their richness in proline, these proteins show promise for skin formulations since they may interact with the skin's creatine epidermis. Prior research has demonstrated the efficacy of gliadin nanoparticles as medication release control mechanisms, particularly for hydrophobic and amphiphilic substances such as amoxicillin, vitamin A, and vitamin E [72,73]. High affinity for binding to the body mucosa is an advantageous characteristic of gliadin [74,75]. Because hydrophobic amino acids and glutamine are present in its structure, Gliadin forms abundant hydrogen bonds with the mucous layer. It engages in hydrophobic interactions with the cell membrane. As a result, Gliadin nanoparticles demonstrate significant potential in formulating oral medications, particularly for the treatment of gastric diseases such as gastric ulcers. Through their interaction with gastric mucus, these nanoparticles effectively remove *Helicobacter pylori*, the cause of gastric ulcers, from the stomach mucosa while simultaneously enhancing bioavailability and extending drug release time [76,77].

3.7 Lectin

Lectins are a broad class of glycoproteins, or proteins with the ability to bind to carbohydrates, include various members, with Wheat Germ Agglutinin (WGA) standing out as a particularly notable plant lectin. WGA has excellent stability, little immunogenicity, toxicity, and resistance to proteolytic breakdown. Its ability to specifically identify and bind to intestinal mucosa's glycosylated components makes it a promising choice for improving the absorption of oral medication formulations [78–81].

Over the past 2 decades, lectins, including WGA, have assumed a leading role in the pharmaceutical industry's two main sectors. The first section focuses on improving current medications with limited bioavailability's absorption, while the second area focuses on developing targeted drug formulations for cancer treatment [82–85]. Furthermore, certain lectins, such as WGA, through triggering apoptosis in cancer cells, have shown noteworthy anticancer benefits. Cell membranes, composed of various proteins and phospholipids, feature different oligosaccharide roots that can specifically bind to lectins. This interaction forms the foundation for lectins' tailored medication delivery, as illustrated in Fig. 5.8.

Since different cells exhibit distinct oligosaccharide patterns on their surfaces, particularly between cancer cells and normal cells of the same kind, distinct lectins can serve as drug delivery vehicles to specific regions and cells, as depicted in Fig. 5.9. Extensive research in this field has resulted in

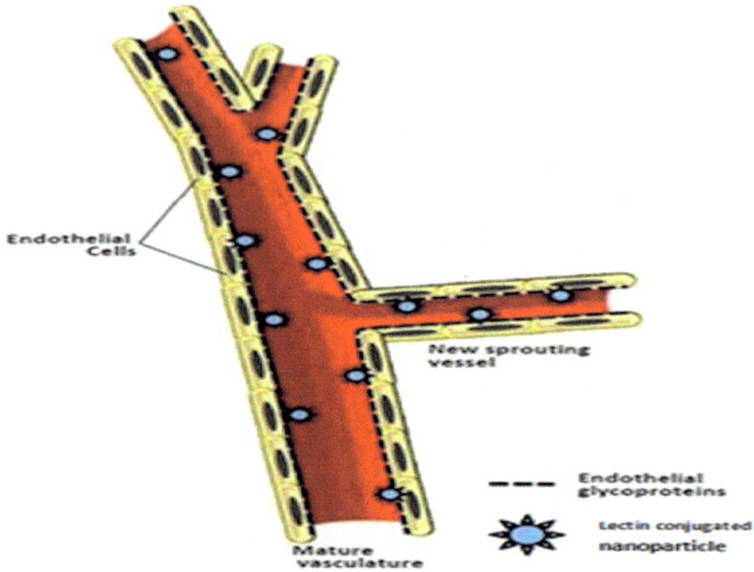

Figure 5.8 A variety of lectin-coated nanoparticles can attach themselves to glycoproteins present on the luminal surface of vascular endothelial cell membranes, offering potential applications in targeted drug delivery [45].

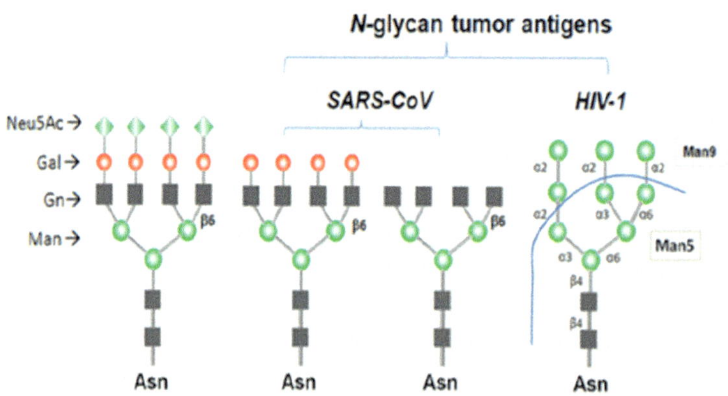

Figure 5.9 Tumors and viruses exhibit distinct sugar sequences compared with normal cells, providing target lectin antigens for use in targeted drug delivery [45].

the development of nanoparticles coated with lectins for creating targeted drug delivery systems. Lectins are the second generation of bioadhesive enhancers because they can increase drug formulations' cellular absorption while simultaneously releasing nanoparticles from the mucosal barrier through processes including clathrin-dependent endocytosis [86].

Lectins can attach to the carbohydrates on the *Helicobacter pylori* surface, which can improve the efficacy of treatment [84,85,87]. Furthermore, lectins are essential for the creation of oral vaccinations. To improve the immune response to oral vaccinations, lectin-coated nanoparticles carrying pathogenic antigens are directed toward the intestinal Peyer's patch surface [88,89]. The gastrointestinal tract is not the only mucosa that lectins may bind to; they can also improve drug delivery through nonoral routes such the nasal mucosa, vagina, lungs, and eyes, as well as through the blood–brain barrier. Interestingly, compared with other lectins, odorranalectin—the smallest member of the lectin family—shows less immunogenicity. It can recognize and attach itself to L-fucose, a sugar that is widely distributed on the surface of the cells that line the nasal mucosa. Drug transport to the brain has been facilitated by the enhanced nose-to-brain transfer shown by nanoparticles containing this lectin [90–94].

4. Microbial protein

Microbial-based protein nanocomposites for biomedical applications have yet to be well researched and reported as of currently. Nevertheless, this protein can be synthesized using different techniques and microbial agents. For instance, Mayer conducted the optimization study of bacteria-based Lysates used in cell-based and cell-free protein synthesis [61]. Another interesting study was on the synthesis of microbial protein from fermented grass. These four stages of producing the microbial protein include [1] lactic acid fermentation of grass juice using *Bacillus coagulans* [2], lactic acid extraction using membrane electrolysis [3], aerobic microbial production by *Cupriavidus necator*, and [4] digestion of the side products. This process produces high-quality food-grade microbial protein and methane as a side product [95]. Another study reported on the production of microbial protein from *Candida utilis* on a medium consisting of enzymatically hydrolyzed brown seaweed and spurs wood. This combination produced a good growth rate and cell yields [96]. Other than that, Zhu et al. converted yellow wine waste into microbial protein using mixed yeast and fungus cultures, which are *Candida utilis* and *Geotrichum candidum*, at a 1:1 ratio. From the reaction, they managed to produce a product with 68.5% protein content with essential amino acid content [97].

5. Biomedical applications

5.1 Biomedical application of nanocomposite

5.1.1 Bone tissues regeneration

As mineral connective tissue, bone is essential to many bodily processes. Still, a number of bone abnormalities, including fractures or deformities brought on by trauma, surgery, or the excision of primary tumors, can impair bone's ability to perform these duties. The complex balance of bone metabolism necessitates efficient regeneration strategies, which has led to the investigation of many therapy alternatives to address the intricacy of clinical bone illnesses [98].

The need for bone regeneration is rising as a result of numerous clinical bone disorders, including infections, malignancies, and bone loss. Bone, being a metabolically active and dynamic organ with unique regenerative capabilities, faces challenges from such disorders [99]. Autografts, allografts, xenografts, and artificial alternatives, such metals and synthetic cement, are common therapies for these problems [100]. Jin et al. prepared porous Chitosan-Hydroxyapatite (CS/HA)-alginate composite scaffolds for bone tissue engineering. By using freeze-drying and in situ co-precipitation, the scaffolds were created. Using this technique, porous materials appropriate for bone regeneration were produced [101].

Bone tissue, consisting mostly of hydroxyapatite and collagen, exhibits a complex microstructure with tropocollagen strands and mineralized formations. On a microscopic level, mineralized strands combine to form fibrils, contributing to the high-level compact bone osteon architectures. The macroscopic bone structure comprises compact bone as the trabecular or spongy bone and the outer shell in the interior [102]. In cases of bone defects resulting from various causes, the imperative is to reconstruct and regenerate bone tissue, necessitating grafts with specific properties such as high biocompatibility, osteoinductivity, osteoconductivity, osseointegrativity, and robust mechanical strength [103]. Trends in bone tissue engineering at the moment focus on biomaterial enhancements that mimic the microstructure, biological attributes, and mechanical resilience of natural bone tissue. Notably, studies by Wu et al. [104] highlight the influence of tailored scaffold pore sizes, demonstrating that specific dimensions promote better in vivo bone regeneration. Clinical applications, such as Dellavia et al. [105] use of titanium scaffolds for guided alveolar bone regeneration and Omar et al. [106] Ca-phosphate bioceramic implants produced by 3D printing for cranial defect reconstruction, showcase successful outcomes, emphasizing the potential of these advancements in bone tissue engineering [107].

Magnesium ions (Mg^{2+}) have demonstrated bioactive properties and play a crucial role in bone tissue regeneration. In the area of tissue engineering for bones, the controlled release of Mg^{2+} has been identified as a significant factor influencing bone regeneration. The use of biodegradable microspheres provides a method for the precise management of bioactive substance release, showcasing additional benefits in various bone regeneration applications such as barrier membranes, cell therapies, grafting, and bioactive substances [108]. Recent research suggests that the controlled release from a core-shell nanofiber structure possesses the capacity to greatly advance the development of bone-healing chemicals and cell therapies [109]. The way the body reacts to bone biomaterials is a critical determinant in the fate of scaffolds and the overall success of the regeneration process. Graphene oxide and nanohydroxyapatite (nHAp) have emerged as promising elements for bone tissue regeneration, prompting increased studies on polymeric nanocomposite scaffolds reinforced with nanohydroxyapatite (nHAp) and graphene oxide (GO). Gelatin—alginate (GA) and GO/nHAp components were used to create a three-dimensional porous polymeric nanocomposite scaffold, which demonstrates a synergistic strategy for encouraging tissue regeneration(nHAp). Hydrogels incorporating hyaluronic acid, tricalcium phosphate, and nanosilver derived from corn silk extract (CSE-Ag NPs) have been innovatively developed through microwave-assisted biosynthesis of spherical nanoparticles of silver in a solution without organic solvent. These thermosensitive hydrogels, which gel at temperatures close to the human body, are designed to encapsulate pharmaceuticals or growth factors, providing a platform to enhance bone repair [110,111].

The mechanism of zinc's impact on bone development remains unclear. Mesenchymal stem cells (MSCs) are crucial for distinguishing various bone forms for repair and replacement. A new bone healing approach uses MSC secretome extracellular vesicles, minimizing risks associated with traditional methods. Multimodal treatment platforms are essential for postsurgery bone loss and recurrent malignant bone cancers. Combining natural polymers with carbon nanotubes creates a nanocomposite material, enabling the development of carbon nanotube-based scaffolds with MSCs, depicted in Fig. 5.10. This facilitates protein absorption and drives MSC differentiation, contributing to bone repair and reconstruction [113—115].

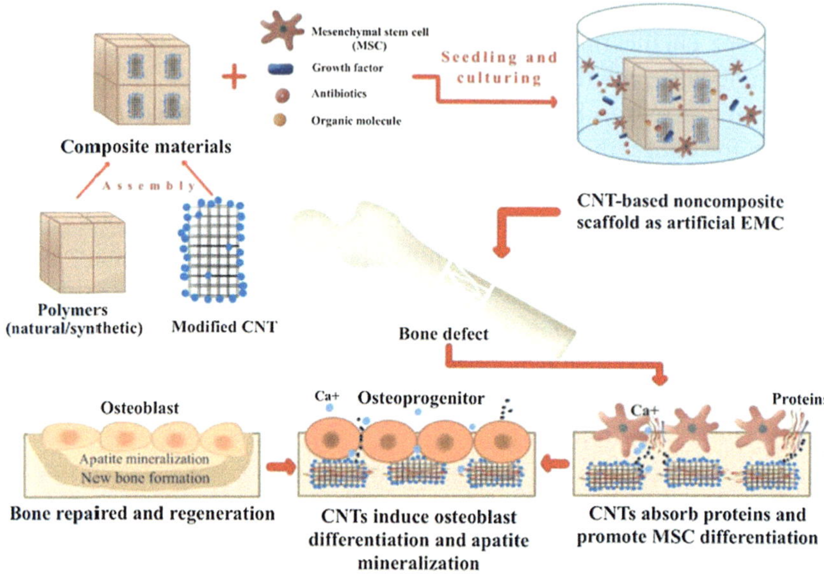

Figure 5.10 The process of bone regeneration using MSCs [112].

5.1.2 Tissue regeneration

Tissue engineering seeks to replace or regenerate biological functions in tissues or organs through the integration of biomaterials, biomolecules, and cells. At the core of this approach are scaffold biomaterials and their manufacturing techniques, driving continuous exploration for novel biomaterial formulations. The emphasis encompasses diverse biomaterial generations, including bioceramics, bioactive glasses, composites made of natural and manmade polymers, playing a vital role in scaffold fabrication—an essential component of tissue engineering. The review thoroughly investigates scaffold fabrication methods and highlights advancements in tissue engineering across various applications such as regeneration of the bone, skin, cartilage, nervous system, and heart. These developments function as preclinical protocols for organ and tissue restoration after injury. The latest trends and issues in this sector thoroughly explain this dynamic subject of biomaterials for tissue regeneration. Tissue regeneration and tissue engineering are commonly used terms in the treatment of diseased tissues and organs. Tissue engineering is a growing biomedical field that aims to repair tissue defects by combining biomaterials with living cells [116–118]. It offers a promising approach for in-situ tissue regeneration by the use of cells in bioactive scaffolds, providing an

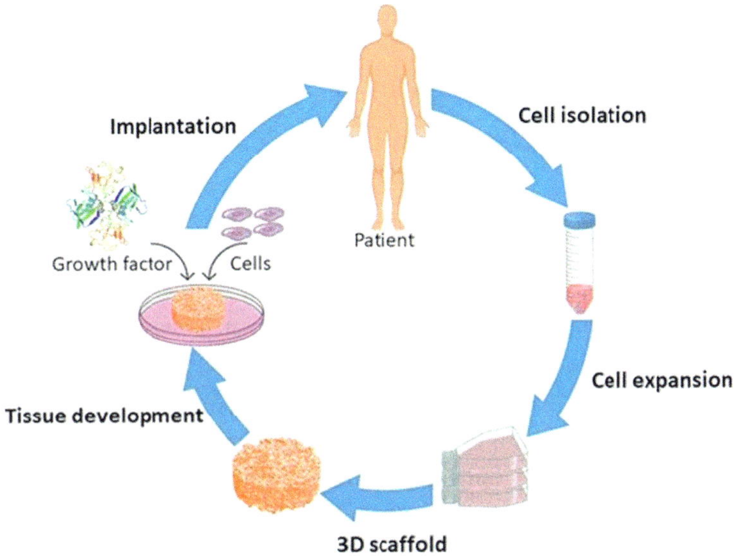

Figure 5.11 Diagram illustrating the tissue engineering method using scaffolds site MDPI [119].

alternative to grafting and transplantation for damaged or diseased tissues. The field has progressed with the development of novel materials designed to restore tissue function. Scaffolds play a crucial role in the tissue regeneration process, featuring a 3D porous structure that supports the movement and adhesion of cells via pore channels, facilitating afterward, tissue growth. Fig. 5.11 illustrates the steps of culturing cells onto scaffolds and the eventual formation of tissue.

5.1.3 Drug delivery

Biopolymers play an important role in biomedical applications due to their excellent biocompatibility and biodegradability [120,121]. Among these, biopolymer-based nanoparticles stand out as highly promising nanocarriers for administering medicinal medications to cancerous cells, particularly those in cell lines of ovarian cancer. This is attributed to their favorable biodistribution and biodegradation within biological systems [122,123]. Furthermore, biopolymers find extensive use in various biomedical applications, spanning gene delivery [120], tissue engineering, and drug delivery [124].

Chitosan (CS), a versatile and readily available biopolymer, has captured significant interest in medical applications due to its unique qualities

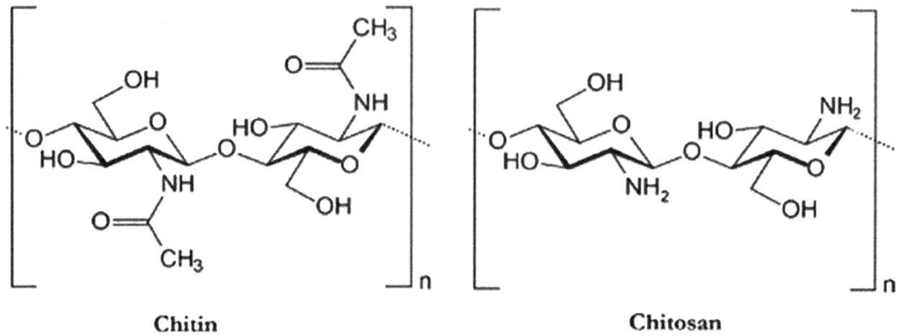

Figure 5.12 Structural composition of chitin and chitosan at the molecular level [130].

[125,126]. It is the second most common copolymer after cellulose and is composed of 2-acetamido-2-deoxy-D-glucopyranose and 2-amino-2-deoxy-D-glucopyranose units [127–129]. Typically obtained from chitin through partial deacetylation in an environment that is alkaline, as illustrated in Fig. 5.12 [131–134], this polymer undergoes digestion by human enzymes. Its role in wound healing involves actively promoting hemostasis and expediting tissue regeneration [135–137]. Notably, chitosan, derived from renewable resources, extends its range of applications [138]. In orthopedics, it finds application in combination with various polymeric biomaterials and inorganic bioactive compounds, showcasing potential as intervertebral discs, bone and cartilage tissue engineering, and alternatives to bone grafts [130,139]. Leveraging its antibacterial properties, chitosan and its nanoparticles (NPs) actively contribute to diverse biological applications, including food preservation [140].

Natural polymers, due to their nontoxicity, biodegradability, sustainability, eco-friendliness, and biocompatibility, are considered suitable host materials for nanoparticles, particularly in biological applications [141,142]. Public health research has prioritized the creation of efficient drug delivery methods to guarantee that bioactive compounds avoid nontarget cells, organs, or tissues and reach their intended location of action [143,144]. Concepts such as drug targeting and controlled drug delivery aim to improve the therapeutic index of medications by improving their localization to particular human body parts, thereby lowering the likelihood of adverse effects under normal conditions [145,146]. This approach offers several advantages, including the ability to easily adjust drug levels after parenteral administration to reach the target illness site, enhanced efficacy in pharmacological treatment, and decreased drug side effects [147,148]. The incorporation of medicines into the systems occurs without undergoing

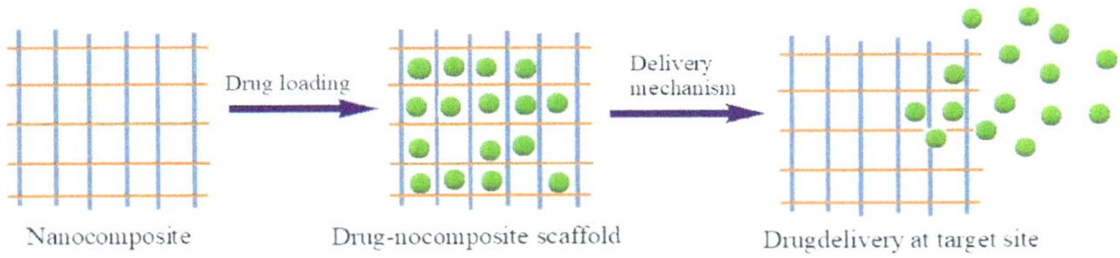

Figure 5.13 The drug loading and delivery system utilized in biopolymer nanocomposites is depicted in the schematic representation [149].

chemical processes, crucial for preserving drug activity. Moreover, the system proves versatile for various administration methods, including parenteral, intraocular, nasal, and oral. Fig. 5.13 shows the drug loading and delivery system utilized in biopolymer nanocomposites is depicted in the schematic representation.

5.1.4 Anticancer

Cancer remains a leading cause of human mortality despite extensive efforts to understand its biology and develop effective therapies. Creating an effective in vitro tumor microenvironment and coming up with efficient ways to test anticancer medications to understand the nature of cancer and develop treatments are the main problems facing researchers studying cancer. Current conventional cancer treatments, such as surgery, radiation, and chemotherapy, have limitations, including the risk of causing harm to healthy tissues or not eliminating cancer. Nanotechnology emerges as a promising avenue for directly and selectively targeting therapies for cancerous cells and neoplasms, guiding surgical tumor resection, and enhancing the efficacy of radiation-based treatments. Moreover, nanotechnology provides tools to address drug resistance and facilitate the use of innovative immunotherapies [150].

Nanotechnology's role in cancer therapeutics has primarily focused on enhancing the pharmacokinetics and reducing the systemic toxicities of chemotherapies by selectively delivering anticancer drugs to tumor tissues. Chemotherapeutic medications can be conjugated or encapsulated on the surface of nanoparticles to create nanoformulations, which can raise the total therapeutic index of the pharmaceuticals that are administered. Through the increased permeability and retention (EPR) effect, passive tumor targeting is necessary for the selective distribution of nanotherapeutic platforms although other mechanisms have also been proposed [150]. Specific nanotechnology research has concentrated on elevating the capabilities of radiotherapy by leveraging the unique properties of nanoscale materials. In particular, nanotechnology platforms designed for radiotherapy treatments make use of the X-ray and nanoparticle interaction, driven by the inherent atomic-level properties of the materials. Researchers are actively investigating the use of nanotechnology to deliver nucleic acids as efficient therapeutic methods for various cancers. These efforts are centered regarding the creation and description of spherical nucleic acids (SNAs) for the delivery of RNA medicines to treat brain cancer [151].

5.1.5 Nanomedicine

The field of biomedical applications of nanoparticles (NPs) is rapidly advancing, and electron microscopy (EM) plays a crucial role in identifying the intracellular locations of these nanoparticles. Electron microscopy (EM) enables the monitoring and quantification of NP dispersion, dissolution, and the internalized dose by cells and tissues. However, the accuracy of these measurements relies on appropriate sample preparation. When preparing cellular material for electron microscopy (EM), It is crucial to take into account the resolution of cellular ultrastructure while preventing the target NPs from being significantly altered or lost.

Various electron microscopy (EM) imaging modes are now available with the necessary spatial resolution and sensitivity to measure and quantify the position and number of nanoparticles (NPs) in a biological matrix. In addition, the determination of the NP composition and ionic concentration inside intracellular compartments is made possible by analytical electron microscopy (EM). These techniques encompass both transmission and scanning electron microscopy (EM) and bridge the traditional boundaries between electron microscopy (EM) for biological and physical scientists [152].

5.2 Sample preparation of cells for electron microscopy

In electron microscopy (EM) of cells, a significant challenge arises due to the high water content of biological specimens, requiring preparatory steps before exposure to the vacuum in an electron microscopy (EM) column. Traditional room temperature preparation protocols exist for cells and tissues, aiming to preserve the biological matrix at scales around 10 nm while maintaining the physicochemical properties of nanoparticles (NPs) within cellular compartments [152].

Nanomaterial-containing commercial products have become ubiquitous in our daily lives, and the dimensional parameters are crucial for identifying nanoparticles. Various techniques exist for measuring particle size and shape, with electron microscopy-based methods often being preferred for characterizing dimensional properties. The reliable measurement of constituent particle size is presented in this work through a novel sample preparation approach using the spin coating technique. This method involves three essential processing steps: (i) extraction from complicated media, (ii) redispersion via probe sonication, and (iii) spin coating deposition. The method takes into account variables that can affect the agglomeration state of nanoparticles, such as pH, zeta potential, time, concentration, sonication, and spin coater parameters [153].

5.3 Quantification of nanoparticles uptake

Quantitative assessment of nanoparticle (NP) uptake, including determining the number of cells containing nanoparticles (NPs) and the quantity and distribution of internalized NPs per cell, is crucial in the realms of nanotoxicology and nanomedicine. Establishing a connection between NP exposure levels and the internalized NP dose is a pivotal step for advancing these fields, and electron microscopy (EM) proves instrumental in quantifying the NP dose despite the challenge of obtaining statistically significant results [154].

In the domains of nanotoxicology and nanomedicine, the quantification of nanoparticles in biological systems (such as cells, tissues, and organs) is increasingly essential. The dose plays a pivotal role in evaluating the behavior and potential risks associated with nanomaterials. While there are numerous methods for measuring nanoparticles in cells and tissues; nevertheless, more research and development is needed to ensure reliable, reproducible, and comparable measurements across different methods. Microscopy, particularly electron microscopy, enables the detection and localization of nanoparticles in cells, and its extensive use in recent years has contributed to characterizing nanoparticles and their pathways in living systems [155–157]. However, for all microscopy techniques to produce quantitative data, strong sampling strategies are needed. Stereology, a well-known sampling technique in various fields, when combined with electron microscopy, proves highly successful in quantifying nanoparticle uptake by cells.

The biomedical application of NPs is a rapidly expanding field, with a strong focus on their utilization for cellular and tissue imaging as well as drug delivery. The established significance of electron microscopy (EM) in assessing nanoparticle behavior at the cellular level has made a substantial contribution to the fields of nanotoxicology and nanomedicine.

6. Conclusion

This chapter provides an overview of various protein nanocomposite systems developed for biomedical applications in recent years. Due to their inherent biocompatibility and biodegradability, proteins have been explored for diverse medical applications, including drug delivery, skin tissue engineering, bone and cartilage engineering, wound healing, and others. Animal-based protein nanocomposites have received the most attention, followed by plant-based proteins. Notably, microbial protein nanocomposites for medical applications have yet to be reported, presenting an intriguing avenue for future exploration. The existing research has yielded valuable insights into protein-based materials for medical applications, laying the groundwork for potential improvements in performance. Opportunities abound for the development of protein-based nanocomposites with exceptional properties that align with the requirements of specific applications. The knowledge gained from reported studies serves as a valuable resource, guiding future steps in enhancing the effectiveness of these materials for biomedical purposes.

Acknowledgments

The authors are thankful to Universiti Sains Malaysia for providing a financial support (short-term grant; 304/PKIMIA/6315580).

References

[1] Wang Z, Kang S, Cao S, Krecker M, Tsukruk VV, Singamaneni S. Protein-based functional nanocomposites. MRS Bull December 2020;45(12):1017–26.

[2] Silva NH, Vilela C, Marrucho IM, Freire CS, Neto CP, Silvestre AJ. Protein-based materials: from sources to innovative sustainable materials for biomedical applications. J Mater Chem B 2014;2(24):3715–40.

[3] Hadidi M, Jafarzadeh S, Forough M, Garavand F, Alizadeh S, Salehabadi A, Khaneghah AM, Jafari SM. Plant protein-based food packaging films; recent advances in fabrication, characterization, and applications. Trends Food Sci Technol February 1, 2022;120:154–73.

[4] Łopusiewicz Ł, Drozłowska E, Trocer P, Kostek M, Śliwiński M, Henriques MH, Bartkowiak A, Sobolewski P. Whey protein concentrate/isolate biofunctional films modified with melanin from watermelon (*Citrullus lanatus*) seeds. Materials September 2, 2020;13(17):3876.

[5] Adams RL, Broughton KS. Insulinotropic effects of whey: mechanisms of action, recent clinical trials, and clinical applications. Ann Nutr Metabol September 2, 2016;69(1):56–63.

[6] Erfan NA, Barakat NA, Muller-Borer BJ. Preparation and characterization of β-lactoglobulin/poly (ethylene oxide) magnetic nanofibers for biomedical applications. Colloids Surf A Physicochem Eng Asp September 5, 2019;576:63–72.

[7] Pino P, Ronchetti S, Mollea C, Sangermano M, Onida B, Bosco F. Whey proteins—zinc oxide bionanocomposite as antibacterial films. Pharmaceutics September 8, 2021;13(9):1426.
[8] Słota D, Głąb M, Tyliszczak B, Douglas TE, Rudnicka K, Miernik K, Urbaniak M, Rusek-Wala P, Sobczak-Kupiec A. Composites based on hydroxyapatite and whey protein isolate for applications in bone regeneration. Materials April 29, 2021;14(9):2317.
[9] Sumathra M, Rajan M, Amarnath Praphakar R, Marraiki N, Elgorban AM. In vivo assessment of a hydroxyapatite/κ-carrageenan—maleic anhydride—casein/doxorubicin composite-coated titanium bone implant. ACS Biomater Sci Eng January 31, 2020;6(3):1650—62.
[10] Joseph M, Nampoori VP, Kailasnath M. Low temperature structure tunability of zinc oxide nanostructures using milk protein casein. Surface Interfac June 1, 2021;24:101157.
[11] Liu S, Yu H, Huang K. Structural characteristics and biocompatibility of a casein-based nanocomposite for potential biomedical applications. J Mater Sci March 2018;53(6):3959—71.
[12] Dumitrescu GD, Serafim A, Ginghina RE, Iovu H, Marinescu R, Olăreț E, Stancu IC. Development of new hybrid casein-loaded PHEMA-PEGDA hydrogels with enhanced mineralisation potential. Materials January 22, 2022;15(3):840.
[13] Raoufinia R, Mota A, Keyhanvar N, Safari F, Shamekhi S, Abdolalizadeh J. Overview of albumin and its purification methods. Adv Pharmaceut Bull December 2016;6(4):495.
[14] Zewde B, Atoyebi O, Gugssa A, Gaskell KJ, Raghavan D. An investigation of the interaction between bovine serum albumin-conjugated silver nanoparticles and the hydrogel in hydrogel nanocomposites. ACS Omega April 22, 2021;6(17):11614—27.
[15] Xu K, Zhao Z, Zhang J, Xue W, Tong H, Liu H, Zhang W. Albumin-stabilized manganese-based nanocomposites with sensitive tumor microenvironment responsivity and their application for efficient SiRNA delivery in brain tumors. J Mater Chem B 2020;8(7):1507—15.
[16] Akbal O, Vural T, Malekghasemi S, Bozdoğan B, Denkbas EB. Saponin loaded montmorillonite-human serum albumin nanocomposites as drug delivery system in colorectal cancer therapy. Appl Clay Sci December 15, 2018;166:214—22.
[17] Elgohary MM, Helmy MW, Abdelfattah EZ, Ragab DM, Mortada SM, Fang JY, Elzoghby AO. Targeting sialic acid residues on lung cancer cells by inhalable boronic acid-decorated albumin nanocomposites for combined chemo/herbal therapy. J Contr Release September 10, 2018;285:230—43.
[18] Ye W, Qin M, Qiu R, Li J. Keratin-based wound dressings: from waste to wealth. Int J Biol Macromol June 30, 2022;211:183—97.
[19] Zhai M, Xu Y, Zhou B, Jing W. Keratin-chitosan/n-ZnO nanocomposite hydrogel for antimicrobial treatment of burn wound healing: characterization and biomedical application. J Photochem Photobiol B Biol March 1, 2018;180:253—8.
[20] Das A, Das A, Basu A, Datta P, Gupta M, Mukherjee A. Newer guar gum ester/chicken feather keratin interact films for tissue engineering. Int J Biol Macromol June 1, 2021;180:339—54.
[21] Keskin Z, Urkmez AS, Hames EE. Novel keratin modified bacterial cellulose nanocomposite production and characterization for skin tissue engineering. Mater Sci Eng C June 1, 2017;75:1144—53.
[22] Arun A, Malrautu P, Laha A, Luo H, Ramakrishna S. Collagen nanoparticles in drug delivery systems and tissue engineering. Appl Sci December 1, 2021;11(23):11369.

[23] Râpă M, Stefan LM, Zaharescu T, Seciu AM, Țurcanu AA, Matei E, Predescu AM, Antoniac I, Predescu C. Development of bionanocomposites based on PLA, collagen and AgNPs and characterization of their stability and in vitro biocompatibility. Appl Sci March 26, 2020;10(7):2265.
[24] Marin MM, Ianchis R, Leu Alexa R, Gifu IC, Kaya MG, Savu DI, Popescu RC, Alexandrescu E, Ninciuleanu CM, Preda S, Ignat M. Development of new collagen/clay composite biomaterials. Int J Mol Sci December 30, 2021;23(1):401.
[25] Salahuddin B, Wang S, Sangian D, Aziz S, Gu Q. Hybrid gelatin hydrogels in nanomedicine applications. ACS Appl Bio Mater March 9, 2021;4(4):2886–906.
[26] Samadian H, Khastar H, Ehterami A, Salehi M. Bioengineered 3D nanocomposite based on gold nanoparticles and gelatin nanofibers for bone regeneration: in vitro and in vivo study. Sci Rep July 6, 2021;11(1):13877.
[27] Ramirez-Barron SN, Sanchez-Valdes S, Betancourt R, Gallardo CA, Puente-Urbina B, Rodriguez-Fernández OS, Carneiro-da Cunha MG, dos Santos-Correia MT, Sanche-zMartinez ZV. Preparation and characterization of gelatin-gallic acid/ZnO nanocomposite with antibacterial properties as a promising multi-functional bioadhesive for wound dressing applications. Int J Adhesion Adhes January 1, 2021;104:102749.
[28] Rakhshaei R, Namazi H, Hamishehkar H, Kafil HS, Salehi R. In situ synthesized chitosan–gelatin/ZnO nanocomposite scaffold with drug delivery properties: higher antibacterial and lower cytotoxicity effects. J Appl Polym Sci June 10, 2019;136(22):47590.
[29] Cheng Y, Morovvati MR, Huang M, Shahali M, Saber-Samandari S, Angili SN, Nejad MG, Shakibaie M, Toghraie D. A multilayer biomimetic chitosan-gelatin-fluorohydroxyapatite cartilage scaffold using for regenerative medicine application. J Mater Res Technol September 1, 2021;14:1761–77.
[30] Yoo SC, Park YK, Park C, Ryu H, Hong SH. Biomimetic artificial nacre: boron nitride nanosheets/gelatin nanocomposites for biomedical applications. Adv Funct Mater December 2018;28(51):1805948.
[31] Shi R, Niu Y, Gong M, Ye J, Tian W, Zhang L. Antimicrobial gelatin-based elastomer nanocomposite membrane loaded with ciprofloxacin and polymyxin B sulfate in halloysite nanotubes for wound dressing. Mater Sci Eng C June 1, 2018;87:128–38.
[32] Samadian H, Salehi M, Farzamfar S, Vaez A, Ehterami A, Sahrapeyma H, Goodarzi A, Ghorbani S. In vitro and in vivo evaluation of electrospun cellulose acetate/gelatin/hydroxyapatite nanocomposite mats for wound dressing applications. Artif Cell Nanomed Biotechnol October 31, 2018;46(Suppl. 1):964–74.
[33] Șerban MV, Nazarie SR, Dinescu S, Radu IC, Zaharia C, Istrătoiu EA, Tănasă E, Herman H, Gharbia S, Baltă C, Hermenean A. Silk ProteinsEnriched nanocomposite hydrogels based on modified MMT clay and poly (2-hydroxyethyl methacrylate-co-2-acrylamido-2-methylpropane sulfonic acid) display favorable properties for soft tissue engineering. Nanomaterials January 31, 2022;12(3):503.
[34] Eivazzadeh-Keihan R, Ahmadpour F, Aliabadi HA, Radinekiyan F, Maleki A, Madanchi H, Mahdavi M, Shalan AE, Lanceros-Méndez S. Pectin-cellulose hydrogel, silk fibroin and magnesium hydroxide nanoparticles hybrid nanocomposites for biomedical applications. Int J Biol Macromol December 1, 2021;192:7–15.
[35] Mehrabani MG, Karimian R, Rakhshaei R, Pakdel F, Eslami H, Fakhrzadeh V, Rahimi M, Salehi R, Kafil HS. Chitin/silk fibroin/TiO2 bio-nanocomposite as a biocompatible wound dressing bandage with strong antimicrobial activity. Int J Biol Macromol September 1, 2018;116:966–76.

[36] Afjeh-Dana E, Naserzadeh P, Nazari H, Mottaghitalab F, Shabani R, Aminii N, Mehravi B, Rostami FT, Joghataei MT, Mousavizadeh K, Ashtari K. Gold nanorods reinforced silk fibroin nanocomposite for peripheral nerve tissue engineering applications. Int J Biol Macromol May 15, 2019;129:1034–9.

[37] Timms JF, Cutillas PR. Overview of quantitative LC-MS techniques for proteomics and activitomics. Methods Mol Biol 2010;658:19–45.

[38] Zhang H, Wu RA. Proteomic profiling of protein corona formed on the surface of nanomaterial. Sci China Chem May 2015;58:780–92.

[39] Trebacz H, Barzycka A. Mechanical properties and functions of elastin: an overview. Biomolecules March 22, 2023;13(3):574.

[40] Hu Z, Zhao L, Zhang H, Zhang Y, Wu RA, Zou H. The on-bead digestion of protein corona on nanoparticles by trypsin immobilized on the magnetic nanoparticle. J Chromatogr A March 21, 2014;1334:55–63.

[41] Fernández-Iglesias N, Bettmer J. Complementary mass spectrometric techniques for the quantification of the protein corona: a case study on gold nanoparticles and human serum proteins. Nanoscale 2015;7(34):14324–31.

[42] Legat J, Matczuk M, Timerbaev A, Jarosz M. CE separation and ICP-MS detection of gold nanoparticles and their protein conjugates. Chromatographia November 2017;80:1695–700.

[43] Kokkinopoulou M, Simon J, Landfester K, Mailänder V, Lieberwirth I. Visualization of the protein corona: towards a biomolecular understanding of nanoparticle-cell-interactions. Nanoscale 2017;9(25):8858–70.

[44] Stewart M, Mulenos M, Steele L, Sayes C. Differences among unique nanoparticle protein corona constructs: a case study using data analytics and multi-variant visualization to describe physicochemical characteristics. Appl Sci 2018;8(12):2669.

[45] Kianfar E. Protein nanoparticles in drug delivery: animal protein, plant proteins and protein cages, albumin nanoparticles. J Nanobiotechnol May 29, 2021;19(1):159.

[46] Chen T, Tang Y, Zhao H, Zhang KQ, Wang X, Meng K. Sustainable wheat gluten foams used in self-expansion medical dressings. Smart Mat Med January 1, 2022;3:329–38.

[47] Nataraj D, Sakkara S, Meenakshi HN, Reddy N. Properties and applications of citric acid crosslinked banana fibre-wheat gluten films. Ind Crop Prod November 15, 2018;124:265–72.

[48] Aziz S, Hosseinzadeh L, Arkan E, Azandaryani AH. Preparation of electrospun nanofibers based on wheat gluten containing azathioprine for biomedical application. Int J Poly Mat Poly Biomat July 24, 2019;68(11):639–46.

[49] Ramakrishnan LS, Unnikrishnan PS, Sabu CK, Krishnan AG, Nair MB. Effect of wheat gluten on improved thermal cross-linking and osteogenesis of hydroxyapatite-gelatin composite scaffolds. Int J Biol Macromol July 31, 2021;183:1200–9.

[50] Tortorella S, Maturi M, Buratti VV, Vozzolo G, Locatelli E, Sambri L, Franchini MC. Zein as a versatile biopolymer: different shapes for different biomedical applications. RSC Adv 2021;11(62):39004–26.

[51] Gough CR, Bessette K, Xue Y, Mou X, Hu X. Air-jet spun corn zein nanofibers and thin films with topical drug for medical applications. Int J Mol Sci August 12, 2020;21(16):5780.

[52] Zhang D, Jiang F, Ling J, Ouyang XK, Wang YG. Delivery of curcumin using a zein-xanthan gum nanocomplex: fabrication, characterization, and in vitro release properties. Colloids Surf B Biointerfaces August 1, 2021;204:111827.

[53] Amjadi S, Gholizadeh S, Ebrahimi A, Almasi H, Hamishehkar H, Taheri RA. Development and characterization of the carvone-loaded zein/pullulan hybrid electrospun nanofibers for food and medical applications. Ind Crop Prod September 1, 2022;183:114964.

[54] Fereydouni N, Movaffagh J, Amiri N, Darroudi S, Gholoobi A, Goodarzi A, Hashemzadeh A, Darroudi M. Synthesis of nano-fibers containing nano-curcumin in zein corn protein and its physicochemical and biological characteristics. Sci Rep January 21, 2021;11(1):1902.
[55] Rad ZP, Mokhtari J, Abbasi M. Fabrication and characterization of PCL/zein/gum Arabic electrospun nanocomposite scaffold for skin tissue engineering. Mater Sci Eng C December 1, 2018;93:356–66.
[56] Rad ZP, Mokhtari J, Abbasi M. Calendula officinalis extract/PCL/Zein/Gum Arabic nanofibrous bio-composite scaffolds via suspension, two-nozzle and multilayer electrospinning for skin tissue engineering. Int J Biol Macromol August 15, 2019;135:530–43.
[57] Ullah A, Haider MK, Wang FF, Morita S, Kharaghani D, Ge Y, Yoshiko Y, Lee JS, Kim IS. "Clay-corn-caprolactone" a novel bioactive clay polymer nanofibrous scaffold for bone tissue engineering. Appl Clay Sci April 1, 2022;220:106455.
[58] Goder D, Matsliah L, Giladi S, Reshef-Steinberger L, Zin I, Shaul A, Zilberman M. Mechanical, physical and biological characterization of soy protein films loaded with bupivacaine for wound healing applications. Int J Poly Mat Poly Biomat March 24, 2021;70(5):345–55.
[59] Unalan I, Fuggerer T, Slavik B, Buettner A, Boccaccini AR. Antibacterial and antioxidant activity of cinnamon essential oil-laden 45S5 bioactive glass/soy protein composite scaffolds for the treatment of bone infections and oxidative stress. Mater Sci Eng C September 1, 2021;128:112320.
[60] Khabbaz B, Solouk A, Mirzadeh H. Polyvinyl alcohol/soy protein isolate nanofibrous patch for wound-healing applications. Progress Biomat September 2019;8:185–96.
[61] Khalid U, Tabassum P, Khan MA, Mohamad N, Akil A, Mohd R. Degradation of organic pollutants using metal-doped TiO2 photocatalysts under visible light: a comparative study. Desalination Water Treat 2019;161:275–82.
[62] Wu M, Wu P, Xiao L, Zhao Y, Yan F, Liu X, Xie Y, Zhang C, Chen Y, Cai L. Biomimetic mineralization of novel hydroxyethyl cellulose/soy protein isolate scaffolds promote bone regeneration in vitro and in vivo. Int J Biol Macromol November 1, 2020;162:1627–41.
[63] Zhao Y, Wang Z, Zhang Q, Chen F, Yue Z, Zhang T, Deng H, Huselstein C, Anderson DP, Chang PR, Li Y. Accelerated skin wound healing by soy protein isolate–modified hydroxypropyl chitosan composite films. Int J Biol Macromol October 15, 2018;118:1293–302.
[64] Patil DA, Tated S, Mhaske ST. Plasticized kafirin-based films: analysis of thermal, barrier and mechanical properties. Polym Bull March 2021;78:1721–33.
[65] Olivera N, Rouf TB, Bonilla JC, Carriazo JG, Dianda N, Kokini JL. Effect of LAPONITE addition on the mechanical, barrier and surface properties of novel biodegradable kafirin nanocomposite films. J Food Eng March 1, 2019;245:24–32.
[66] Li X, Maldonado L, Malmr M, Rouf TB, Hua Y, Kokini J. Development of hollow kafirin-based nanoparticles fabricated through layer-by-layer assembly as delivery vehicles for curcumin. Food Hydrocolloids November 1, 2019;96:93–101.
[67] Sooväli L, Rõõm E-I, Kütt A, Kaljurand I, Leito I. Uncertainty sources in UV–Vis spectrophotometric measurement. Accred Qual Assur 2006;11(5):246–55.
[68] Cedervall T, Lynch I, Lindman S, et al. Understanding the nanoparticle–protein corona using methods to quantify exchange rates and affinities of proteins for nanoparticles. Proc Natl Acad Sci USA 2007;104(7):2050–5.
[69] Xu L, Jiang S, Wu J, Zou Q. An in silico approach to identification, categorization and prediction of nucleic acid binding proteins. Briefings Bioinf 2021;22(3). https://doi.org/10.1093/bib/bbaa171.

[70] Xian-Fang W, Peng G, Yi-Feng L, Hong-Fei L, Fan L. Predicting thermophilic proteins by machine learning. Curr Bioinf 2020;15:493. https://doi.org/10.2174/1574893615666200207094357.
[71] Zou Q, Xing P, Wei L, Liu B. Gene2vec: gene subsequence embedding for prediction of mammalian N6-methyladenosine sites from mRNA. RNA 2019;25(2):205–18. https://doi.org/10.1261/rna.069112.118.
[72] Xue C, Bei J, Dengkui W, Guoli L, et al. Gate-tunable the interface properties of GaAs–WSe2 (1D–2D) vdWs heterojunction for high-responsivity, self-powered photodetector. Appl Phys Lett 2021;118:041102. https://doi.org/10.1063/5.0035275.
[73] Kianfar E. Production and identification of vanadium oxide nanotubes. Indian J Sci Technol 2015;8(S9):455–64.
[74] Kari OK, Rojalin T, Salmaso S, et al. Multi-parametric surface plasmon resonance platform for studying liposome–serum interactions and protein corona formation. Drug Deliv Transl Res 2017;7(2):228–40.
[75] Sen R, Dasgupta D. Simple fluorescence assays probing conformational changes of *Escherichia coli* RNA polymerase during transcription initiation. In: Adhya S, Garges S, editors. Methods in enzymology. The Netherlands: Elsevier; 2003. p. 598–605.
[76] Wang Y, Li M, Xu X, Tang W, Xiong L, Sun Q. Formation of protein corona on nanoparticles with digestive enzymes in simulated gastrointestinal fluids. J Agric Food Chem 2019;67(8):2296–306.
[77] Mukherjee S, Chowdhury D, Kotcherlakota R, Patra S, et al. Potential theranostics application of bio-synthesized silver nanoparticles (4-in-1 system). Theranostics 2014;4(3):316.
[78] Clemments AM, Botella P, Landry CC. Protein adsorption from biofluids on silica nanoparticles: corona analysis as a function of particle diameter and porosity. ACS Appl Mater Interfaces 2015;7(39):21682–9.
[79] Cedervall T, Lynch I, Foy M, et al. Detailed identification of plasma proteins adsorbed on copolymer nanoparticles. Angew Chem Int Ed 2007;46(30):5754–6.
[80] Docter D, Distler U, Storck W, et al. Quantitative profiling of the protein coronas that form around nanoparticles. Nat Protoc 2014;9(9):2030.
[81] Mukherjee S, Dasari M, Priyamvada S, Kotcherlakota R, Bollu VS, Patra CR. A green chemistry approach for the synthesis of gold nanoconjugates that induce the inhibition of cancer cell proliferation through induction of oxidative stress and their in vivo toxicity study. J Mater Chem B 2015;3(18):3820–30.
[82] Safian MT, Umar K, Parveen T, Yaqoob AA, Ibrahim MN. Biomedical applications of smart polymer composites. In: Smart polymer nanocomposites. Woodhead Publishing; January 1, 2021. p. 183–204.
[83] Yaqoob AA, Safian MT, Rashid M, Parveen T, Umar K, Ibrahim MN. Introduction of smart polymer nanocomposites. In: Smart polymer nanocomposites. Woodhead Publishing; January 1, 2021. p. 1–25.
[84] Kianfar E. Gas hydrate: applications, structure, formation, separation processes, Thermodynamics. In: Taylor JC, editor. Chapter 8: Advances in chemistry research. vol 62. USA: Nova Science Publishers, Inc.; 2020.
[85] Kianfar M, Kianfar F, Kianfar E. The effect of nano-composites on the mechanic and morphological characteristics of NBR/PA6 blends. Am J Oil Chem Technol 2016;4(1):29–44.
[86] Pelaz B, Del Pino P, Maffre P, et al. Surface functionalization of nanoparticles with polyethylene glycol: effects on protein adsorption and cellular uptake. ACS Nano 2015;9(7):6996–7008.

[87] Kianfar E. The effect of nano-composites on the mechanic and morphological characteristics of NBR/PA6 blends. Am J Oil Chem Technol 2016;4(1):27–42.
[88] Kianfar F, Moghadam SRM, Kianfar E. Energy optimization of ilam gas refinery unit 100 by using HYSYS refinery software (2015). Indian J Sci Technol 2015;8(S9):431–6.
[89] Jietao H, Jing L, Yayu Z, Zekai L, Zhiwei Q, Zili L, Wei Y, et al. A new anti-biofilm strategy of enabling arbitrary surfaces of materials and devices with robust bacterial anti-adhesion via a spraying modified microsphere method. J Mater Chem A 2019;7:26039–52.
[90] Abdullah A, Abdullah AZ, Ahmed M, Khan J, Shahadat M, Umar K, Alim MA. A review on recent developments and progress in sustainable acrolein production through catalytic dehydration of bio-renewable glycerol. J Clean Prod March 20, 2022;341:130876.
[91] Santos-Martinez MJ, Inkielewicz-Stepniak I, Medina C, et al. The use of quartz crystal microbalance with dissipation (QCM-D) for studying nanoparticle-induced platelet aggregation. Int J Nanomed 2012;7:243.
[92] Ahmad H, Umar K, Ali SG, Singh P, Islam SS, Khan HM. Preconcentration and speciation of arsenic by using a graphene oxide nanoconstruct functionalized with a hyperbranched polyethyleneimine. Microchim Acta June 2018;185:1–7.
[93] Brewer SH, Glomm WR, Johnson MC, Knag MK, Franzen S. Probing BSA binding to citrate-coated gold nanoparticles and surfaces. Langmuir 2005;21(20):9303–7.
[94] Chen H, Wang J, Cheng Y, Wang C, Liu H, Bian H, Pan Y, Sun J, Han W. Application of protein-based films and coatings for food packaging: a review. Polymers December 9, 2019;11(12):2039.
[95] Sakarika M, Delmoitié B, Ntagia E, Chatzigiannidou I, Gabet X, Ganigué R, Rabaey K. Production of microbial protein from fermented grass. Chem Eng J April 1, 2022;433:133631.
[96] Sharma S, Hansen LD, Hansen JØ, Mydland LT, Horn SJ, Øverland M, Eijsink VG, Vuoristo KS. Microbial protein produced from brown seaweed and spruce wood as a feed ingredient. J Agric Food Chem July 13, 2018;66(31):8328–35.
[97] Zhu W, He Q, Gao H, Nitayavardhana S, Khanal SK, Xie L. Bioconversion of yellow wine wastes into microbial protein via mixed yeast-fungus cultures. Bioresour Technol March 1, 2020;299:122565.
[98] Gordeladze JO, Haugen HJ, Lyngstadaas SP, Reseland JE. Bone tissue engineering: state of the art, challenges, and prospects. Tissue engineering for artificial organs: regenerative medicine. Smart Diag Personal Med May 8, 2017;2:525–51.
[99] Mir NA, Haque MM, Khan A, Umar K, Muneer M, Vijayalakshmi S. Semiconductor mediated photocatalysed reaction of two selected organic compounds in aqueous suspensions of Titanium dioxide. J Adv Oxid Technol July 1, 2012;15(2): 380–91.
[100] Vijaya Bhaskar Reddy A, Yusop Z, Jaafar J, Bin Aris A, Abdul Majid Z, Umar K, Talib J. Simultaneous determination of three organophosphorus pesticides in different food commodities by gas chromatography with mass spectrometry. J Separ Sci June 2016;39(12):2276–83.
[101] Jin HH, Kim DH, Kim TW, Shin KK, Jung JS, Park HC, Yoon SY. In vivo evaluation of porous hydroxyapatite/chitosan–alginate composite scaffolds for bone tissue engineering. Int J Biol Macromol December 1, 2012;51(5):1079–85.
[102] Mir NA, Khan A, Umar K, Muneer M. Photocatalytic study of a xanthene dye derivative, phloxine B in aqueous suspension of TiO2: adsorption isotherm and decolourization kinetics. Energy Environ Focus September 1, 2013;2(3):208–16.

[103] Daculsi G, Fellah BH, Miramond T, Durand M. Osteoconduction, osteogenicity, osteoinduction, what are the fundamental properties for a smart bone substitutes. Irbm November 1, 2013;34(4–5):346–8.

[104] Wu R, Li Y, Shen M, Yang X, Zhang L, Ke X, Yang G, Gao C, Gou Z, Xu S. Bone tissue regeneration: the role of finely tuned pore architecture of bioactive scaffolds before clinical translation. Bioact Mater May 1, 2021;6(5):1242–54.

[105] Dellavia C, Canciani E, Pellegrini G, Tommasato G, Graziano D, Chiapasco M. Histological assessment of mandibular bone tissue after guided bone regeneration with customized computer-aided design/computer-assisted manufacture titanium mesh in humans: a cohort study. Clin Implant Dent Relat Res August 2021;23(4):600–11.

[106] Omar O, Engstrand T, Kihlström Burenstam Linder L, Åberg J, Shah FA, Palmquist A, Birgersson U, Elgali I, Pujari-Palmer M, Engqvist H, Thomsen P. In situ bone regeneration of large cranial defects using synthetic ceramic implants with a tailored composition and design. Proc Natl Acad Sci USA October 27, 2020;117(43): 26660–71.

[107] Farag MM. Recent trends on biomaterials for tissue regeneration applications. J Mater Sci January 2023;58(2):527–58.

[108] Yuan Z, Wei P, Huang Y, Zhang W, Chen F, Zhang X, Mao J, Chen D, Cai Q, Yang X. Injectable PLGA microspheres with tunable magnesium ion release for promoting bone regeneration. Acta Biomater February 1, 2019;85:294–309.

[109] Cheng G, Yin C, Tu H, Jiang S, Wang Q, Zhou X, Xing X, Xie C, Shi X, Du Y, Deng H. Controlled co-delivery of growth factors through layer-by-layer assembly of core–shell nanofibers for improving bone regeneration. ACS Nano June 11, 2019;13(6):6372–82.

[110] Makvandi P, Ali GW, Della Sala F, Abdel-Fattah WI, Borzacchiello A. Hyaluronic acid/corn silk extract based injectable nanocomposite: a biomimetic antibacterial scaffold for bone tissue regeneration. Mater Sci Eng C February 1, 2020;107:110195.

[111] Jeong J, Kim JH, Shim JH, Hwang NS, Heo CY. Bioactive calcium phosphate materials and applications in bone regeneration. Biomater Res December 2019;23(1):1.

[112] Abbas M, Alqahtani MS, Alhifzi R. Recent developments in polymer nanocomposites for bone regeneration. Int J Mol Sci February 7, 2023;24(4):3312.

[113] O'Connor JP, Kanjilal D, Teitelbaum M, Lin SS, Cottrell JA. Zinc as a therapeutic agent in bone regeneration. Materials January 2020;13(10):2211.

[114] Huang CC, Kang M, Lu Y, Shirazi S, Diaz JI, Cooper LF, Gajendrareddy P, Ravindran S. Functionally engineered extracellular vesicles improve bone regeneration. Acta Biomater June 1, 2020;109:182–94.

[115] Yang Q, Yin H, Xu T, Zhu D, Yin J, Chen Y, Yu X, Gao J, Zhang C, Chen Y, Gao Y. Engineering 2D mesoporous Silica@ MXene-integrated 3D-printing scaffolds for combinatory osteosarcoma therapy and NO-augmented bone regeneration. Small April 2020;16(14):1906814.

[116] Khan MA, Ahmad A, Umar K, Nabi SA. Synthesis, characterization, and biological applications of nanocomposites for the removal of heavy metals and dyes. Ind Eng Chem Res January 14, 2015;54(1):76–82.

[117] Umar K, Dar AA, Haque MM, Mir NA, Muneer M. Photocatalysed decolourization of two textile dye derivatives, Martius Yellow and Acid Blue 129, in UV-irradiated aqueous suspensions of Titania. Desalination Water Treat August 1, 2012;46(1–3): 205–14.

[118] Hutmacher DW. Scaffold design and fabrication technologies for engineering tissues—state of the art and future perspectives. J Biomater Sci Polym Ed 2001;12:107–24.

[119] Asadian M, Chan KV, Norouzi M, Grande S, Cools P, Morent R, De Geyter N. Fabrication and plasma modification of nanofibrous tissue engineering scaffolds. Nanomaterials January 8, 2020;10(1):119.
[120] Gheorghita R, Anchidin-Norocel L, Filip R, Dimian M, Covasa M. Applications of biopolymers for drugs and probiotics delivery. Polymers August 15, 2021;13(16): 2729.
[121] Zhao D, Yu S, Sun B, Gao S, Guo S, Zhao K. Biomedical applications of chitosan and its derivative nanoparticles. Polymers April 23, 2018;10(4):462.
[122] Rao KS, Reddy PR, Rao KM, Kumar SP. A green approach to synthesize silver nanoparticles from natural polymer for biomedical application. Indian J Adv Chem Sci 2015;5:340−4.
[123] Ribeiro LN, Alcântara AC, Darder M, Aranda P, Araújo-Moreira FM, Ruiz-Hitzky E. Pectin-coated chitosan−LDH bionanocomposite beads as potential systems for colon-targeted drug delivery. Int J Pharm March 10, 2014;463(1):1−9.
[124] Rebitski EP, Darder M, Carraro R, Aranda P, Ruiz-Hitzky E. Chitosan and pectin core−shell beads encapsulating metformin−clay intercalation compounds for controlled delivery. New J Chem 2020;44(24):10102−10.
[125] Sharma K, Porat ZE, Gedanken A. Designing natural polymer-based capsules and spheres for biomedical applications—a review. Polymers December 9, 2021;13(24): 4307.
[126] Khan A, Alamry KA. Recent advances of emerging green chitosan-based biomaterials with potential biomedical applications: a review. Carbohydr Res August 1, 2021;506:108368.
[127] Yaqoob AA, Al-Zaqri N, Yaakop AS, Umar K. Potato waste as an effective source of electron generation and bioremediation of pollutant through benthic microbial fuel cell. Sustain Energy Technol Assessments October 1, 2022;53:102560.
[128] Mahmood MA, Madni A, Rehman M, Rahim MA, Jabar A. Ionically cross-linked chitosan nanoparticles for sustained delivery of docetaxel: fabrication, post-formulation and acute oral toxicity evaluation. Int J Nanomed December 20, 2019:10035−46.
[129] Noshirvani N, Ghanbarzadeh B, Gardrat C, Rezaei MR, Hashemi M, Le Coz C, Coma V. Cinnamon and ginger essential oils to improve antifungal, physical and mechanical properties of chitosan-carboxymethyl cellulose films. Food Hydrocolloids September 1, 2017;70:36−45.
[130] Younes I, Rinaudo M. Chitin and chitosan preparation from marine sources. Structure, properties and applications. Mar Drugs March 2, 2015;13(3):1133−74.
[131] Soni B, Mahmoud B, Chang S, El-Giar EM. Physicochemical, antimicrobial and antioxidant properties of chitosan/TEMPO biocomposite packaging films. Food Packag Shelf Life September 1, 2018;17:73−9.
[132] Hu YL, Qi W, Han F, Shao JZ, Gao JQ. Toxicity evaluation of biodegradable chitosan nanoparticles using a zebrafish embryo model. Int J Nanomed December 2011;14:3351−9.
[133] Qu B, Luo Y. A review on the preparation and characterization of chitosan-clay nanocomposite films and coatings for food packaging applications. Carbohydrate Poly Technol Appl December 25, 2021;2:100102.
[134] Upadhyaya L, Singh J, Agarwal V, Tewari RP. The implications of recent advances in carboxymethyl chitosan based targeted drug delivery and tissue engineering applications. J Contr Release July 28, 2014;186:54−87.
[135] Burkatovskaya M, Castano AP, Demidova-Rice TN, Tegos GP, Hamblin MR. Effect of chitosan acetate bandage on wound healing in infected and noninfected wounds in mice. Wound Repair Regen May 2008;16(3):425−31.

[136] Granata G, Stracquadanio S, Leonardi M, Napoli E, Malandrino G, Cafiso V, Stefani S, Geraci C. Oregano and thyme essential oils encapsulated in chitosan nanoparticles as effective antimicrobial agents against foodborne pathogens. Molecules July 2, 2021;26(13):4055.

[137] Martău GA, Mihai M, Vodnar DC. The use of chitosan, alginate, and pectin in the biomedical and food sector—biocompatibility, bioadhesiveness, and biodegradability. Polymers November 8, 2019;11(11):1837.

[138] Valencia Zapata ME, Mina Hernandez JH, Grande Tovar CD, Valencia Llano CH, Diaz Escobar JA, Vázquez-Lasa B, San Román J, Rojo L. Novel bioactive and antibacterial acrylic bone cement nanocomposites modified with graphene oxide and chitosan. Int J Mol Sci June 15, 2019;20(12):2938.

[139] de Salamanca AE, Diebold Y, Calonge M, García-Vazquez C, Callejo S, Vila A, Alonso MJ. Chitosan nanoparticles as a potential drug delivery system for the ocular surface: toxicity, uptake mechanism and in vivo tolerance. Invest Ophthalmol Vis Sci April 1, 2006;47(4):1416–25.

[140] Gomes LP, Paschoalin VM, Del Aguila EM. Chitosan nanoparticles: production, physicochemical characteristics and nutraceutical applications. Rev Virtual Quim January 1, 2017;9(1):387–409.

[141] Reddy MS, Ponnamma D, Choudhary R, Sadasivuni KK. A comparative review of natural and synthetic biopolymer composite scaffolds. Polymers March 30, 2021;13(7):1105.

[142] Muvva A, Chacko IA, Ghate V, Lewis SA. Modified pectins for colon-specific drug delivery. J Indian J Pharmaceut Edu Res April 1, 2020;54(2).

[143] Han J, Zhao D, Li D, Wang X, Jin Z, Zhao K. Polymer-based nanomaterials and applications for vaccines and drugs. Polymers January 2, 2018;10(1):31.

[144] Kiadeh SZ, Ghaee A, Farokhi M, Nourmohammadi J, Bahi A, Ko FK. Electrospun pectin/modified copper-based metal–organic framework (MOF) nanofibers as a drug delivery system. Int J Biol Macromol March 15, 2021;173:351–65.

[145] Tiwari G, Tiwari R, Sriwastawa B, Bhati L, Pandey S, Pandey P, Bannerjee SK. Drug delivery systems: an updated review. Int J Pharm Investig January 2012;2(1):2.

[146] Hassan ME, Bai J, Dou DQ. Biopolymers; definition, classification and applications. Egypt J Chem September 1, 2019;62(9):1725–37.

[147] Gursoy M, Sargin I, Mujtaba M, Akyuz B, Ilk S, Akyuz L, Kaya M, Cakmak YS, Salaberria AM, Labidi J, Erdem N. False flax (Camelina sativa) seed oil as suitable ingredient for the enhancement of physicochemical and biological properties of chitosan films. Int J Biol Macromol July 15, 2018;114:1224–32.

[148] Vunain E, Mishra AK, Mamba BB. Fundamentals of chitosan for biomedical applications. In: Chitosan based biomaterials. vol 1. Woodhead Publishing; January 1, 2017. p. 3–30.

[149] Kedir WM, Abdi GF, Goro MM, Tolesa LD. Pharmaceutical and drug delivery applications of chitosan biopolymer and its modified nanocomposite: a review. Heliyon August 15, 2022.

[150] Zheleznyak A, Shokeen M, Achilefu S. Nanotherapeutics for multiple myeloma. Wiley Interdiscipl Rev Nanomed Nanobiotechnol November 2018;10(6):e1526.

[151] Kumthekar P, Ko CH, Paunesku T, Dixit K, Sonabend AM, Bloch O, Tate M, Schwartz M, Zuckerman L, Lezon R, Lukas RV. A first-in-human phase 0 clinical study of RNA interference–based spherical nucleic acids in patients with recurrent glioblastoma. Sci Transl Med March 10, 2021;13(584):eabb3945.

[152] Boyd RD, Pichaimuthu SK, Cuenat A. New approach to inter-technique comparisons for nanoparticle size measurements; using atomic force microscopy, nanoparticle tracking analysis and dynamic light scattering. Colloids Surf A Physicochem Eng Asp August 20, 2011;387(1–3):35–42.

[153] De la Calle I, Menta M, Séby F. Current trends and challenges in sample preparation for metallic nanoparticles analysis in daily products and environmental samples: a review. Spectrochim Acta B Atom Spectrosc November 1, 2016;125:66–96.
[154] Choi J, Zheng Q, Katz HE, Guilarte TR. Silica-based nanoparticle uptake and cellular response by primary microglia. Environ Health Perspect May 2010;118(5): 589–95.
[155] Elsaesser A, Taylor A, de Yanés GS, McKerr G, Kim EM, O'Hare E, Howard CV. Quantification of nanoparticle uptake by cells using microscopical and analytical techniques. Nanomedicine November 2010;5(9):1447–57.
[156] Zhou X, Dorn M, Vogt J, Spemann D, Yu W, Mao Z, Estrela-Lopis I, Donath E, Gao C. A quantitative study of the intracellular concentration of graphene/noble metal nanoparticle composites and their cytotoxicity. Nanoscale 2014;6(15): 8535–42.
[157] Brandelli A. The interaction of nanostructured antimicrobials with biological systems: cellular uptake, trafficking and potential toxicity. Food Sci Hum Wellness March 1, 2020;9(1):8–20.

CHAPTER 6

Silk fibroin-based nanocomposites for tissue engineering

Abhishek Kumar[1,2], Anant Narayan Bhatt[2] and Mohd Saquib Ansari[1]

[1]Department of Biomedical Sciences, Shaheed Rajguru College of Applied Sciences for Women, University of Delhi, Delhi, New Delhi, India; [2]Institute of Nuclear Medicine and Allied Sciences, Defence Research and Development Organization, Delhi, New Delhi, India

1. Introduction

Tissue engineering (TE) is a multidisciplinary field that employs biopolymers extensively in treating and regenerating damaged tissues by applying their scaffold-forming abilities that provide a suitable mesh-like anchorage for nearby cells to migrate toward, adhere, and proliferate for tissue repair. Tissue injury caused by trauma and degenerative diseases necessitates using donor tissue, such as allografts, which have a low success rate. For such applications, the biomaterial must be highly biocompatible, have well-optimized 3D structure-forming mechanical properties, have degradation kinetics corresponding to the tissue regeneration time, and be simultaneously metabolized for efficient clearance from the host body. The process includes seeding cells and growth factors in biomaterial scaffolds to support faster tissue regeneration [1].

TE-related applications have utilized various natural and synthetic polymeric materials as porous scaffolds. Synthetic polymers are highly modifiable and have exceptional mechanical properties, but they lack the biocompatibility and immunocompatibility that natural polymers offer [2,3]. Many natural biopolymers like alginate [4,5], cellulose [6,7], chitosan [8−10], gum tragacanth [11], and collagen [12,13] have been used for TE and related applications like wound healing with much success, but the main drawback these natural polymers face is their poor mechanical strength and batch-to-batch variations [2]. Because of these complications,

Protein-Based Nanocomposites for Tissue Engineering
ISBN 978-0-323-99357-9
https://doi.org/10.1016/B978-0-323-99357-9.00007-7

there has been an increase in research on TE applications based on silk protein. This dependence on silk fibroins is caused by silk's exceptional in vitro and in vivo biocompatibility [14,15] and silk fiber's rigid and elastic character [16].

The textile industry makes extensive use of silk. Silk-producing arthropods (including silkworms, spiders, and bees) contain silk in their glands, which they transform into fibers during metamorphosis. Silk generated by silkworms is favored for industrial and biomedical applications due to its relative homogeneity and high fiber yield (600–1500 m per cocoon) [17]. Silk has been approved by the Food and Drug Administration (FDA), has a long history of more than 2 decades of biological uses as sutures, and is presently used to treat skin lesions, lips, eyes, mouth surgeries, and oral surgeries [18]. Silk fibroin (SF), a natural protein extracted from silkworm silk, can potentially be utilized in TE due to silk fibroin's numerous desirable physiochemical properties, which include exceptional biocompatibility, biodegradability, bioresorbability, minimal immunogenicity, and adaptable mechanical properties [14].

This chapter examines current research in the field of tissue regeneration that has been founded on silk fibroin, and it evaluates the possibilities for further development of silk fibroin's use in therapeutically related applications. This chapter also discusses a short description of the silk protein and the mechanical characteristics of the SF, which are highly pertinent to the applications of silk biomaterials in tissue regeneration. While also summarizing the current advancements and applications of silk in TE.

2. Sources and properties of silk fibroin

Silk proteins are biosynthesized in the epithelial cells of the glands of silk-producing families such as silkworms, spiders, and mites. These families weave the silk into threads during the stage of their metamorphosis, known as cocoon development. The most commonly produced silk is derived from *Bombyx mori* (*B. mori*, mulberry silk moth), which was domesticated from an ancestral species in China that fed on mulberry, producing one of the finest quality silk fibers compared with most other species. The silk produced by *B. mori* silkworms has 75%–83.3% SF and 16.7%–25% of sericin [19] (Fig. 6.1A). SF has a semicrystalline structure which primarily strengthens the silk by providing it with a load-bearing capacity. In contrast, sericin is an irregular protein polymer that functions as a gummifying substance [20].

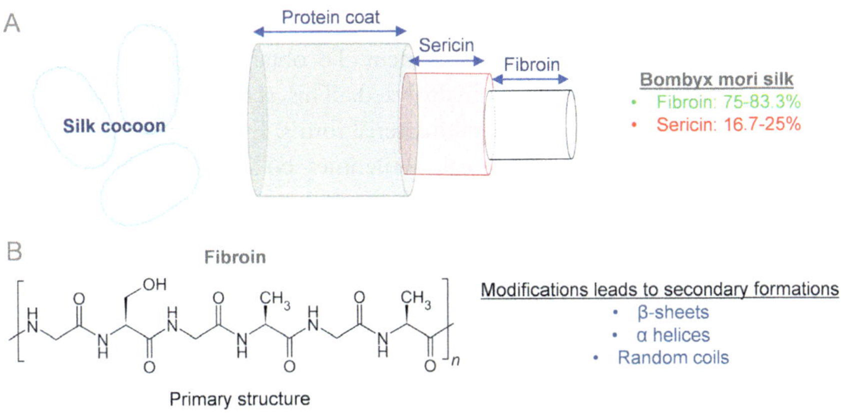

Figure 6.1 The figure illustrates (A) Silk from *B. mori* and its composition, (B) Primary structure of fibroin and its secondary formations. *(Figure made using bioRender.com.)*

Silk fibroin (SF) fibers have a diameter between 10 and 25 m and are composed of two categories of proteins: a light chain and a heavy chain in the ratio 1:1 connected by a solitary disulfide bond. SFs are composed of hydrophobic (ordered, highly conserved) and hydrophilic (less ordered, relatively more complex) block copolymers. Fig. 6.1B illustrates the primary structure of the fibroin. The elasticity and toughness of SF are the product of the mixture of these two kinds of blocks [15]. The silk structure can be modified appropriately during the spinning or regeneration processes to produce a range of secondary structures. These secondary formations can then be used to manipulate the physical characteristics of the material [21].

Silk has a well-established reputation for being hypoallergenic due to its extensive history of use in sutures [22]. As with other nonautologous biomaterials that can elicit a foreign body response, it is difficult to rule out the possibility that silk proteins will induce adverse immunological reactions [23]. This is particularly accurate, considering that silk does not come from a mammalian source. There have been isolated instances of delayed hypersensitivity to silk sutures [24], and it is hypothesized that these reactions are caused by the presence of a gum-like silk protein called sericin.

It has been discovered that fibroin fibers that do not contain any sericin have superior mechanical characteristics to fibroin fibers that contain sericin. It has been reported that sericin can induce inflammation, whereas sericin-free fibroin fibers have shown improved in vitro and in vivo biocompatibility. As a result, the sericin proteins found in SF are frequently eliminated through a degumming procedure to guarantee their biocompatibility in TE applications.

The first step of silk strand processing is known as "degumming," and it includes removing the glue protein sericin. To obtain silk solution, degummed silk thread must first be hydrolyzed. This stage is required for the manufacture of a range of other silk material forms. Even when the fibers are challenging to dissolve, fibroin can sometimes be extracted directly from silkworm glands using the appropriate buffer solution [25].

3. Silk fibroin nanocomposites

Silk fibroin is a highly adaptable protein that is capable of taking on a variety of conformations. Its mechanical properties can be easily enhanced by the addition of various inorganic materials into its network [26]. Nanocomposites are typically designed for engineering target tissues that have stringent mechanical requirements. Incorporating inorganic phases, which can increase the scaffold's electrical [27], mechanical [28], thermal [29], and biological performance [30,31], has been the primary focus in creating nanocomposites.

As a potential biomaterial for filling bone defects, a nanocomposite composed of strontium-doped hydroxyapatite and silk fibroin has been created by a research group [32]. During the course of the research, it was shown that the addition of strontium to the material did not have any effect on the biocompatibility of the substance; nonetheless, an improvement in the viability of mesenchymal stem cells was accomplished. In another study, a nerve conduit was constructed by adsorbing gold nanoparticles onto silk fibers and electrospinning them into a nanocomposite sheet, which was given a tubular form by rolling on a stainless steel mandrel [33]. In vitro research showed that the conduits encouraged the adhesion and multiplication of Schwann cells. Similarly, in vivo testing revealed that the conduits did not produce any immunogenic or toxic responses. The animals that were implanted with Schwann cell-filled nerve conduits for the purpose of the study were able to carry out sophisticated locomotory tasks such as stretching and jumping, and they had an outstanding sciatic function index (SFI) with an average lifespan (Table 6.1).

For the purpose of replicating heterogeneous complicated tissue structures such as the osteochondral interface, a research group has investigated the possibilities of generating strontium-doped nano-apatites as multifunctional silk-based cartilage and bone bio-inks. Strontium's involvement in downregulating cyclooxygenase-2 by inhibiting the prostaglandins (PGE2) pathway facilitated anti-osteoclastic activity while favoring M2

Table 6.1 Various silk nanocomposites and their characteristics.

Silk source	Inorganic composite	Scaffold type	Target organ/ tissue	Ref.
Bombyx mori	Calcium carbonate, hydroxyapatite	Particles	Bone	[32,34]
Bombyx mori	Gold, molybdenum disulphide	Electrospun mat	Peripheral nerve, cardiac tissue	[33,35]
Bombyx mori	Hydroxyapatite, magnetite	Hydrogel	Osteochondral tissue, bone	[36,37]
Bombyx mori	Calcium phosphate, diopside ceramic	Sponge	Osteochondral tissue, maxillofacial bone	[38,39]

macrophage. Which further validated the nanocomposite's potential for fabricating clinically viable prostheses for osteoporosis-related osteochondral defect repair [36]. In another study, the biological efficacy of silk-nano calcium-phosphate scaffolds was evaluated. In vitro results of enzymatic degradation demonstrated that the incorporation of calcium phosphate enhanced the biostability of the scaffold. Furthermore, the human adipose-derived stromal cells (hASCs) were cultured onto the scaffolds, and the scanning electron microscopy revealed that the microporous structure was advantageous for cell adhesion, whereas the macroporous structure was advantageous for cell migration and proliferation [38]. The histological analysis of the cell-cultured scaffolds also revealed an abundance of extracellular matrix within the scaffolds.

4. Different forms of silk biomaterials for TE

4.1 Silk fibers/electrospun mats

Regardless of the differences in their chemical makeup and mechanical properties, the cells that make up human tissues and organs discharge their extracellular matrix in the shape of nanoscale fibers. Natural polymers are commonly preferred over synthetic polymers due to their enhanced biocompatibility and bio-functionality [40]. Their structural similarity to native extracellular matrix components like collagen, hyaluronic acid, and elastin provides an advantage for adequate chemical signaling. Silk fibroin frameworks that have been electrospinned into nanofibers have shown promise in a variety of applications involving the regeneration of tissue [41]. Endothelial cell responses to silk fibers have been studied in terms of cell morphology, proliferation, formation of intercellular contact, and expression of adhesion molecules, with successful activation of signal transduction to increase cell attachment, polarization, and thus migration [42]. In addition, many different mixtures of silk fibroin with other types of biopolymers have been extensively researched. For example, in one experiment, chitin and silk fibroin mixtures with varying proportions were electrospinned into nanofibrous structures and tested for their ability to promote initial cell attachment and dissemination [43].

4.2 Silk hydrogels

Silk protein hydrogels with various properties have been developed in recent years. Researchers have developed silk fibroin hydrogels with high strength, injectability, self-healing ability, binding property, conductivity, and other properties by designing and controlling the multiscale structure of silk fibroin at the molecular level. Since an injectable hydrogel can be injected into a tissue defect with a slightly invasive injection, it can solidify in situ and replace the defect in the body, proving its promise for use in TE [44]. The silk fibroin hydrogels have qualities such as high drug loading and the ability to biodegrade. In addition, it has been demonstrated that SF protein hydrogels are capable of realizing the functions of injectability, thixotropy, and in situ gelation. As a result, silk fibroin functional hydrogels have received a considerable amount of attention in the field of medication release [45]. Silk hydrogels have also been extensively used in wound healing due to their capacity to collect wound exudate, load drugs, and keep a moist environment. As a result, the silk hydrogels enriched with anti-inflammatory, antimicrobial, and antioxidant properties can accelerate the wound repair process [46].

4.3 Silk porous scaffolds/sponges

Porous three-dimensional sponges make excellent frames for TE substrates because they closely mimic the physiological microenvironment found in living tissue. The silk-based scaffolds have proven to be excellent candidates for TE. These scaffolds must be made and sterilized, as the manufacturing process affects the scaffold's surface and bulk characteristics, and sterilization is a crucial component of in vivo TE [47]. Incorporating inorganic or organic additives into the preparation of composite silk three-dimensional structures is done with the intention of achieving favorable outcomes in terms of both mechanical and biological properties. The manufacturing procedure usually includes the addition of fillers to ensure that the fillers are spread equally throughout the scaffold. Silk-based composites provide a significant amount of support for epithelialization. When compared to other therapeutic materials, it has been discovered that fibroin-alginate sponges and films provide the best environment for appropriate skin wound recovery [48].

4.4 Silk particles

Microspheres or microparticles made of silk fibroin can be produced through a number of processes, including spray drying, salting out, electrostatic fields, lipid templating, water-in-oil emulsion, electrostatic fields, and break up of laminar aqueous flow, among others [49,50]. Because the particles generated have a size range of 0.2–20 μm, these techniques have proven to be especially useful in the context of drug distribution uses. In one study, a scaffold made by SF microparticle aggregation demonstrated compression modulus comparable to the natural cancellous bone while retaining the appropriate porosities and interconnected pore architecture for bone TE [51]. The following figure provides a brief sketch of the different forms of engineered silk for TE application (Fig. 6.2).

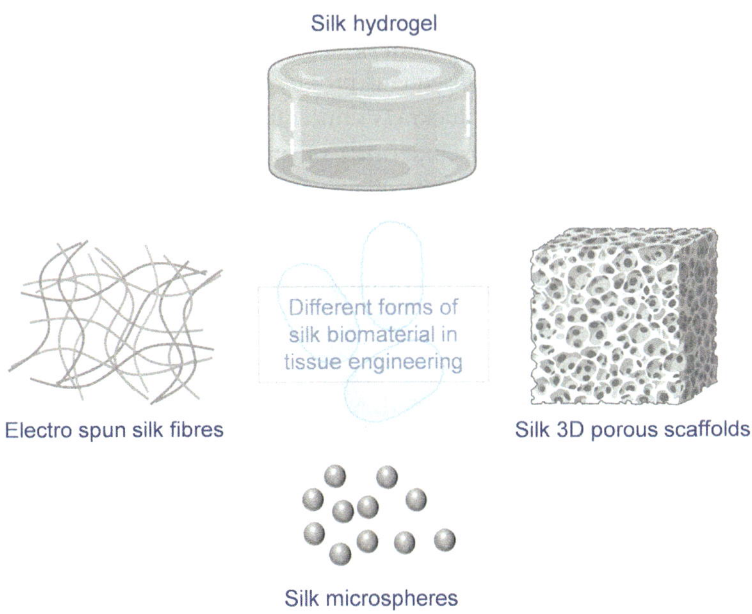

Figure 6.2 The diagram illustrates the various types of engineered silk used in TE applications. *(Figure made using bioRender.com.)*

5. Different applications of silk biomaterials in TE

5.1 Vascular tissue generation

Large tissues and tissue-engineered constructs necessitate an increased supply of oxygen and nutrients to reach the central regions. The currently available bypass vascular grafts lack the necessary properties for the fabrication of healthy autologous vessels. The main challenges are replicating the biological blood-material interface and producing vessels at the microvascular scale (<6 mm inner diameter). Researchers have attempted to create nanofibrous SF scaffolds that are nonwoven, tubular, and e-spun for developing tissue-engineered vascular grafts due to high biodegradability and compatibility [52]. To attain greater patency, as demonstrated by SF vascular grafts, it is essential for the model of the vascular graft to have anti-thrombogenic as well as antiatherogenic properties. Moreover, rapid endothelialization helps to improve the patency of the graft and reduces the risk of infection [53].

5.2 Skin tissue regeneration

Multiple research has highlighted silk's effect on cell migration and shown that it promotes healing by modulating the production of well-known indicators of cell proliferation, such as vimentin, cyclin D1, VEGF, and fibronectin [54]. The technique most usually applied for the fabrication of a bilayer skin construct is the use of porous matrices. This technique involves first populating the silk scaffold with fibroblasts, followed by the placement of keratinocytes and their subsequent proliferation [55]. In one study, the generation of a trilayer full-thickness skin equivalent was achieved by first generating a bilayer (dermo-epidermal) of pristine collagen gel and then depositing it on top of a previously generated hypodermal layer made up of pristine silk scaffold [56].

5.3 Bone and ligament tissue regeneration

Porous scaffolds composed of silk may operate as a guide for the adhesion, proliferation, and migration of osteocytes to achieve functional bone repair in three dimensions. Furthermore, they may stimulate stem cell osteogenic differentiation [57]. Adipose-derived mesenchymal stem cells, or ADSCs, are being widely explored as a potential new cell source in the field of bone TE. Silk scaffolds supplemented with ADSCs have the potential to enhance matrix mineralization and bone growth [58].

Other than bones, ligaments are composed of collagen-rich, well-aligned proteins, with the principal function of stabilizing the joints.

Researchers have constructed a silk collagen sponge scaffold woven with sheets of ligament-derived stem/progenitor cells (LSPCs), which has demonstrated the appropriate development of composite fibers following implantation. Silk collagen sponge scaffolds infused with LSPCs have also shown promising results in cell proliferation and differentiation, ligament fiber regeneration, and ligament bone interface healing [59].

5.4 Tracheal tissue regeneration

The trachea, or windpipe, is a cartilaginous tube that connects the larynx to the bronchi of the lungs, allowing air to travel through. Scaffolds made of SF have been utilized in cartilage TE, with applications in the regeneration of tracheal tissue. Experiments conducted in vitro using scaffolds made of SF and chitosan revealed chondrocyte adhesion, proliferation, and differentiation. While in vivo experiments in nude mouse models displayed that cell scaffolds wrapped in perichondrium significantly improved chondrogenesis and produced mechanically sound structures [60]. SF has the potential to support the formation of an epithelial lining resulting engineered trachea with characteristics similar to those of a fully functional trachea. The figure below provides a scope for the broad application of silk in TE (Fig. 6.3).

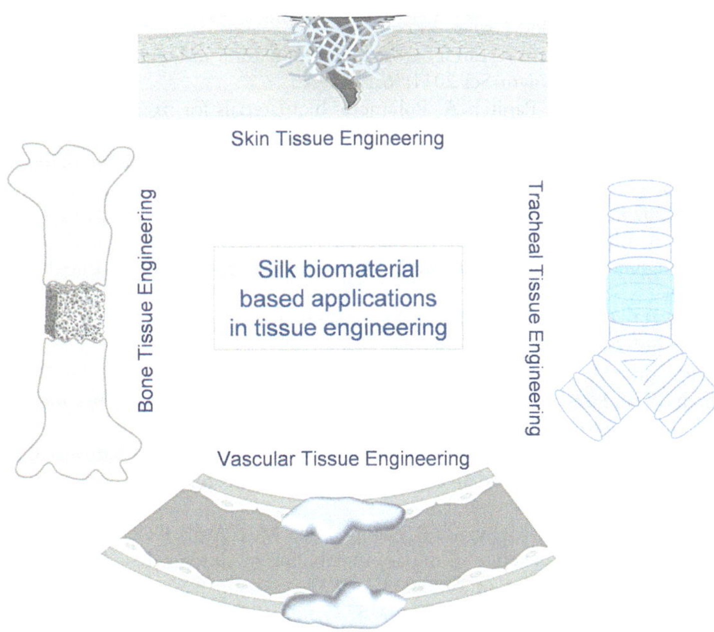

Figure 6.3 The diagram demonstrates the substantial application of silk in the field of tissue engineering. *(Figure made using bioRender.com.)*

6. Conclusion and prospects

The use of SF made from silkworm cocoons as surgical sutures date back many years. Because of its accessibility, outstanding mechanical characteristics, biodegradability, varied processability, and biocompatibility, SF is an intriguing polymeric biomaterial for a wide range of biomedical applications, particularly for guided tissue repair and functional TE. Recent advancements have focused on bionanotechnology-based technologies such as micropatterning and 3D bioprinting to build SF multilevel structures with high structural definition down to the nanoscale. Several studies have concluded that this benefits cellular proliferation, differentiation, migration, and adhesion. Silk-based designs permit easy control over matrix morphology, degradation rate, and conformal attachment to underlying tissues while posing minimal risk to the immune system and exhibiting exceptional biocompatibility. Silk systems will particularly benefit applications requiring delayed biodegradation and robust mechanical properties, such as bone, ligament, and musculoskeletal tissues.

References

[1] Howard D, Buttery LD, Shakesheff KM, Roberts SJ. Tissue engineering: strategies, stem cells and scaffolds. J Anat 2008;213:66–72.
[2] Sionkowska A. Current research on the blends of natural and synthetic polymers as new biomaterials. Prog Polym Sci 2011;36:1254–76.
[3] Seal BL, Otero TC, Panitch A. Polymeric biomaterials for tissue and organ regeneration. Mater Sci Eng R Rep 2001;34:147–230.
[4] Kumar A, Sah DK, Khanna K, Rai Y, Yadav AK, Ansari MS, et al. A calcium and zinc composite alginate hydrogel for pre-hospital hemostasis and wound care. Carbohydr Polym 2023;299:120186.
[5] Kumar A, Bhatt AN, Singh LRK, Karim Z, Ansari MS. Alginate-based hydrogels for tissue engineering. Polysacch Based Nanocompos Gene Deliv Tissue Eng 2021:59–69. Elsevier.
[6] Hickey RJ, Pelling AE. Cellulose biomaterials for tissue engineering. Front Bioeng Biotechnol 2019;7:45.
[7] Kanikireddy V, Varaprasad K, Jayaramudu T, Karthikeyan C, Sadiku R. Carboxymethyl cellulose-based materials for infection control and wound healing: a review. Int J Biol Macromol 2020;164:963–75.
[8] Ahsan SM, Thomas M, Reddy KK, Sooraparaju SG, Asthana A, Bhatnagar I. Chitosan as biomaterial in drug delivery and tissue engineering. Int J Biol Macromol 2018;110:97–109.
[9] Moeini A, Pedram P, Makvandi P, Malinconico M, d'Ayala GG. Wound healing and antimicrobial effect of active secondary metabolites in chitosan-based wound dressings: a review. Carbohydr Polym 2020;233:115839.
[10] Gupta I, Kumar A, Bhatt AN, Sapra S, Gandhi S. Green synthesis-mediated silver nanoparticles based biocomposite films for wound healing application. J Inorg Organomet Polym Mater 2022:1–18.

[11] Kalonia A, Sharma AK, Shaw P, Kumar A, Bhatt AN, Shukla A, et al. Ascorbate formulation improves healing efficacy in excisional wound mice model through interplay between pro and anti-inflammatory cytokines and angiogenic markers. Cytokine 2023;164:156158.
[12] Dong C, Lv Y. Application of collagen scaffold in tissue engineering: recent advances and new perspectives. Polymers 2016;8:42.
[13] Mathew-Steiner SS, Roy S, Sen CK. Collagen in wound healing. Bioengineering 2021;8:63.
[14] Vepari C, Kaplan DL. Silk as a biomaterial. Prog Polym Sci 2007;32:991–1007.
[15] Kasoju N, Bora U. Silk fibroin in tissue engineering. Adv Healthc Mater 2012;1:393–412.
[16] Vollrath F. Strength and structure of spiders' silks. Rev Mol Biotechnol 2000;74:67–83.
[17] Kundu B, Rajkhowa R, Kundu SC, Wang X. Silk fibroin biomaterials for tissue regenerations. Adv Drug Deliv Rev 2013;65:457–70.
[18] Omenetto FG, Kaplan DL. New opportunities for an ancient material. Science (80-) 2010;329:528–31.
[19] Sun W, Gregory DA, Tomeh MA, Zhao X. Silk fibroin as a functional biomaterial for tissue engineering. Int J Mol Sci 2021;22:1499.
[20] Liu B, Song Y, Jin L, Wang Z, Pu D, Lin S, et al. Silk structure and degradation. Colloids Surf B Biointerfaces 2015;131:122–8.
[21] Shao Z, Vollrath F. Surprising strength of silkworm silk. Nature 2002;418:741.
[22] Holland C, Numata K, Rnjak-Kovacina J, Seib FP. The biomedical use of silk: past, present, future. Adv Healthc Mater 2019;8:1800465.
[23] Thurber AE, Omenetto FG, Kaplan DL. In vivo bioresponses to silk proteins. Biomaterials 2015;71:145–57.
[24] Rossitch E, Bullard DE, Oakes WJ. Delayed foreign-body reaction to silk sutures in pediatric neurosurgical patients. Child's Nerv Syst 1987;3:375–8.
[25] Mandal BB, Kundu SC. A novel method for dissolution and stabilization of non-mulberry silk gland protein fibroin using anionic surfactant sodium dodecyl sulfate. Biotechnol Bioeng 2008;99:1482–9.
[26] Zuluaga-Vélez A, Quintero-Martinez A, Orozco LM, Sepúlveda-Arias JC. Silk fibroin nanocomposites as tissue engineering scaffolds – a systematic review. Biomed Pharmacother 2021;141:111924.
[27] Li Y, Zhao Y, Ma C, Zhao Y. Novel solvent-thermal preparation of a SnO_2 nanoparticles/expanded graphite multiscale composite with extremely enhanced electrical performances for Li-ion batteries. Electrochim Acta 2016;218:191–8.
[28] Mehrasa M, Asadollahi MA, Nasri-Nasrabadi B, Ghaedi K, Salehi H, Dolatshahi-Pirouz A, et al. Incorporation of mesoporous silica nanoparticles into random electrospun PLGA and PLGA/gelatin nanofibrous scaffolds enhances mechanical and cell proliferation properties. Mater Sci Eng C 2016;66:25–32.
[29] Tsai CY, Chien HT, Ding PP, Chan B, Luh TY, Chen PH. Effect of structural character of gold nanoparticles in nanofluid on heat pipe thermal performance. Mater Lett 2004;58:1461–5.
[30] Kumar Janakiraman A, Yin Wong Z, Cheng Z, Khanna K, Begum MY, Djearamane S, et al. Fabrication, characterization and in vitro cell cytotoxicity of ZnO nanoparticles on MDA-MB 231 breast cancer cell line. Chem Select 2023;8. e202302669.
[31] Al-Suwayyid LSA, Janakiraman AK, Thiagarajah S, Gunasekaran B, Khanna K, Kumar A, et al. Green synthesis of ginger-encapsulated zinc oxide nanoparticles: unveiling their characterization and selective cytotoxicity on MDA-MB 231 breast cancer cells. J Adv Pharm Technol Res 2023;14:325–31.

[32] Wang L, Pathak JL, Liang D, Zhong N, Guan H, Wan M, et al. Fabrication and characterization of strontium-hydroxyapatite/silk fibroin biocomposite nanospheres for bone-tissue engineering applications. Int J Biol Macromol 2020;142:366–75.
[33] Das S, Sharma M, Saharia D, Sarma KK, Sarma MG, Borthakur BB, et al. In vivo studies of silk based gold nano-composite conduits for functional peripheral nerve regeneration. Biomaterials 2015;62:66–75.
[34] Shi P, Abbah SA, Chuah YJ, Li J, Zhang Y, He P, et al. Yolk shell nanocomposite particles as bioactive bone fillers and growth factor carriers. Nanoscale 2017;9:14520–32.
[35] Nazari H, Heirani-Tabasi A, Hajiabbas M, Khalili M, Shahsavari Alavijeh M, Hatamie S, et al. Incorporation of two-dimensional nanomaterials into silk fibroin nanofibers for cardiac tissue engineering. Polym Adv Technol 2020;31:248–59.
[36] Moses JC, Saha T, Mandal BB. Chondroprotective and osteogenic effects of silk-based bioinks in developing 3D bioprinted osteochondral interface. Bioprinting 2020;17:e00067.
[37] Tanasa E, Zaharia C, Hudita A, Radu I-C, Costache M, Galateanu B. Impact of the magnetic field on 3T3-E1 preosteoblasts inside SMART silk fibroin-based scaffolds decorated with magnetic nanoparticles. Mater Sci Eng C 2020;110:110714.
[38] Yan L, Oliveira JM, Oliveira AL, Reis RL. In vitro evaluation of the biological performance of macro/micro-porous silk fibroin and silk-nano calcium phosphate scaffolds. J Biomed Mater Res Part B Appl Biomater 2015;103:888–98.
[39] Ghorbanian L, Emadi R, Razavi SM, Shin H, Teimouri A. Fabrication and characterization of novel diopside/silk fibroin nanocomposite scaffolds for potential application in maxillofacial bone regeneration. Int J Biol Macromol 2013;58:275–80.
[40] Amini S, Salehi H, Setayeshmehr M, Ghorbani M. Natural and synthetic polymeric scaffolds used in peripheral nerve tissue engineering: advantages and disadvantages. Polym Adv Technol 2021;32:2267–89.
[41] Zhang X, Reagan MR, Kaplan DL. Electrospun silk biomaterial scaffolds for regenerative medicine. Adv Drug Deliv Rev 2009;61:988–1006.
[42] Bondar B, Fuchs S, Motta A, Migliaresi C, Kirkpatrick CJ. Functionality of endothelial cells on silk fibroin nets: comparative study of micro-and nanometric fibre size. Biomaterials 2008;29:561–72.
[43] Park KE, Jung SY, Lee SJ, Min B-M, Park WH. Biomimetic nanofibrous scaffolds: preparation and characterization of chitin/silk fibroin blend nanofibers. Int J Biol Macromol 2006;38:165–73.
[44] Zheng H, Zuo B. Functional silk fibroin hydrogels: preparation, properties and applications. J Mater Chem B 2021;9:1238–58.
[45] Mandal BB, Kapoor S, Kundu SC. Silk fibroin/polyacrylamide semi-interpenetrating network hydrogels for controlled drug release. Biomaterials 2009;30:2826–36.
[46] Sonamuthu J, Cai Y, Liu H, Kasim MSM, Vasanthakumar VR, Pandi B, et al. MMP-9 responsive dipeptide-tempted natural protein hydrogel-based wound dressings for accelerated healing action of infected diabetic wound. Int J Biol Macromol 2020;153:1058–69.
[47] Tandon S, Kandasubramanian B, Ibrahim SM. Silk-based composite scaffolds for tissue engineering applications. Ind Eng Chem Res 2020;59:17593–611.
[48] Gholipourmalekabadi M, Sapru S, Samadikuchaksaraei A, Reis RL, Kaplan DL, Kundu SC. Silk fibroin for skin injury repair: where do things stand? Adv Drug Deliv Rev 2020;153:28–53.
[49] Qu J, Wang L, Hu Y, Wang L, You R, Li M. Preparation of silk fibroin microspheres and its cytocompatibility. 2013.

[50] Rajkhowa R, Gil ES, Kluge J, Numata K, Wang L, Wang X, et al. Reinforcing silk scaffolds with silk particles. Macromol Biosci 2010;10:599–611.

[51] Nisal A, Sayyad R, Dhavale P, Khude B, Deshpande R, Mapare V, et al. Silk fibroin micro-particle scaffolds with superior compression modulus and slow bioresorption for effective bone regeneration. Sci Rep 2018;8:7235.

[52] Kiritani S, Kaneko J, Ito D, Morito M, Ishizawa T, Akamatsu N, et al. Silk fibroin vascular graft: a promising tissue-engineered scaffold material for abdominal venous system replacement. Sci Rep 2020;10:1–9.

[53] Haga M, Yamamoto S, Okamoto H, Hoshina K, Asakura T, Watanabe T. Histological reactions and the in vivo patency rates of small silk vascular grafts in a canine model. Ann Vasc Dis 2017;10:132–8.

[54] Park YR, Sultan MT, Park HJ, Lee JM, Ju HW, Lee OJ, et al. NF-κB signaling is key in the wound healing processes of silk fibroin. Acta Biomater 2018;67:183–95.

[55] MacNeil S. Progress and opportunities for tissue-engineered skin. Nature 2007;445:874–80.

[56] Bellas E, Seiberg M, Garlick J, Kaplan DL. In vitro 3D full-thickness skin-equivalent tissue model using silk and collagen biomaterials. Macromol Biosci 2012;12:1627–36.

[57] Ding Z, Cheng W, Mia MS, Lu Q. Silk biomaterials for bone tissue engineering. Macromol Biosci 2021;21:2100153.

[58] Chen H, Qian Y, Xia Y, Chen G, Dai Y, Li N, et al. Enhanced osteogenesis of ADSCs by the synergistic effect of aligned fibers containing collagen I. ACS Appl Mater Interfaces 2016;8:29289–97.

[59] Ruan D, Zhu T, Huang J, Le H, Hu Y, Zheng Z, et al. Knitted silk-collagen scaffold incorporated with ligament stem/progenitor cells sheet for anterior cruciate ligament reconstruction and osteoarthritis prevention. ACS Biomater Sci Eng 2019;5:5412–21.

[60] Zang M, Zhang Q, Davis G, Huang G, Jaffari M, Ríos CN, et al. Perichondrium directed cartilage formation in silk fibroin and chitosan blend scaffolds for tracheal transplantation. Acta Biomater 2011;7:3422–31.

CHAPTER 7

Collagen-based nanocomposites for tissue engineering

Nasir Adamu[1], Khalid Umar[2], Tabassum Parveen[3], Nur Farhana Jaafar[2] and Ilham Maulana[4]
[1]Science Laboratory Technology, Federal Polytechnic Daura, Daura, Katsina State, Nigeria; [2]School of Chemical Sciences, Universiti Sains Malaysia, Penang, Malaysia; [3]Department of Botany, Aligarh Muslim University, Aligarh, Uttar Pradesh, India; [4]Department of Chemistry, Faculty of Mathematics and Natural Sciences, Universitas Syiah Kuala, Banda Aceh, Indonesia

1. Introduction

In recent years, advancements in collagen-based biomaterials have significantly progressed, enabling a broad spectrum of applications, including injectable collagen matrices and scaffolds for bone regeneration. Improved production and cross-linking techniques have been pivotal in making collagen widely utilized in research and medical settings. Its prevalence throughout the human body, coupled with its numerous advantages such as biodegradability, biocompatibility, accessibility, and adaptability, further contribute to its popularity. However, the proteinaceous nature of collagen poses a challenge in terms of sterilization, as altering its structure can be challenging [1]. A study by Recker and Barger-Lux [2] indicates that human bones comprise approximately 30%–35% organic material, 67%–70% hydroxyapatite (HA), various inorganic materials, and around 20% water. The organic components primarily consist of collagenous fibers, mainly type I collagen, chondroitin sulfate, hyaluronic acid, and keratan sulfate. Among these, collagen type I is a crucial structural element, supporting complete integration within bone tissue and contributing to its strength and hemostatic qualities.

It should be noted that collagen type I while offering strength does not possess the ability to swell [3]. Hydroxyapatite (HA), a complex calcium phosphate, forms bones alongside the collagenous framework. According to Swetha et al. [4], it is commonly utilized in developing tissue engineering products for treating bone abnormalities through bone grafting,

Protein-Based Nanocomposites for Tissue Engineering
ISBN 978-0-323-99357-9
https://doi.org/10.1016/B978-0-323-99357-9.00004-1

replacement, and restoration. These bioceramics are also recommended for the implantation of bone tissue due to their osteoconductivity, reabsorbability, short time of implantation, cellular invasion, and significant bone ingrowth [5]. Polymer nanocomposites have been developed to enhance synthetic bone substitutes' mechanical and functional properties. These substitutes can be made of materials such as collagen or hydroxyapatite and can be impregnated with bone marrow or designed to promote the growth of blood cells before implantation. In a study by Fujii et al. hydroxyapatite was utilized as a biomineral scaffolding material in combination with human hair protein to create a fully biodegradable material with an appropriate immunological response, resulting in improved mechanical properties in the final bone-substitute products [6]. In this field of research, investigators have explored various natural and synthetic polymers, including Pluronic F127, cellulose, carboxymethyl cellulose, atelocollagen, gelatin, collagen, hyaluronan, poly(L-lactic acid), chitosan, cellulose graft polyacrylamide, low-density polyethylene, poly(-caprolactone), poly(methyl methacrylate), poly(acrylamide), polysulfone, keratin, poly(vinyl alcohol), amphiphilic copolymers derived from polyethylene glycol-block-poly(D, L-lactic acid) [7], pullulan/dextran, and poly(xylitol-co-dodecanedioate) [8], as well as silk fibroin [9].

Collagen is the most prevalent protein, constituting nearly all soft and hard tissues in mammals and comprising about one-third of the body's protein tissue mass [10]. Various tissues, such as bones, skin, tendons, and teeth, house collagen [11]. Researchers have identified 28 different collagen types, with type I being the most widespread in the extracellular matrix (ECM) and extensively found in tendons and bones [12]. Collagens consist of three interconnected (α-polypeptide) chains forming homotrimers or heterotrimers, and their specific structure depends on the collagen type. Each chain adopts a polyalanine type II shape, and the repeating Gly-X-Y triplet forms a tightly packed triple helix configuration, with X often being a proline (or any amino acid) and Y typically hydroxyproline [13]. The amino acid sequence requires glycine in every third position due to its small size and ability to occupy the confined space within the triple helix center. Previous studies have highlighted collagen's desirability as a biomaterial due to its favorable properties, including strong biocompatibility, degradability, adhesion, osteogenic induction capabilities, and low immunogenicity [14]. Therefore, collagen's limited mechanical strength across physical, chemical, and mechanical qualities constrains its potential applications.

Therefore, to improve the performance of collagen, researchers either modify it or combine it with scaffolding materials. Collagen is an effective matrix for various cell types, facilitating 3D cell culturing within a hydrogel. Research has demonstrated the biological advantages of collagen-based matrices, promoting cell migration within scaffolds [15]. Enhanced collagen can be integrated into a titanium scaffold to offer structural integrity without sacrificing other aspects [16].

2. Methods of preparation and processing of collagen structure

Collagen is a complex molecule comprising three polypeptide chains designated by Arabic numerals. All three chains must be identical to create homotrimers, whereas heterotrimers necessitate different chains. The fibrils consist of three collagen chains constructed from polyprotein II helices, with three of these helices exhibiting a left-handed twist. These left-handed helices intertwine to create three right-handed triple helices, with a residue interwoven between them. Studies conducted by both [17,18] indicate that collagen chains exhibit high glycine hydroxyproline and proline concentrations. Every third residue participates in an interchain hydrogen bond and electrostatic attraction between lysine and aspartic acid. A residue shift involving three chains is necessary to accommodate glycine residues in the core. Each trimerization domain in collagen can select and organize three separate strands [19]. In most collagen types, the trimerization domain is located at the carboxyl terminus of the nontriple helix domain. Numerous collagen trimerization domains have been found, including the multiplexin trimerization domain in types XV and XVIII, the NC1 domain in type IV collagen, the C1q-type domain in types VIII and X, and the C-propeptide in fibrillar collagens (types I, II, III, V, and XI). It has been determined that these four types of collagen trimerization domains exist [20]. Cattle are the primary source of collagen and have a diverse range of origins [21]. Cattle tissues, such as tendons, bones, and lung tissues, can make collagen. Pigs are also a typical root or form of collagen. Porcine collagen is frequently utilized for hernia repair and wound healing because it resembles human collagen and has no immunological limitations [22]. Collagen, characterized by minimal immunogenicity, reduces the risk of rejection when administered or ingested by a foreign entity. Even with its minimal antigenicity, the molecule can be alterable to prevent immune response. Collagen's immunogenicity can be reduced by adding cross-linking or by using protease specificity to remove the nonhelical portion of the collagen molecules [23]. Cross-linking serves two purposes: minimizing antigen-antibody reactivity and screening antigen locations [24].

Collagen is an insoluble protein in organic solvents due to its high affinity for water. The covalent bonds within collagen are crucial in maintaining the quaternary structure and preventing molecules from deviating from their fibrous shape. The extraction conditions employed can directly affect the degree of collagen dissociation. Only Type I collagen can be extracted from adult tissues under nondenaturing conditions, while other collagen types are not recovered under identical conditions [25]. When exposed to ultraviolet light, metal nanoparticles can activate physical and photochemical cross-linking activities [26,27]. Previous studies have demonstrated that incorporating polyvinylpyrrolidone-capped zinc oxide nanoparticles into the collagen matrix can induce gelation, reducing the need for chemical cross-linking agents [28].

Collagen requires specific processing to provide the precise functions needed for scaffold tissue regeneration. Several physicochemical processes can cross-link it to enhance its stability chemically and mechanically. Aldehydes are the most used chemical reagents, including poly epoxy and glutaraldehyde [29]. In addition, physical therapy like heat treatment and dehydration can also efficiently stimulate collagen cross-linking (ultraviolet, gamma, and microwave). Although it has been shown to reduce biocompatibility, aldehydes, isocyanates, and carbodiimide can be used for chemical cross-linking [30]. Collagen can also be used to incorporate drugs into the system through simple covalent bonds. The capacity of collagen to absorb water can be decreased through cross-linking, and the diffusion of any linking molecules can be slowed down [31]. In addition, the interaction between collagen and drugs can lengthen the duration of drug release. Fig. 7.1 depicts the illustration of the collagen structure in the diagram below [32].

3. The biological characteristics of collagen in bone tissue engineering

Although the precise function of collagen in the development of bone is still unknown, it is well known that collagen is essential for the proliferation and differentiation of osteoclasts and bone mesenchymal stem cells (BMSCs). This ultimately results in an overall improvement in osteogenesis. In addition essential to promoting the mechanisms involved in bone

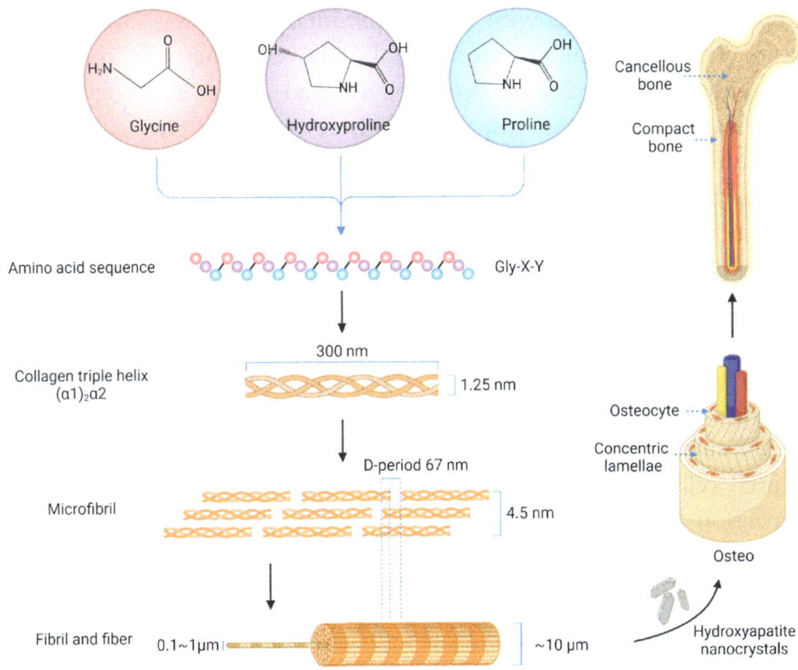

Figure 7.1 The hierarchical structure of type I collagen fiber and its relationship to human bone is evident [32].

regeneration is mineralized collagen. The extensive interactions between collagen and bone cells contribute significantly to the intricate and dynamic process of bone formation, establishing collagen as a crucial component for sustaining and promoting skeletal tissue growth [33].

3.1 Collagen-based hydrogel in bone regeneration

A hydrogel composed of raw collagen was generated through three-dimensional culturing. The use of collagen has repeatedly demonstrated its capacity to maintain the chondrocyte phenotype, which is essential for developing new cartilage-like tissue. Studies have shown that chondrocytes can synthesize extracellular matrix (ECM) and distribute uniformly in three-dimensional space to create new cartilage-like tissue [34]. In a survey by Ochi et al. knee cartilage defects were treated using cartilage cells propagated in collagen hydrogel. The results indicated that the transplanted tissue gradually assimilated into the neighboring subchondral bone, suggesting that the interface between the transplanted chondrocyte gel complex and the bone with the subchondral defect was challenging to discern. In another study, Katsube et al. discovered that locations restored using collagen gel-cultured chondrocytes had higher histological scores than those repaired with suspension culture 6 months after surgery. In a separate study, Kaizawa et al. utilized collagen extracted from human tendons to create hydrogels to address nonunion following rotator cuff injuries. The results demonstrated a considerable improvement in collagen content and bone mass during the repair process, indicating that adequate tendon-bone connection leads to increased bone mass at the tendon insertion location [34,35]. According to research on the cytoskeletal elements of bone cells, 3D cultures of bone cells resulted in more acting fiber than 2D culture [36]. Amorphous mineralized granules were also visible in the 3D-cultured cells, but mineralized nodules were only visible in 2D-cultured cells, demonstrating a volume difference. Another study found a connection between osteoblast activity and collagen contraction during bone repair. In this study, inherent mechanical stress changed gene expression [37]. Osteocytes engage the collagen fracture callus during this process, mineralizing the matrix to aid in fracture repair. Before pre-coacervation, the first step of cartilage development, BMSCs strongly express type I collagen, and this expression decreases during chondrocyte differentiation [38]. According to studies, BMSCs can develop into cartilage when cultivated in collagen with the proper density. However, in the 3D collagen culture, low-density cells did not develop into cartilage [39]. This culture technique generates several gradient cartilage tissues that are excellent candidates for tissue engineering. In a 14-day experiment, bone marrow mesenchymal stem cells (BMSCs) and human umbilical vein endothelial cells (HUVECs) were cultured in a collagen hydrogel to explore how collagen shear stress affects the osteogenic and angiogenic properties of these cell types. Within the initial 2 days, no observable responses related to osteogenesis or angiogenesis were detected. However, dynamic coculture under stress leads to increased expression of vascular endothelial growth factor (VEGF) and bone morphogenetic protein-2 (BMP-2) genes in human umbilical vein endothelial cells (HUVECs). This implies that human bone marrow mesenchymal stem cells (hMSCs) grow before initiating osteogenesis and angiogenesis. In a separate investigation, Paduano et al. examined dental pulp stem cells using a hydrogel composed of demineralized bovine bone and collagen [40]. This study revealed that collagen did not significantly affect the differentiation capability of dental pulp stem cells.

3.2 Collagen application in various biomedical uses

Collagen is a very useful material in the dental, pharmaceutical, and medical fields. It can be made into lattice-like gels or compressed solids that are cross-linked [41]. Collagen is primarily used in materials for osteogenesis and bone filling, antithrombogenic surfaces, burn and wound cover dressings, and the immobilization of therapeutic enzymes. Lately, there has been a global surge in the interest of researchers in using collagen as a medication delivery vehicle. Collagen-based drug delivery systems include collagen-and synthetic polymer-infused injectable microspheres made of gelatin, a degraded form of collagen, and collagen-and synthetic polymer-interpenetrating networks implanted in hydrogels. Furthermore, collagen membranes are used in the delivery of drugs to the eyes [42].

3.3 Collagen-based drug used in sheet/disc/film

Collagen films play a crucial role as barrier membranes in biomaterial applications, with thickness ranging from 0.01 to 0.5 mm. These films are produced by air-drying a casted collagen preparation, akin to ophthalmological shields, using biodegradable materials. The incorporation of drugs into collagen membranes is achieved through hydrogen bonding, covalent bonding, or simple entrapment. Hydroxylation allows for sterilization, rendering the membranes pliable while maintaining adequate strength to resist manipulation. Collagen films, sheets, and discs find application in treating tissue infections, such as infected corneal tissue or liver cancer, and serve as carriers for antibiotics like tetracycline [43]. In the realm of gene delivery to stimulate bone formation, collagen films, and matrices have been utilized as carriers. A study [44] employed collagen film and matrix as gene delivery carriers to enhance bone formation, creating a composite with recombinant human bone morphogenetic protein 2 (rhBMP-2) and collagen. This facilitated monitoring bone development and observing changes in the absorbency of the carrier collagen. Biodegradable collagen films or matrices have proven effective as scaffolds, supporting the survival of transfected fibroblasts in another study [45]. Combining collagen with other polymers, such as adding atelocollagen matrix to the surface of polyurethane films, enhanced the attachment and proliferation of fibroblasts, providing robust support for cell growth [46].

3.4 Collagen shields are used in drug delivery systems

The collagen shield, designed specifically for use as bandage contact lenses, gradually dissolves in the cornea, offering the advantage of applying the formulation to the ocular surface and potential for self-administration [47]. The mechanical properties of the shield protect the healing corneal epithelium from the blinking action of the eyelids. Drug delivery through collagen shields depends on loading the shield with medication and subsequent release [48]. In this process, the collagen matrix functions as a reservoir, entrapping drugs in its interstices. As the shield dissolves, tears flush through, creating a biologically compatible collagen solution layer. This layer lubricates the eye's surface, reduces lid rubbing on the cornea, prolongs the contact time between the drug and the cornea, and enhances epithelial healing. The bolus release of the drug from the lenses amplifies the drug effect [49].

3.5 Collagen sponges are used in drug delivery systems

Collagen sponges are made from the collagen found in cow's skin. Because of their adaptable qualities, they are frequently mixed with other materials to increase their durability. Because of their ability to absorb substances, adherence to moist wound beds, and protective qualities, they are used in the management of wounds, particularly severe burns and different kinds of wounds. Collagen sponges also help administer medicinal substances, such steroids and growth factors, for improved wound healing in a variety of applications, such as intravaginal administration for cervical dysplasia [45,50].

3.6 Collagen-based drug delivery systems: gels, hydrogels, and liposomes

Collagen gels offer a flowable consistency, suggesting the potential for an easily injectable and biocompatible drug delivery matrix. These gels are primarily utilized in injectable systems, with available forms including injectable suspensions of collagen fibers and nonfibrillar, viscous solutions in aqueous media. Specifically designed formulations for ophthalmic use start as liquids but transform into gels after administration, ensuring prolonged retention in the eye's cul-de-sac. This feature enables sustained delivery of nonsteroidal anti-inflammatory drugs or antibiotics [50]. Collagen gels, with their injectable and biocompatible nature, find applications in drug delivery systems. They are used in ophthalmic formulations for sustained drug release, as carriers for chondrocytes in cartilage repair, and in combination with polyhydroxyethylmethacrylate (PHEMA) for anticancer drug delivery. A unique system incorporating liposomes in a collagen gel showcases controlled release profiles for insulin and growth hormone [45,51,52].

3.7 Collagen-based drug delivery systems utilizing nanoparticles and nanospheres

The combination of electrostatic and entropic forces results in the formation of nanospheres, with sodium sulfate playing a role as a dissolving reagent to boost charge—charge interactions between plasmid DNA and collagen. Nanoparticles, which the reticuloendothelial system can absorb, enhance the uptake of exogenous compounds, including anti-HIV drugs, into various cells, especially macrophages. This characteristic positions collagen-based nanoparticles as advantageous carriers for systemic drug delivery. Consequently, nanoparticles function as parenteral carriers for cytotoxic agents and therapeutic compounds like camptothecin and hydrocortisone [53].

3.8 Different materials for making nanocomposite with collagen

Several types of collagen exist, but only a select few are utilized to create collagen-based materials. Notably, fibril-forming collagens, with type I collagen most abundant in mammals, are extensively employed in producing collagen-based biomaterials for various applications such as tissue engineering and wound healing. Due to its remarkable versatility, collagen is a crucial component in fabricating scaffolds that can be three-dimensional printed using modern 3D bioprinting technology [54].

Collagen obtained the sourced from various animal tissues, including skin, tendons, gut, bladder mucosa, rat tails, sponges, and even corals from invertebrates. The features of extracted collagen may vary slightly depending on the animal and tissue source. Noteworthy research [55—59] indicates that collagen derived from marine species offers several advantages compared with collagen from terrestrial organisms. These benefits include environmental sustainability, high collagen production, nontoxic properties, and easy absorption owing to its smaller molecular mass. To address potential concerns associated with collagen obtained from animal sources, researchers propose using recombination technology to create recombinant collagens through transfection of yeast and *Escherichia coli*.

However, the widespread application of collagen from animal sources may be limited due to potential downsides such as allergies and disease transmission [60].

4. Nano-collagen synthesis

The term "nano-collagen" refers to collagen that has been reduced to the nanoscale, combining the advantageous properties of collagen, known for its biomaterial-based wound-healing abilities, with nanoparticles, including a high volume-to-surface ratio. The downsizing of collagen fibers offers advantages in terms of wound accessibility and penetration, initiating the healing process effectively [61]. Various manufacturing methods utilize chemical, physical, and self-assembly processes to create nano-collagen. These methods encompass emulsification, complex coacervation, phase separation, nano-spray drying, desolvation, and several others. The generation of nano-collagen fibers involves the following procedures: (a) Electrospraying deposition, (b) Electrospinning, (c) Nano-emulsion, and (d) Milling.

4.1 Electrospraying deposition

The electrospray deposition procedure involves spraying a solution of nano-collagen onto a specific target. This technique finds widespread application in the biomedical field, particularly in utilizing nanoparticles for pharmaceutical purposes. This method's use of collagen in particle form is a crucial aspect. Collagen particles are expelled in a fine mist from a nozzle onto a target surface that is charged with a strong opposing (negative) voltage. This process is well-suited for pharmaceutical applications, primarily due to the tendency of the solvent in collagen particles to evaporate upon deposition onto the target surface. Consequently, the resulting nano-collagen particles are uniformly dispersed. The evaporation during deposition facilitates drug delivery applications and minimizes the risk of molecular agglomeration, reducing the likelihood of contamination. It is widely used in the automotive, pharmaceutical, and agricultural industries [62–64]. Fig. 7.2 shows the electrospray deposition setup.

4.2 Electrospinning

Electrospinning was utilized for the production of nanocollagen fibers. This method transforms a polymeric liquid into nanofibers in an electric

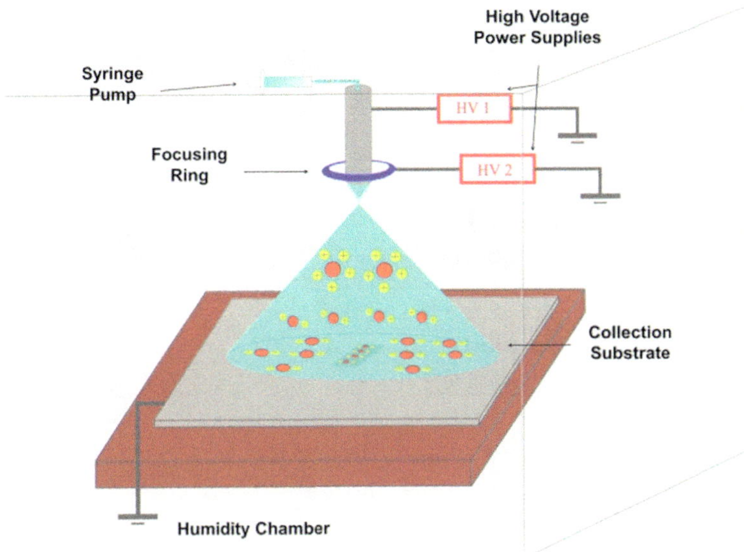

Figure 7.2 The electrospray deposition setup illustrates a schematic diagram [65].

field. These are achieved by charging a spinneret at high voltages and low currents to introduce droplets of the polymeric solution into electrospinning. Because of the high charge, the droplet surface elongates into a conical shape known as the Taylor cone. The creation of this shape is due to the electrostatic friction between the charged droplet surface and the columbic forces of the spinneret. When the electrostatic forces surpass the surface tension that maintains the stability of the Taylor cone, the cone extends and whips, ultimately forming fibers [66]. Electrospinning is a cost-effective and versatile method for producing nanofibers. It is a preferred choice for creating nanocollagen scaffolds for various applications including tissue engineering, tissue healing, regeneration, and matrices replicating the original extracellular matrix (ECM). The resulting fibers were collected on a metallic collector, which allowed for control over their shape as they dried and lost solvent molecules. Over time, electrospun collagen nanofibers have developed "smart" properties that enhance their applicability. Some of these smart capabilities, as detailed in Nagarajan et al. [67], include responsiveness to external stimuli, such as pH changes, exposure to light, and magnetic fields, as well as the ability to retain shapes or even self-cleaning. Structure of spinning as shown in Fig. 7.3.

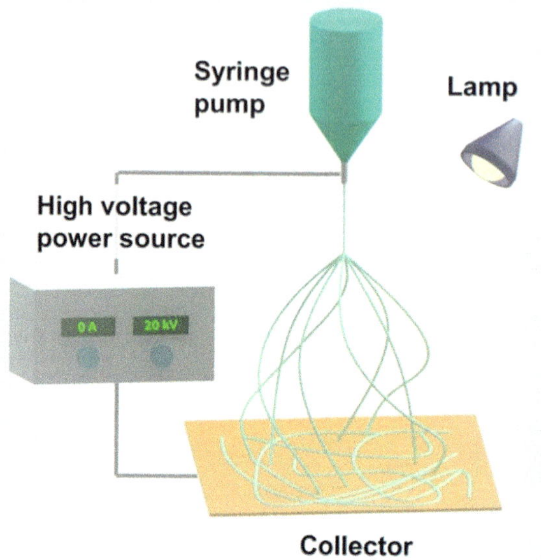

Figure 7.3 Structure of electrospinning [68].

4.3 Milling

Milling a polymeric collagen solution involves subjecting the material to significant mechanical stress, forming nanoscale collagen particles. This technology is considered one of the most cost-effective methods for large-scale production of nano-collagen [69,70]. However, the mechanical and kinetic energy produced during milling also generates significant heat, which may cause collagen to become denatured [71]. To prevent denaturation and protect the structural integrity of collagen, the process is carried out using liquid nitrogen at cryogenic temperatures to reduce the heat generated. Fig. 7.4 depicts the mechanical structure of the milling process.

4.4 Nanoemulsion

Collagen and nanoparticles were combined as droplets via the nanoemulsion technique. When two immiscible liquids combine in two separate phases, water in the oil phase and oil in the water phase, they create an emulsion known as an emulsion. The size ranges of the nanoemulsions were set apart from those of the emulsions. Compared with a typical emulsion droplet, a nanoemulsion droplet can range in size from 20 to

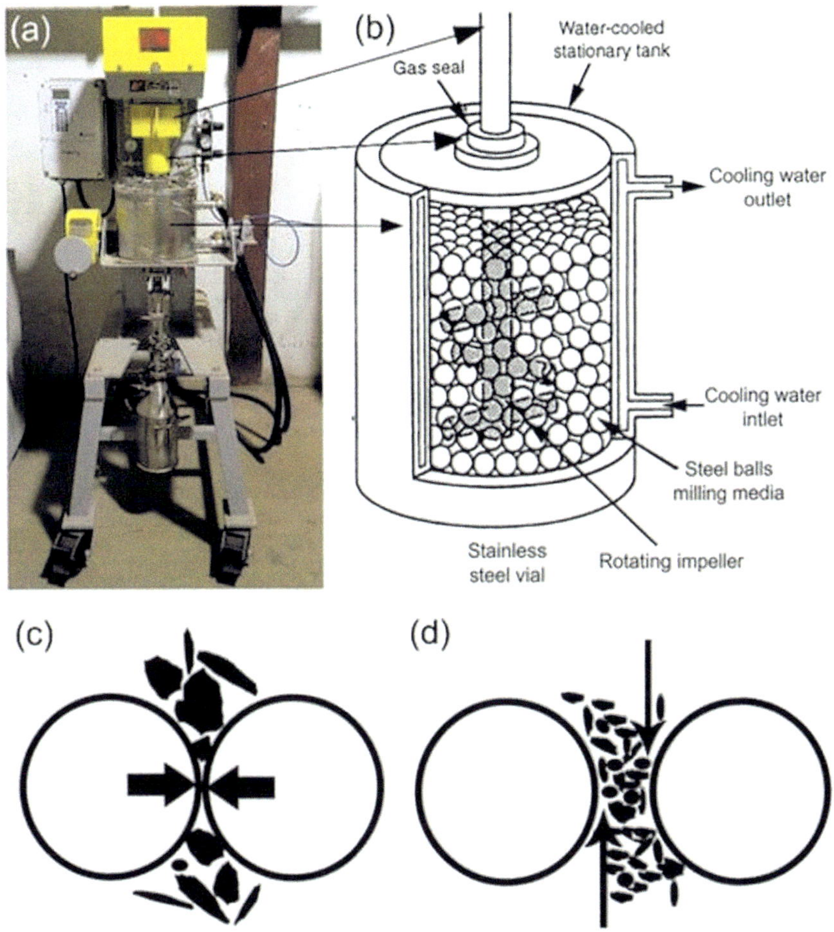

Figure 7.4 (A) An attritor ball mill is captured in a photograph, while sketches actively portray (B) the movement of balls within the attritor ball mill, (C) the impact forces, and (D) the shear forces generated by the ball milling media [72].

200 nm [73]. To create a homogeneous emulsion system, an organic phase comprising a lipophilic surfactant in an immiscible solvent was mixed with an aqueous phase containing collagen and a hydrophilic surfactant in water. The mixture was stirred continuously at room temperature. This emulsion system was mixed with heated oil to create nano-collagen emulsion particles [74]. Nanoemulsions have a natural tendency to deposit active ingredients deep within the tissues. This feature has been utilized in culinary, cosmetic, and drug industries for drug delivery. Many qualities shared by

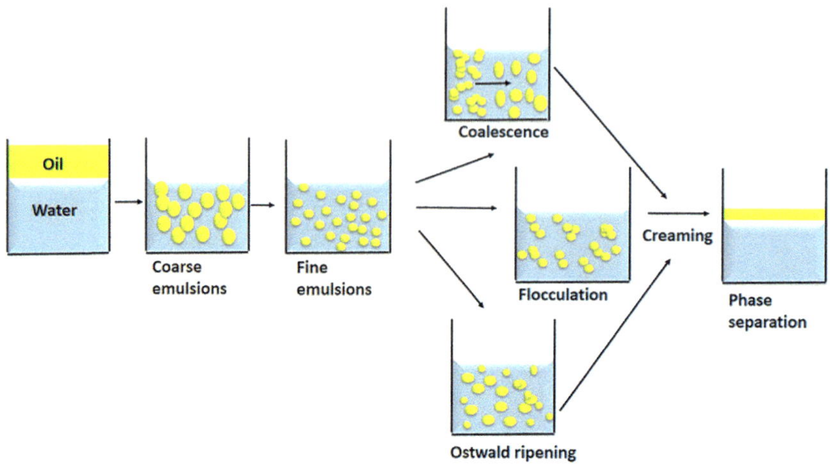

Figure 7.5 Nanoemulsion formation and the mechanisms leading to destabilization [76].

collagen nanoemulsion droplets can help speed up and improve wound healing. Because of the technological benefits that they provide to producers, the synthesis of collagen nanoemulsions has increased dramatically. This increase corresponds to the growing applications of collagen nanoemulsions, particularly in cosmetics and medical applications [75]. Fig. 7.5 illustrates various mechanisms of nanoemulsion formation.

5. Applications

5.1 Bone grafting

The matrix of bones contains a substantial amount of collagen, which is essential for the formation of bones. The osteoblasts play a crucial role in synthesizing the type I collagen protein, which is necessary for the formation of bones. The extracellular matrix (ECM) comprises collagen fibers ranging in size from 50 to 500 nm and are produced by osteoblasts. Subsequently, hydroxyapatite crystals are deposited onto these collagen fibers, causing the bone to harden and mature [75]. This process is helpful for restoration in severe bone damage, such as complicated fractures. A collagen scaffold can be placed on the injured tissue area to provide a stable foundation for the growth of apatite crystals, accelerating and enhancing the process of new bone formation. Therefore, the collagen scaffold must resemble natural collagen fibers to facilitate successful bone grafting and promote optimal bone regrowth. Recognizing the difficulty of bone healing, particularly in cases of nonsterile wound bone loss, it is difficult and time-consuming to manage injuries to the bone-related tissues.

Furthermore, such circumstances increase the risk and susceptibility to illnesses. Cardoso et al. supported using nanocollagen biomaterials (AgNPcol), composed of silver nanoparticles stabilized with type I collagen, as an effective method for accelerating bone reconstruction. This was recognized as a viable answer to infection problems caused by the non-sterility of bone lesions.

In addition, collagen silver nanoparticles demonstrated antimicrobial efficacy against various bacteria, proving their ability to accelerate wound healing. Furthermore, the generated cells did not exhibit any toxicity [77]. Sun et al. conducted another study where they infused AgNPs and bone morphogenic protein BMP2 into collagen scaffolds to enhance bone repair. Fortunately, the inclusion of bone morphogenic proteins increased the expression of crucial proteins such as osteopontin, osteonectin, and runt-related transcription factor two. Mesenchymal stromal cells derived from bone marrow exhibit faster differentiation in the presence of these stimuli [78]. These results demonstrated that nano-collagen holds therapeutic promise for bone grafting and healing. Most dental patients often grapple with insufficient alveolar ridge formation after tooth extraction, which can be attributed to poor oral hygiene or a lack of awareness. To address this problem, Wang et al. proposed the employment of synthetic nanocollagen bone implants for the preservation of the alveolar ridge after tooth extraction. After the implantation of the nanocollagen bone, a CT scan was conducted to observe any changes in bone mineral density. The findings revealed that the nanocollagen bone implant had successfully fused with the natural alveolar ridge, significantly increasing bone mineral density [79,80]. Fig. 7.6 shows the application of bone grafting in collagen.

5.2 Articular cartilage

Articular cartilage, a specialized connective tissue covering the bone edges within synovial joints, is crucial in facilitating smooth joint movement by providing a low-friction surface. Any damage to this cartilage can result in significant discomfort during joint motion. Unfortunately, unlike many other bodily tissues, articular cartilage lacks the ability to regenerate new cells to repair damaged areas. This limitation is primarily attributed to the absence of a direct blood supply, making it challenging to address with

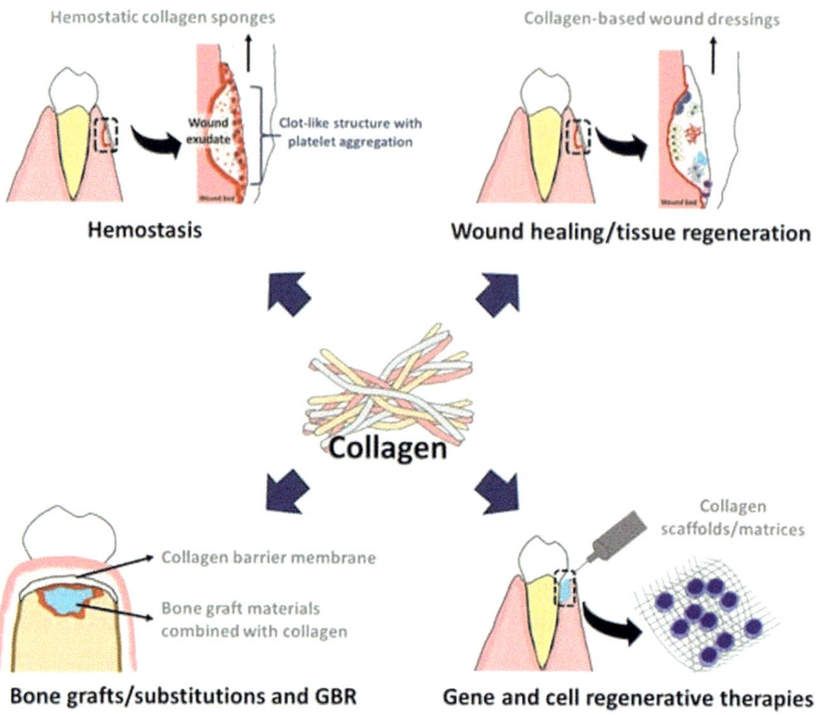

Figure 7.6 The application of bone grafting in collagen [81].

medications designed for targeted therapeutic conditions. The current treatment options for articular cartilage damage involve surgical interventions like chondrocyte implantation and osteochondral transplant. However, these procedures have a high cost and additional patient risk factors. Recognizing these challenges, ongoing research efforts focus on advancing cartilage tissue engineering [10]. 3D collagen scaffolds are created using 3D bioprinting and then changed in vitro to make them acceptable for transplantation in cartilage tissue engineering. Using three-dimensional bioprinting techniques in conjunction with nano-collagen scaffolds dramatically eliminates the requirement for donor cartilage transplants and less effective surgical treatments. For example, a collagen-hydroxyapatite hydrogel nanocomposite was successfully used in a study, providing encouraging results. In addition to being suitable for facilitating fluid transfer, hydrogel composite was also discovered to be stable up to a temperature of 90°C [82]. Jiang et al. presented an alternative strategy for promoting chondrocyte differentiation in articular cartilage to start

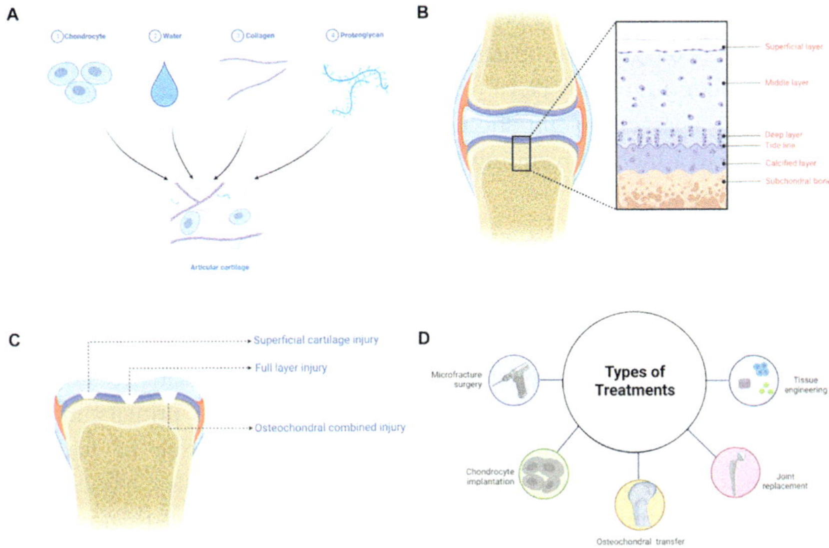

Figure 7.7 The application of collagen treatment in articular cartilage [84].

restoration mechanisms. The usage of nano-hydroxyapatite collagen scaffolds allowed for the suppression of chondrocyte dedifferentiation [83]. Fig. 7.7, the application of collagen treatment in articular cartilage.

5.3 Nerve tissue

Researchers actively explore treatments for damaged nerve tissues due to the nervous system's crucial role in overseeing and coordinating the body's operations. The lack of cell division in terminally differentiated neurons underscores the urgency of addressing nerve tissue injuries. While nerve tissue autografts have been performed in some instances, challenges such as a shortage of donor locations or abnormalities have made this approach more difficult. As a result, there is a growing interest in seeking viable alternative treatments or materials for nerve damage. Extensive research has investigated the effectiveness of collagen as a scaffold for promoting cell adherence and rapid growth in both standard and nanoscale collagen research [85]. Collagen, employed to create neural guiding conduits, facilitates the regrowth of neurons across small gaps of 2−3 cm in peripheral nerve tissue. Furthermore, collagen hydrogels have successfully treated lesions in the central nervous system, as evidenced by Zhang et al. [86].

In addressing nerve tissue degeneration, researchers can actively implant collagen nanospheres to transport therapeutic drugs and other stem cells for structural support [87]. Zhang et al. actively demonstrated tricalcium phosphate, collagen nanoparticles, nerve growth factors, and specific collagen fibers in treating facial nerve regeneration and repair. The observed growth of a larger myelin sheath and increased muscle action potential make this area highly promising for future research and investigations into nerve regeneration [88].

5.4 Skin wound healing

The text explores the intricacies of wound healing, delineating the four distinct phases involved: hemostasis, inflammation, growth, and remodeling as shown in Fig. 7.8. Any disruption in these sequential processes can significantly protract the overall healing timeline [89]. A primary impediment to successful wound healing is the pervasive issue of pathogen infection, which not only triggers inflammation but also hampers the natural healing trajectory [90]. Schimek et al. devised full-thickness skin equivalents (ftSEs) to facilitate advanced cell culture techniques. These innovations provide a conducive environment for studying wound healing processes at a cellular level, particularly within a 96-well cell culture system [91].

Collagen emerges as a pivotal player in wound healing, functioning as a slow-biodegrading component of the extracellular matrix (ECM). Its role as a dermal substitute becomes apparent, especially when infused with nanoparticles [90]. Noteworthy applications include using collagen granules infused with gold nanoparticles (AuNPs) in therapies. Studies, such as one focusing on diabetic foot ulcers, indicate that employing collagen in wound

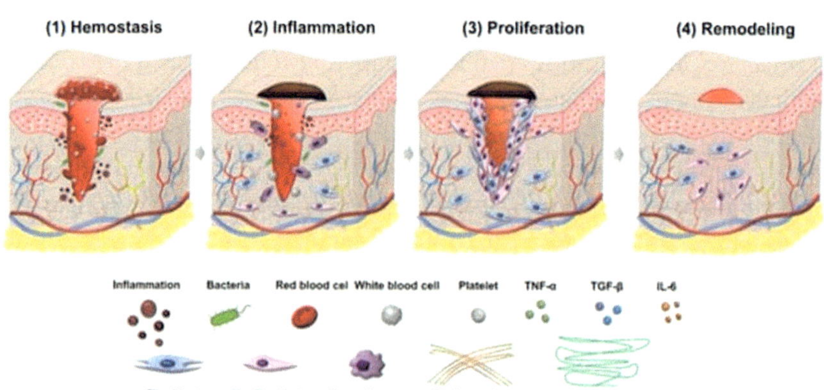

Figure 7.8 Illustrates the process of wound healing [94].

treatment results in expedited healing compared with traditional saline dressing. The integration of gold nanoparticles (AuNPs) into collagen scaffolds, as demonstrated by Akturk et al. showcases a novel approach [92]. This combination enhances tensile strength and bolsters stability against enzymatic degradation. AuNPs, with their unique properties, offer advantages such as promoting wound healing without triggering rejection and reducing inflammation in the surrounding wound area.

Furthermore, the text delves into the recent attention garnered by silver nanoparticles (AgNPs) as potent antibacterial agents. Their demonstrated efficacy in treating burns and infections stems from their interference with bacterial quorum sensing systems. Notably, the text suggests a lower likelihood of bacterial resistance to silver nanoparticles, adding to their appeal in wound healing applications. Silver nanoparticles are applied to collagen-based dermal scaffolds to serve as antimicrobial dressings without posing harmful risks. Nanosilver exhibits antimicrobial effects on Gram-positive and Gram-negative bacteria, damaging their intracellular structures. The negatively charged surfaces of bacteria interact with the positively charged silver nanoparticles, leading to the rupture of the inner membrane. In wound healing, silver nanoparticles (AgNPs) are incorporated with collagen nanofibers during electrospinning. In vitro data suggest that both gold nanoparticles (AuNPs) and silver nanoparticles (AgNPs) can provide the antibacterial conditions necessary for promoting wound healing. Compared with collagen nanofiber collagen, the collagen composite nanofiber mat's rate of wound healing was noticeably higher [93]. The process of wound healing is shown in Fig. 7.8.

6. Conclusions

Collagen-based biomaterials have a low immunogenicity and excellent biocompatibility; they are essential in tissue engineering and regenerative medicine. Since collagen can be isolated from a variety of tissue sources and mixed with other molecules, it is still the protein of choice for the creation of biomaterials. Collagen is used in laboratory settings as a decellularized extracellular matrix (ECM) for basic research and as a substitute material for tissue in medical applications. The goal of current research is to improve the mechanical strength, biodegradability, and transport properties of collagen-based biomaterials to optimize them for medical applications. Notable advancements have been made in the use of collagen type I for bone tissue creation. Collagen with maximum natural structure and minimal immunogenicity or antigenicity can now be prepared thanks to advancements in the exploration of various collagen sources and the optimization of extraction and purification techniques. Collagen alterations have been a major area of progress in bone tissue engineering, resulting in improved mechanical characteristics and biological resistance. For a variety of uses in bone grafting, collagens are frequently altered or mixed with other materials to form a variety of bone substitute materials, such as hydrogels, collagen sponges, nanofibers/microfibers, and nanoparticles/microspheres.

Acknowledgments

This article was financially supported by Universiti Sains Malaysia, (Malaysia) under short term grant; 304/PKIMIA/6315580.

References

[1] Parenteau-Bareil R, Gauvin R, Berthod F. Collagen-based biomaterials for tissue engineering applications. Materials March 16, 2010;3(3):1863–87.
[2] Recker RR, Barger-Lux J. Embryology, anatomy, and microstructure of bone. Disorders of bone and mineral metabolism. New York: Raven; 1992. p. 219.
[3] Kalfas IH. Principles of bone healing. Neurosurg Focus April 1, 2001;10(4):1–4.
[4] Swetha M, Sahithi K, Moorthi A, Srinivasan N, Ramasamy K, Selvamurugan N. Biocomposites containing natural polymers and hydroxyapatite for bone tissue engineering. Int J Biol Macromol July 1, 2010;47(1):1–4.
[5] Hayashi M, Muramatsu H, Sato M, Tomizuka Y, Inoue M, Yoshimoto S. Surgical treatment of facial fracture by using unsintered hydroxyapatite particles/poly L-lactide composite device (OSTEOTRANS MX): a clinical study on 17 cases. J Cranio-Maxillofacial Surg December 1, 2013;41(8):783–8.
[6] Fujii T, Tanaka T, Ohkawa K. Biomineralization of calcium phosphate on human hair protein film and formation of a novel hydroxyapatite–protein composite material. J Biomed Mater Res Part B November 2009;91(2):528–36.
[7] Kutikov AB, Song J. An amphiphilic degradable polymer/hydroxyapatite composite with enhanced handling characteristics promotes osteogenic gene expression in bone marrow stromal cells. Acta Biomater September 1, 2013;9(9):8354–64.
[8] Wang CY, Zhao Y, Yang M, Wang SF. Nano-collagen artificial bone for alveolar ridge preservation in the Kazakh from Xinjiang Tacheng Region. Chinese J Tissue Eng Res March 19, 2015;19(12):1864.
[9] Kim H, Che L, Ha Y, Ryu W. Mechanically-reinforced electrospun composite silk fibroin nanofibers containing hydroxyapatite nanoparticles. Mater Sci Eng C July 1, 2014;40:324–35.
[10] Kim Y, Kim G. Collagen/alginate scaffolds comprising core (PCL)–shell (collagen/alginate) struts for hard tissue regeneration: fabrication, characterisation, and cellular activities. J Mater Chem B 2013;1(25):3185–94.
[11] El-Fiqi A, Lee JH, Lee EJ, Kim HW. Collagen hydrogels incorporated with surface-aminated mesoporous nanobioactive glass: improvement of physicochemical stability and mechanical properties is effective for hard tissue engineering. Acta Biomater December 1, 2013;9(12):9508–21.

[12] Avila Rodríguez MI, Rodríguez Barroso LG, Sánchez ML. Collagen: a review on its sources and potential cosmetic applications. J Cosmet Dermatol February 2018;17(1):20–6.
[13] Persikov AV, Ramshaw JA, Kirkpatrick A, Brodsky B. Electrostatic interactions involving lysine make major contributions to collagen triple-helix stability. Biochemistry February 8, 2005;44(5):1414–22.
[14] Fallas JA, Gauba V, Hartgerink JD. Solution structure of an ABC collagen heterotrimer reveals a single-register helix stabilized by electrostatic interactions. J Biol Chem September 25, 2009;284(39):26851–9.
[15] Boudko SP, Engel J, Bächinger HP. The crucial role of trimerization domains in collagen folding. Int J Biochem Cell Biol January 1, 2012;44(1):21–32.
[16] Boudko SP, Bächinger HP. Structural insight for chain selection and stagger control in collagen. Sci Rep November 29, 2016;6(1):37831.
[17] León-López A, Morales-Peñaloza A, Martínez-Juárez VM, Vargas-Torres A, Zeugolis DI, Aguirre-Álvarez G. Hydrolyzed collagen—sources and applications. Molecules November 7, 2019;24(22):4031.
[18] Abraham GA, Murray J, Billiar K, Sullivan SJ. Evaluation of the porcine intestinal collagen layer as a biomaterial. J Biomed Mater Res September 5, 2000;51(3):442–52.
[19] Silvipriya KS, Kumar KK, Bhat AR, Kumar BD, John A. Collagen: animal sources and biomedical application. J Appl Pharmaceut Sci March 28, 2015;5(3):123–7.
[20] Chevallay B, Herbage D. Collagen-based biomaterials as 3D scaffold for cell cultures: applications for tissue engineering and gene therapy. Med Biol Eng Comput March 2000;38:211–8.
[21] Lynn AK, Yannas IV, Bonfield W. Antigenicity and immunogenicity of collagen. J Biomed Mater Res Part B November 15, 2004;71(2):343–54.
[22] Andonegi M, Peñalba M, de la Caba K, Guerrero P. ZnO nanoparticleincorporated native collagen films with electro-conductive properties. Mater Sci Eng C 2020;108:110394.
[23] Prasert A, Sontikaew S, Sriprapai D, Chuangchote S. Polypropylene/ZnO nanocomposites: mechanical properties, photocatalytic dye degradation, and antibacterial property. Materials February 19, 2020;13(4):914.
[24] Agban Y, Lian J, Prabakar S, Seyfoddin A, Rupenthal ID. Nanoparticle cross-linked collagen shields for sustained delivery of pilocarpine hydrochloride. Int J Pharm March 30, 2016;501(1–2):96–101.
[25] Li H, Qu R, Li C, Guo W, Han X, He F, Ma Y, Xing B. Selective removal of polycyclic aromatic hydrocarbons (PAHs) from soil washing effluents using biochars produced at different pyrolytic temperatures. Bioresour Technol July 1, 2014;163:193–8.
[26] Pietrucha K, Safandowska M. Dialdehyde cellulose-crosslinked collagen and its physicochemical properties. Process Biochem December 1, 2015;50(12):2105–11.
[27] Radu FA, Bause M, Knabner P, Lee GW, Friess WC. Modeling of drug release from collagen matrices. J Pharmaceut Sci April 1, 2002;91(4):964–72.
[28] Murata D, Fujimoto R, Nakayama K. Osteochondral regeneration using adipose tissue-derived mesenchymal stem cells. Int J Mol Sci May 19, 2020;21(10):3589.
[29] Katsube K, Ochi M, Uchio Y, Maniwa S, Matsusaki M, Tobita M, Iwasa J. Repair of articular cartilage defects with cultured chondrocytes in atelocollagen gel: comparison with cultured chondrocytes in suspension. Arch Orthop Trauma Surg February 2000;120:121–7.
[30] Moreno-Manzano V, Zaytseva-Zotova D, López-Mocholí E, Briz-Redón Á, Løkensgard Strand B, Serrano-Aroca Á. Injectable gel form of a decellularized bladder induces adipose-derived stem cell differentiation into smooth muscle cells in vitro. Int J Mol Sci November 15, 2020;21(22):8608.

[31] Kaizawa Y, Leyden J, Behn AW, Tulu US, Franklin A, Wang Z, Abrams G, Chang J, Fox PM. Human tendon–derived collagen hydrogel significantly improves biomechanical properties of the tendon-bone interface in a chronic rotator cuff injury model. J Hand Surg October 1, 2019;44(10):899.

[32] Fan L, Ren Y, Emmert S, Vučković I, Stojanovic S, Najman S, Schnettler R, Barbeck M, Schenke-Layland K, Xiong X. The use of collagen-based materials in bone tissue engineering. Int J Mol Sci February 13, 2023;24(4):3744.

[33] Li Y, Liu Y, Li R, Bai H, Zhu Z, Zhu L, Zhu C, Che Z, Liu H, Wang J, Huang L. Collagen-based biomaterials for bone tissue engineering. Mater Des November 15, 2021;210:110049.

[34] Kihara T, Umezu C, Sawada K, Furutani Y. Osteogenic cells form mineralized particles, a few μm in size, in a 3D collagen gel culture. PeerJ October 23, 2019;7:e7889.

[35] Yoneno K, Ohno S, Tanimoto K, Honda K, Tanaka N, Doi T, Kawata T, Tanaka E, Kapila S, Tanne K. Multidifferentiation potential of mesenchymal stem cells in three-dimensional collagen gel cultures. J Biomed Mater Res Part A December 1, 2005;75(3):733–41.

[36] Paduano F, Marrelli M, Alom N, Amer M, White LJ, Shakesheff KM, Tatullo M. Decellularized bone extracellular matrix and human dental pulp stem cells as a construct for bone regeneration. J Biomater Sci Polym Ed May 24, 2017;28(8):730–48.

[37] Murphy CM, Haugh MG, O'brien FJ. The effect of mean pore size on cell attachment, proliferation and migration in collagen–glycosaminoglycan scaffolds for bone tissue engineering. Biomaterials January 1, 2010;31(3):461–6.

[38] Cortes DH, Jacobs NT, DeLucca JF, Elliott DM. Elastic, permeability and swelling properties of human intervertebral disc tissues: a benchmark for tissue engineering. J Biomech June 27, 2014;47(9):2088–94.

[39] O'brien FJ. Biomaterials and scaffolds for tissue engineering. Mater Today March 1, 2011;14(3):88–95.

[40] Chan BP, Leong KW. Scaffolding in tissue engineering: general approaches and tissue-specific considerations. Eur Spine J December 2008;17:467–79.

[41] Patino MG, Neiders ME, Andreana S, Noble B, Cohen RE. Collagen as an implantable material in medicine and dentistry. J Oral Implantol October 1, 2002;28(5):220–5.

[42] Panduranga Rao K. Recent developments of collagen-based materials for medical applications and drug delivery systems. J Biomater Sci Polym Ed January 1, 1996;7(7):623–45.

[43] Minabe M, Uematsu A, Nishijima K, Tomomatsu E, Tamura T, Hori T, Umemoto T, Hino T. Application of a local drug delivery system to periodontal therapy: I. Development of collagen preparations with immobilized tetracycline. J Periodontol February 1989;60(2):113–7.

[44] Murata M, Huang BZ, Shibata T, Imai S, Nagal N, Arisue M. Bone augmentation by recombinant human BMP-2 and collagen on adult rat parietal bone. Int J Oral Maxillofac Surg June 1, 1999;28(3):232–7.

[45] Nakagawa T, Tagawa T. Ultrastructural study of direct bone formation induced by BMPs-collagen complex implanted into an ectopic site. Oral Dis May 2000;6(3):172–9.

[46] Park JC, Hwang YS, Lee JE, Park KD, Matsumura K, Hyon SH, Suh H. Type I atelocollagen grafting onto ozone-treated polyurethane films: cell attachment, proliferation, and collagen synthesis. J Biomed Mater Res December 15, 2000;52(4):669–77.

[47] Lee VH. New directions in the optimization of ocular drug delivery. J Ocul Pharmacol Therapeut 1990;6(2):157–64.

[48] Leaders FE, Hecht G, VanHoose M, Kellog M. New polymers in drug delivery. Ann Ophthalmol May 1, 1973;5(5):513–6.
[49] Podos SM, Becker B, Asseff C, Hartstein J. Pilocarpine therapy with soft contact lenses. Am J Ophthalmol March 1, 1972;73(3):336–41.
[50] Nair R, Sevukarajan M, Mohammed T, Badivaddin CK, Kumar A. Collagen based drug delivery systems: a review. J Innov Trends Pharm Sci. 2010;1:288–304.
[51] Uchio Y, Ochi M, Matsusaki M, Kurioka H, Katsube K. Human chondrocyte proliferation and matrix synthesis cultured in Atelocollagen gel. J Biomed Mater Res 2000;50(2):138–43.
[52] Khan MA, Ahmad A, Umar K, Nabi SA. Synthesis, characterization, and biological applications of nanocomposites for the removal of heavy metals and dyes. Ind Eng Chem Res January 14, 2015;54(1):76–82.
[53] Bender AR, Von Briesen H, Kreuter J, Duncan IB, Rübsamen-Waigmann H. Efficiency of nanoparticles as a carrier system for antiviral agents in human immunodeficiency virus-infected human monocytes/macrophages in vitro. Antimicrob Agents Chemother June 1996;40(6):1467–71.
[54] Ehrlich H, Deutzmann R, Brunner E, Cappellini E, Koon H, Solazzo C, Yang Y, Ashford D, Thomas-Oates J, Lubeck M, Baessmann C. Mineralization of the metre-long biosilica structures of glass sponges is templated on hydroxylated collagen. Nat Chem December 2010;2(12):1084–8.
[55] Orgel JP, Sella I, Madhurapantula RS, Antipova O, Mandelberg Y, Kashman Y, Benayahu D, Benayahu Y. Molecular and ultrastructural studies of a fibrillar collagen from octocoral (Cnidaria). J Exp Biol September 15, 2017;220(18):3327–35.
[56] Tziveleka LA, Ioannou E, Tsiourvas D, Berillis P, Foufa E, Roussis V. Collagen from the marine sponges Axinella cannabina and Suberites carnosus: isolation and morphological, biochemical, and biophysical characterization. Mar Drugs May 29, 2017;15(6):152.
[57] Rahman MA. An overview of the medical applications of marine skeletal matrix proteins. Mar Drugs September 12, 2016;14(9):167.
[58] Afridi SK, Umar K, Parveen T, Razali MR. Nanocomposites in the degradation of organic pollutants. In: Nanocomposites-advanced materials for energy and environmental aspects. Woodhead Publishing; January 1, 2023. p. 321–47.
[59] Olsen D, Yang C, Bodo M, Chang R, Leigh S, Baez J, Carmichael D, Perälä M, Hämäläinen ER, Jarvinen M, Polarek J. Recombinant collagen and gelatin for drug delivery. Adv Drug Deliv Rev November 28, 2003;55(12):1547–67.
[60] Onuma-Ukegawa M, Bhatt K, Hirai T, Kaburagi H, Sotome S, Wakabayashi Y, Ichinose S, Shinomiya K, Okawa A, Enomoto M. Bone marrow stromal cells combined with a honeycomb collagen sponge facilitate neurite elongation in vitro and neural restoration in the hemisected rat spinal cord. Cell Transplant July 2015;24(7):1283–97.
[61] Xue J, Wu T, Dai Y, Xia Y. Electrospinning and electrospun nanofibers: methods, materials, and applications. Chem Rev March 27, 2019;119(8):5298–415.
[62] Mhetar SK, Ashok Nerle A, Patil RL, Pawar RA, Patil MM, Shinde HT. Cost effective ball milling machine for producing nanopowder. Int Res J Eng Technol 2017;4:330–4.
[63] Makkithaya KN, Nadumane S, Zhuo GY, Chakrabarty S, Mazumder N. Nanoparticle based collagen biomaterials for wound healing.
[64] Haseen U, Umar K, Ahmad H, Parveen T, Mohamad Ibrahim MN. Graphene and its composites: applications in environmental remediation. Modern age waste water problems: Solutions using applied nanotechnology. 2020. p. 85–91.

[65] Lei L, Gamboa AR, Kuznetsova C, Littlecreek S, Wang J, Zou Q, Zahn JD, Singer JP. Self-limiting electrospray deposition on polymer templates. Sci Rep October 14, 2020;10(1):17290.
[66] Sundaramurthi D, Krishnan UM, Sethuraman S. Electrospun nanofibers as scaffolds for skin tissue engineering. Polym Rev April 3, 2014;54(2):348–76.
[67] Nagarajan U, Kawakami K, Zhang S, Chandrasekaran B, Nair BU. Fabrication of solid collagen nanoparticles using electrospray deposition. Chem Pharm Bull May 1, 2014;62(5):422–8.
[68] Nguyen TD, Lee JS. Electrospinning-based carbon nanofibers for energy and sensor applications. Appl Sci June 14, 2022;12(12):6048.
[69] Kumar M, Xiong X, Wan Z, Sun Y, Tsang DC, Gupta J, Gao B, Cao X, Tang J, Ok YS. Ball milling as a mechanochemical technology for fabrication of novel biochar nanomaterials. Bioresour Technol September 1, 2020;312:123613.
[70] Umar K. Water contamination by organic-pollutants: TiO 2 photocatalysis. Modern age environmental problems and their remediation. 2018. p. 95–109.
[71] Yukuyama MN, Ghisleni DD, Pinto TD, Bou-Chacra NA. Nanoemulsion: process selection and application in cosmetics—a review. Int J Cosmet Sci February 2016;38(1):13–24.
[72] El-Eskandarany MS, Al-Hazza A, Al-Hajji LA, Ali N, Al-Duweesh AA, Banyan M, Al-Ajmi F. Mechanical milling: a superior nanotechnological tool for fabrication of nanocrystalline and nanocomposite materials. Nanomaterials September 24, 2021;11(10):2484.
[73] Singh AN, Yethiraj A. Liquid–liquid phase separation as the second step of complex coacervation. J Phys Chem B March 18, 2021;125(12):3023–31.
[74] Musazzi UM, Franzè S, Minghetti P, Casiraghi A. Emulsion versus nanoemulsion: how much is the formulative shift critical for a cosmetic product? Drug Deliv Transl Res April 2018;8:414–21.
[75] Katsimbri P. The biology of normal bone remodelling. Eur J Cancer Care November 2017;26(6):e12740.
[76] Aswathanarayan JB, Vittal RR. Nanoemulsions and their potential applications in food industry. Front Sustain Food Syst November 13, 2019;3:95.
[77] Sun CY, Che YJ, Lu SJ. Preparation and application of collagen scaffold-encapsulated silver nanoparticles and bone morphogenetic protein 2 for enhancing the repair of infected bone. Biotechnol Lett February 2015;37:467–73.
[78] Mohamadi F, Ebrahimi-Barough S, Reza Nourani M, Ali Derakhshan M, Goodarzi V, Sadegh Nazockdast M, Farokhi M, Tajerian R, Faridi Majidi R, Ai J. Electrospun nerve guide scaffold of poly (ε-caprolactone)/collagen/nanobioglass: an in vitro study in peripheral nerve tissue engineering. J Biomed Mater Res July 2017;105(7):1960–72.
[79] Orive G, Anitua E, Pedraz JL, Emerich DF. Biomaterials for promoting brain protection, repair and regeneration. Nat Rev Neurosci September 2009;10(9):682–92.
[80] Abdullah A, Abdullah AZ, Ahmed M, Khan J, Shahadat M, Umar K, Alim MA. A review on recent developments and progress in sustainable acrolein production through catalytic dehydration of bio-renewable glycerol. J Clean Prod March 20, 2022;341:130876.
[81] Binlateh T, Thammanichanon P, Rittipakorn P, Thinsathid N, Jitprasertwong P. Collagen-based biomaterials in periodontal regeneration: current applications and future perspectives of plant-based collagen. Biomimetics March 24, 2022;7(2):34.
[82] Jiang X, Zhong Y, Zheng L, Zhao J. Nano-hydroxyapatite/collagen film as a favorable substrate to maintain the phenotype and promote the growth of chondrocytes cultured in vitro. Int J Mol Med December 2020;46(6):2282.
[83] Wallace HA, Basehore BM, Zito PM. Wound healing phases. StatPearls [Internet]. Treasure Island (FL): StatPearls Publishing; 2022.

[84] Wang R, Wang Y, Yang H, Zhao C, Pan J. Research progress of self-assembling peptide hydrogels in repairing cartilage defects. Front Mat October 10, 2022;9:1022386.
[85] Ucar B, Humpel C. Collagen for brain repair: therapeutic perspectives. Neural Regener Res April 2018;13(4):595.
[86] Zhang Z, Li X, Li Z, Bai Y, Liao G, Pan J, Zhang C. Collagen/nano-sized β-tricalcium phosphate conduits combined with collagen filaments and nerve growth factor promote facial nerve regeneration in miniature swine: an in vivo study. Oral Surg Oral Med Oral Pathol Oral Radiol November 1, 2019;128(5):472−8.
[87] Armiento AR, Stoddart MJ, Alini M, Eglin D. Biomaterials for articular cartilage tissue engineering: learning from biology. Acta Biomater January 1, 2018;65:1−20.
[88] Kaviani A, Zebarjad SM, Javadpour S, Ayatollahi M, Bazargan-Lari R. Fabrication and characterization of low-cost freeze-gelated chitosan/collagen/hydroxyapatite hydrogel nanocomposite scaffold. Int J Polym Anal Char April 3, 2019;24(3):191−203.
[89] Lo S, Fauzi MB. Current update of collagen nanomaterials—fabrication, characterisation and its applications: a review. Pharmaceutics February 28, 2021;13(3):316.
[90] Schimek K, Hsu HH, Boehme M, Kornet JJ, Marx U, Lauster R, Pörtner R, Lindner G. Bioengineering of a full-thickness skin equivalent in a 96-well insert format for substance permeation studies and organ-on-a-chip applications. Bioengineering June 7, 2018;5(2):43.
[91] Munish T, Ramneesh G, Sanjeev S, Jasdeep S, Jaspal S, Nikhil G. Comparative study of collagen based dressing and standard dressing in diabetic foot ulcer. J Evol Med Dent Sci March 12, 2015;4(21):3614−22.
[92] Akturk O, Kismet K, Yasti AC, Kuru S, Duymus ME, Kaya F, Caydere M, Hucumenoglu S, Keskin D. Collagen/gold nanoparticle nanocomposites: a potential skin wound healing biomaterial. J Biomater Appl August 2016;31(2):283−301.
[93] You C, Li Q, Wang X, Wu P, Ho JK, Jin R, Zhang L, Shao H, Han C. Silver nanoparticle loaded collagen/chitosan scaffolds promote wound healing via regulating fibroblast migration and macrophage activation. Sci Rep September 5, 2017;7(1):10489.
[94] Trinh XT, Long NV, Van Anh LT, Nga PT, Giang NN, Chien PN, Nam SY, Heo CY. A comprehensive review of natural compounds for wound healing: targeting bioactivity perspective. Int J Mol Sci August 24, 2022;23(17):9573.

CHAPTER 8

Keratin-based nanocomposites for tissue engineering

Mohammad Mushaf[1], Khalid Umar[2], Tabassum Parveen[3], Mohd R. Razali[2] and Khairi Suhud[4]

[1]Institute of Eminence Teaching Fellow, Talent Development Center, Indian Institute of Science, Challakere, Karnataka, India; [2]School of Chemical Sciences, Universiti Sains Malaysia, Penang, Malaysia; [3]Department of Botany, Aligarh Muslim University, Aligarh, Uttar Pradesh, India; [4]Department of Chemistry, Faculty of Mathematics and Natural Sciences, Universitas Syiah Kuala, Banda Aceh, Indonesia

1. Introduction

Tissue engineering (TE) aims to improve or repair diseased or damaged tissues by assembling the right cells and growth signaling molecules onto biomaterial scaffolds [1]. The process of further modifying such biomaterials to improve or impart a biological function and stimulation while still allowing them to function biologically is known as biofunctionalization [2]. In bone prostheses, for example, titanium implants have good mechanical stability and biocompatibility but little osteogenic action to promote better integration with bone [3,4]. Thus, immobilizing natural and synthetic biopolymers to biofunctionalize implant surfaces has been a major field of research. Since the 16th century, keratin—a fibrous protein present in hair, nails, wool, feathers, horns, and hooves—has been used as a biomaterial to promote hemostasis and wound healing [5]. Its potential as a covering for vascular grafts was also shown by early tissue engineering research conducted in the 1980s [6].

The word "keratin" originally referred to a comprehensive class of insoluble proteins that form intermediate filaments (IFs), which are the main building blocks of cytoplasmic epithelium and epidermal appendages, including hair, wool, horns, hooves, and nails. Based on their structure, function, and regulation, mammalian keratins have been divided into two classes by subsequent research endeavors. "Hard" keratins contribute to the muscular system of epidermal appendages by generating arrays of IFs that are well-organized and embedded in a matrix of cystine-rich proteins. On

Protein-Based Nanocomposites for Tissue Engineering
ISBN 978-0-323-99357-9
https://doi.org/10.1016/B978-0-323-99357-9.00014-4

the contrary, "soft" keratins provide mechanical robustness to epithelial cells by forming loosely packed bundles of cytoplasmic IFs.

Schweizer et al. categorized the 54 functional keratin genes as either epithelium or hair keratins in 2006, and they also created a new consensual terminology for hard and soft keratin products [7]. Epithelial and hair keratins have chains of differing molecular weights and compositions (types I and II), each containing nonhelical end-terminal domains and a highly conserved central alpha-helical domain. These chains interact to form heterodimers, which further polymerize into 10-nm intermediate filaments. Distinct differences in amino acid sequences, particularly in the nonhelical domains, contribute to measurable variations in filamentous structures. Hair keratins, characterized by a higher cysteine content, form tougher and more durable structures through intermolecular disulfide bond formation [8–10].

Despite the similar secondary structures of hard and soft keratins, there have been endeavors to decrease reliance on petroleum-based polymers. The shift toward using renewable, environmentally friendly, biodegradable, and biocompatible polymers like cellulose, chitin, starch, pectin, alginate, xanthan, soy protein, and guar gum is gaining prominence for environmental protection and sustainable development [11–14]. The research focus has intensified on exploring biopolymers derived from waste resources or industrial byproducts, with keratin emerging as a promising natural protein extracted from sources such as chicken feathers or low-quality raw wool [15,16]. Therefore, keratin, the principal component of feathers, wools, nails, hair, and horns, is a nonfood protein characterized by its widespread availability and exceptional biocompatible and biodegradable qualities [17]. Among all natural biodegradable polymers, keratin-based materials have significantly advanced modern biomaterials due to its outstanding biodegradability, biocompatibility, and mechanical strength. These materials can be manufactured in various forms, such as hydrogels, films, and sponges, making them adaptable to various biological uses [18].

2. History of keratin study and its current status

Li Shi-Zhen, a Chinese herbalist, pioneered keratin use in medical applications in the sixteenth century; this marked the initial recorded keratin use for such purposes [19]. The scientific community initially employed the term "keratin" in 1850 to describe the material isolated from the hard tissues of animals, such as their horns and hooves [20]. A patent from 1905 disclosed the use of lime solution to remove keratin from horns. During the 1920s, researchers shifted their focus from extraction to better understanding keratin's structure, function, and characteristics. The Council for Scientific and Industrial Research (CSIRO) in Australia achieved a significant breakthrough in the field by creating a comprehensive diagram of a hair strand [21].

Recent research conducted in the United Kingdom has shed light on the microstructural composition of keratin fibers, specifically identifying the inner cortex and outer cuticle The production of keratin-based films and textile fibers from horse hoof has resulted in patent awards for Dutch researchers. The foundational work on squamous cells between 1940 and 1970 laid the groundwork for the principles of biomaterials. Since the 1970s, substantial advancements have been made in isolating and characterizing keratins and their derivatives in various forms, consisting of films, fibers, foam, gels, and coatings [22–24].

In recent decades, keratin-based polymers have attracted considerable for a range of biological purposes, such as medication administration, tissue engineering, and wound repair. A study describing the function of keratin coatings on vascular graft surfaces to inhibit blood clotting was published in 1982 by researchers in Japan. Biocompatibility tests have also been performed on keratins. As a result, these investigations have laid a strong basis for subsequent studies and provided new perspectives on the many uses of keratin-based biomaterials in various domains [6,25].

3. Structure and characteristics of keratin

Most cytoskeletal and epidermal appendageal structures, such as hair, horns, feathers, wool, and nails, comprise keratin, a fibrous protein rich in cysteine and linked to intermediate filaments (IFs) [19]. The degree of sulfur in keratin determines its hardness or softness. Hard keratin with a higher percentage of sulfur crosslinks is responsible for the robust epidermal structure, which consists of intermediate filaments arranged in an orderly fashion and embedded in a crosslinked matrix [7,26]. Soft keratins with low sulfur content, generated by loosely packed bundles of cytoplasmic filaments, provide the epithelial tissues (epidermis) with elasticity [26]. Alpha- and beta-keratin structures are commonly discussed in the literature. Over the past 3 decades, extensive in vitro and in vivo research has been conducted to exploit these hard keratins to develop biomaterials. Feathers,

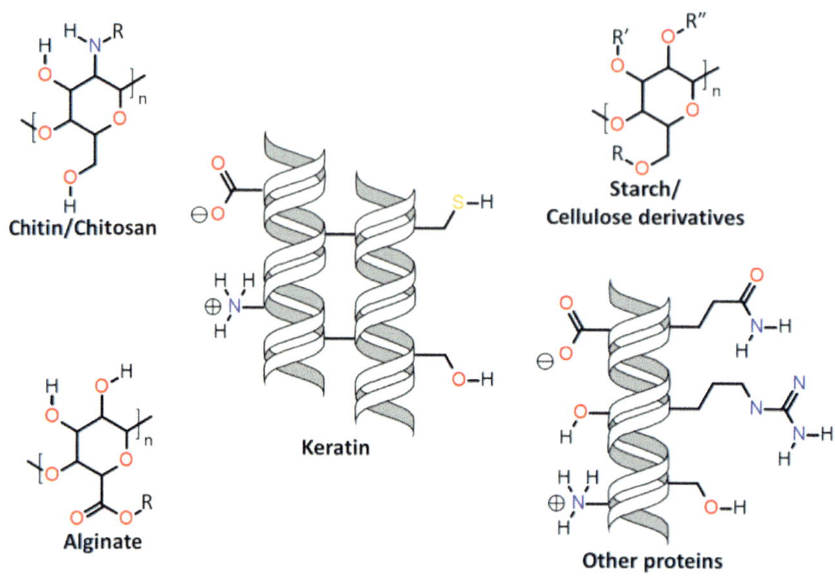

Figure 8.1 A diagrammatic representation of the keratin structure is shown [27].

beaks, reptile claws, feathers, and scales are the main sources of beta-keratin. On the contrary, wool, hair, hooves, nails, horns, and the stratum corneum—the outermost layer of skin—are the main sources of alpha-keratin [7,26]. A diagrammatic representation of the keratin structure is possible, as Fig. 8.1 illustrates [27].

The polypeptide chains form pleated beta-sheets in beta-keratin and alpha-helices in alpha-keratin. Alpha-keratin is a coiled-coil structure made up of two twisted polypeptide chains. Wool has garnered a lot of attention lately as a substitute for alpha-keratin. Alpha- and beta-keratin filament-matrix topologies are carefully and vividly demonstrated at the nanoscale. The alpha-keratin filament is larger than the beta-keratin filament, with a diameter of 3.4–5 nm [28–30].

Wool keratin consists of approximately 95% proteins, 0.5% minerals, and 0.1% lipids, and it boasts a distinct three-dimensional structure [31,32]. The keratin structure primarily comprises polypeptide chains of various amino acids, which form the backbone and are held together through inter- and intramolecular bonding. Keratin has ionic, hydrogen, and disulfide bonds that strengthen and stabilize its structure [33,34]. Protein-degrading enzymes like trypsin and pepsin, water, alkaline solutions, mild acids, and organic solvents are among the solvents in which these proteins are insoluble. Wool keratin contains significant amounts of glycine, proline, serine, and cysteine but only traces of lysine, methionine, and histidine. The physicochemical properties of wool keratin, such as its increased stability and lower solubility, distinguish it from other proteins. Additional ionic, hydrogen, and hydrophobic connections also affect wool keratin's stability and other aspects. The strongest ionic connection between carboxylic anions and ammonium cations is found at pH 4.9, also known as the isoelectric point. In very acidic or basic environments, these ionic interactions significantly weaken. The carboxylic group can be protonated to reduce these bonds at low pH levels, while the amine group can be deprotonated to minimize them at high pH levels [35]. Keratin's disulfide bonds are responsible for its remarkable stability, resistance to disintegration in a variety of solvents, and three-dimensional mesh structure. The main factor affecting the structure of wool is the disturbance of the intricate structure of keratin [35]. Fig. 8.2 shows how the keratinocytes, nails, and stratum corneum (SC) are organized in a complex way. This covers the arrangement of keratin filaments in a hierarchical fashion as well as the kind of lipids that make up these structures. Also shown is the chemical makeup of the lipids present in the SC, nails, and keratinocytes.

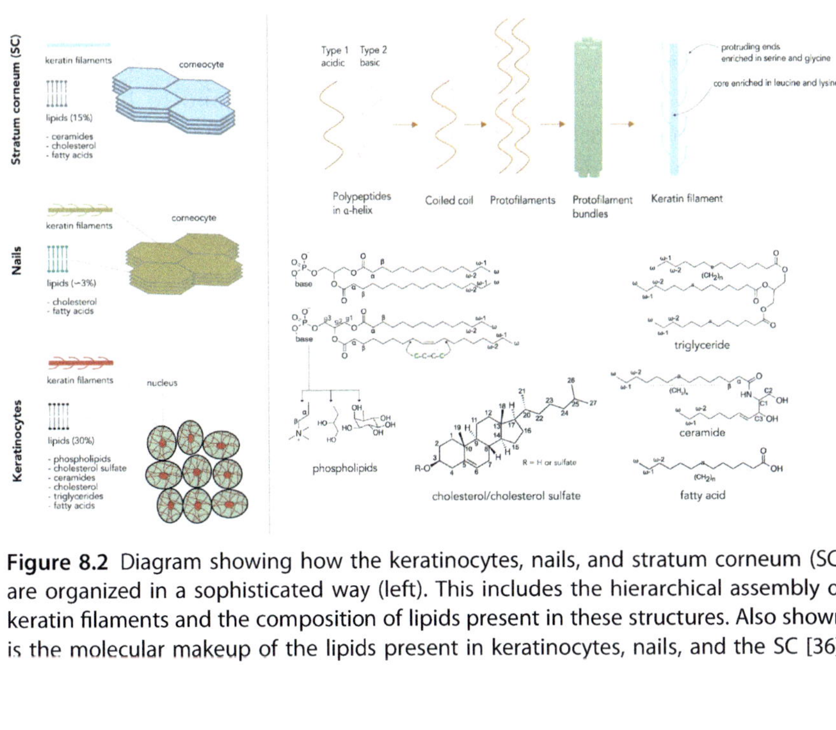

Figure 8.2 Diagram showing how the keratinocytes, nails, and stratum corneum (SC) are organized in a sophisticated way (left). This includes the hierarchical assembly of keratin filaments and the composition of lipids present in these structures. Also shown is the molecular makeup of the lipids present in keratinocytes, nails, and the SC [36].

4. Extraction techniques for keratin

Various methods are commonly employed to extract keratin from materials abundant in this protein. These methods encompass reduction [37], oxidation [38], alkali extraction [39], microwave irradiation [40], steam explosion [41], and the utilization of ionic liquids [42].

4.1 Extracting keratin using the reduction method

The thiol group-containing compounds can extract keratin from keratin-rich materials, weakening the disulfide bonds in stable keratin structures. Early studies utilized various concentrations of sodium thioglycolate and thioglycolic acid to reduce wool keratin, and it was observed that pH levels affected the amount of keratin reduction. Using thiols and a temperature range of 50–60°C, significant protein extraction was seen at pH 2 [43]. Keratin has often been denaturized using urea to increase its solubility in water. The hydrophobic bondings in the polypeptide chain structure diminish as the concentration of urea increases. As a surfactant, sodium dodecyl sulfate (SDS) improved the stability and extraction rate of the extracted keratin. SDS and other anionic surfactants are more efficient than neutral and cationic surfactants. By mixing MEC with urea and thiourea, Nakamura et al. adapted Yamauchi's keratin extraction process and produced a yield of more than 65%, higher than Yamauchi's 5%–12% yield. Because cysteine is environmentally friendly, it was used as the reducing agent instead of MEC. The finished product was found to have higher mechanical properties because of the controlled breakdown of disulfide bonds brought about by using cysteine [37,44].

4.2 Keratin extraction using the alkaline technique

Wool can become soluble in hot, alkaline solutions because the exposure breaks down the sulfur nucleus and cystine residues. This method cannot be utilized commercially because of the damage done to the polypeptide chain structure of keratin and the large number of alkali reagents needed. The amount of NaOH needed for keratin extraction can be reduced by using strong alkaline solutions. When 1% sodium sulfide was added to NaOH solution (0.065 N), Harris et al. observed that wool deteriorated more quickly than when NaOH solution was used alone [45]. Regrettably, the combination of NaOH and sodium sulfide resulted in wool with a high sulfur content. The keratin in wool and feathers contains 11%–17% and 7% of cysteine, respectively [39,46].

It is essential to preserve key amino acids, such as cystine, throughout the entire extraction process, as they are susceptible to breakdown in the presence of strong alkaline solutions [47]. Cystine degradation primarily produces oxalic and pyruvic acids. Nagai et al. evaluated the recovery yield of proteins after alkali treatment [48], noting a 50 percent loss of the initial material during the procedure. Subsequently, he subjected feathers to a 0.1 N NaOH solution for 15 min at 90°C, revealing a distinct amino acid composition in the final product compared with untreated feather samples. This method resulted in keratin with reduced serine, arginine, and cystine levels while exhibiting elevated lysine, methionine, and glutamic acid [48]. Jiangtao et al. have recently introduced a two-step alkali-reduction method for extracting keratin from hair samples [49]. The selected samples were initially treated for 5 h with a solution containing 0.1 mol/L of Na_2SO_3, SDS, and urea. The resulting keratin retained its alpha-helix and beta-sheet structure. However, harsh chemical conditions during the alkaline treatment process limit keratin's industrial application [48].

4.3 Keratin extraction using the oxidation method

Earland et al. conducted pioneering research on keratin extraction from wool and hair, employing HCl, ammonia, and 2% peracetic acid [50]. The findings revealed complete alpha-keratin solubility and beta-keratin insolubility in all experiments. Weston's experiments demonstrated that treating wool with 2% peracetic acid for 30 h led to the oxidation of disulfide links into sulfonate groups [51]. Using infrared research, subsequent validation by Strasheim and Buijs identified cystine monoxide, dioxide, and sulfonate groups. The conversion of disulfite to sulfonate emerged as the most significant aspect of these oxidation processes. Keratin samples treated with peracetic acid were categorized as alpha, beta, or gamma keratoses based on their solubility at different pH levels. Alexander and Earland developed the "keratose" classification method. It involved raising the oxidized sample's alkalinity to separate beta-keratose and reducing it to 4 pH to produce alpha-keratose [52]. In contrast to other techniques, keratin's oxidation (keratosis) using peracetic acid produced distinct physicochemical features because bisulfite linkages were converted into sulfonic acids [53]. Nevertheless, the partial oxidation of cystine to cysteic acid by peracetic acid and the loss of certain aminoacyls are two significant disadvantages of the oxidation approach for keratin extraction [54].

4.4 Discusses the utilization of ionic liquids in the extraction of keratin

Ionic liquids are a class of solvents characterized by their large cations and either organic or inorganic anions. They are distinguished by their high melting and boiling points, chemical stability, and high ion conductivity, among other properties. Ionic liquids have been widely used as catalysts and solvents for various polymers and are considered an environmentally friendly solvent option [55]. Xie et al.'s study discovered that, compared with other ionic liquids, PF6 chloride-containing ionic liquid was the most efficient in dissolving keratin, a protein in wool and feathers. After that, the keratin was separated by precipitation using water or ethanol, changing its structural makeup [42]. Compared with wool, the extracted keratin showed higher heat resistance. Because of their strong nucleophilic activity and high Cl content, ionic liquids containing chloride were the best solvents for removing keratin from feathers in a different investigation by Ji et al. They recommended [Bmim]Cl and got a 75% keratin output since it was less expensive [56]. When Ghosh et al. looked into how temperature affected keratin disintegration, they discovered that utilizing [Bmim]Cl, the highest yield of 57% was achieved at 120°C. Nevertheless, the lower yields seen at higher temperatures could have been caused by the water-soluble amino acids of the ionic liquid. Notably, the extraction procedure needs to be carried out in an inert environment since ionic liquids are hygroscopic [57]. Fig. 8.3 shows the investigation of ionic liquid recovery.

4.4.1 Examine the role of temperature in the context of ionic liquid extraction during the mechanism of keratin dissolution

The surface of wool fibers is coated with a lipid layer primarily composed of 18-methyleicosanoic acids [57]. These acids are linked to the inner protein layers through thioester linkages. The thioesters are cleaved upon the introduction of Cl^- ions, allowing the ionic liquid to penetrate the cortical layer. Hydroxyl protons form complexes with BMIM ions, leading to the disruption of hydrogen bonds during dissociation. Simultaneously, Cl- anions bond with hydroxyl protons, initiating the disintegration of keratin [59,60]. Temperature increases influence keratin dissolution, which enhance ion mobility at low viscosity [57]. However, this process results in a more disorganized final product structure. Therefore, careful temperature and keratin yield selection is crucial based on the desired product qualities. Ghosh et al. observed that increasing the temperature from 120 to 180°C decreased the average cysteine concentration from 8.91 to 0.99 mol%,

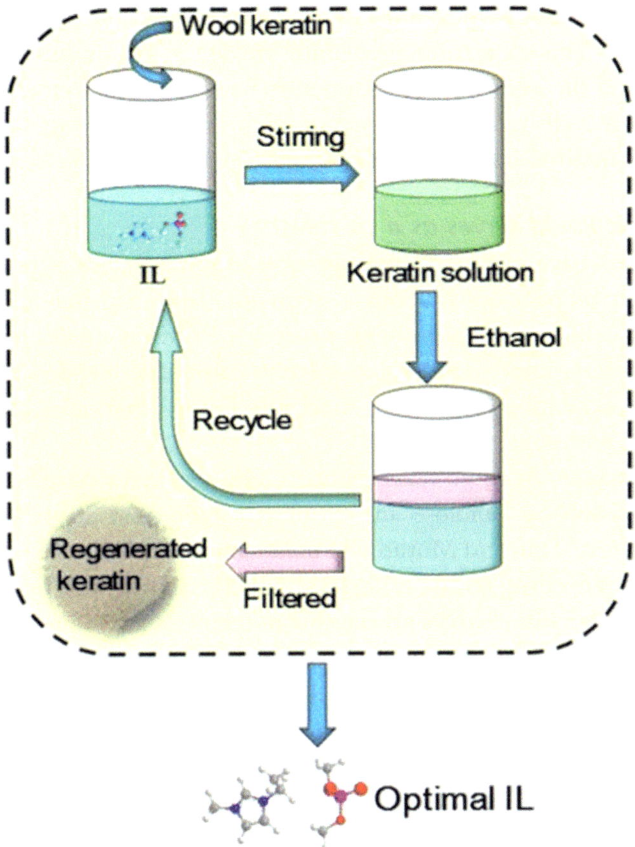

Figure 8.3 The diagram depicts the investigation of ionic liquid recovery. After extensive analysis of dissolution capacity and regenerated keratin properties, dimethyl phosphate ionic liquids (DPILs) have been selected as the most suitable [58].

which should be avoided if the product requires these amino acids. Dissolving wool in the ionic liquid is a time-consuming procedure, typically involving the addition of only 1% wool to the solution until complete dissolution [42,61]. Idris et al. evaluated the solubilization capability of thioglycolate ionic liquids on wool [62]. Choline thioglycolate resulted in the breakdown of wool fibers due to weakened disulfide bonds. Thermogravimetric analysis indicated that the thermal stability of regenerated keratin was lower than that of natural wool [61].

However, Xie et al. contradicted this finding, reporting that regenerated keratins exhibited greater thermal stability [42]. Wang and Cao utilized 1-hydroxyethyl-3-methylimidazolium bis (trifluoroethylsulfonyl) amide to extract keratin from chicken feathers. $NaHSO_3$ was added to break disulfide bonds. This extraction procedure yielded a maximum of 21.5% in 4 hours, and the ionic liquid was found to be reusable up to five times. The ability to recycle ionic liquids may present an advantage of this keratin-dissolving method compared with others [63].

4.4.2 Ionic liquid serves as a co-solvent

Researchers have explored the utilization of ionic liquids as potential co-solvents in biphasic or aqueous systems for dissolving polymers such as wool and cellulose in co-synthesis processes. Previous studies have shown that employing ionic liquids as co-solvents can create blended biopolymer materials exhibiting enhanced mechanical and thermal characteristics compared with separate parts [64].

For instance, At room temperature, a film was created by Hameed and Guo by dissolving cellulose and wool at a ratio of 1:20 in [BMIM]Cl. Similar to this, Tran and Mututuvari used chitosan, cellulose, and keratin to create a film for drug release using [BMIM]Cl [65]. It was observed that the inclusion of keratin played a crucial role in regulating the drug release, with the concentration of keratin being a key determinant [66]. Further investigations have revealed that isolated ionic liquid keratin exhibits a weak alpha structure XRD band [61,67,68]. The regeneration of the beta-sheet structure of the polypeptide chain can be induced by methanol treatment rather than ethanol or water, mirroring the behavior of the original keratin [61,69,70].

4.5 Extracting keratin using steam explosion and supercritical water technology

The steam explosion method, developed by Manson in 1928 [71], is influenced by various variables, including temperature, residence time, particle size, and moisture, all of which can impact the outcome [72–74]. Steam flash explosion (SFE), considered an eco-friendly hydrolysis technique, has found widespread application in producing bio-based products such as delignification of wood, bioconversion of barley [75], pulping of lignocellulosic biomasses [76], and sugar extraction from maize starch [77].

In 1982, Miyamoto et al. utilized SFE to extract keratin from wool, converting approximately 80% of the wool into pepsin-digestible compounds using saturated steam at 164.2°C (6 kg/cm^2) [78]. However, the resulting product contained a lower cysteine content than the original wool. Demonstrating the impact of pressure, Xu et al. showed that increasing pressure reduced wool crystallinity, leading to damage to disulfide bridges while preserving disulfide or hydrogen bonds [79]. Tonin et al. subjecting wool to saturated steam at 220°C for 10 min, achieved a solid product yield of 62.4%, sediment yield of 1.1%, and water-soluble fraction yield of 18.8% [41]. Despite the decrease in cysteine concentration due to intense heating, the chemical structure of keratin was fragmented. Suggesting the use of SFE over conventional steam explosion (CSE) for wool keratin extraction, Zhao et al. highlighted its advantages, including faster processing time, improved digestibility and solubility, and the use of a lower temperature range. It was also noted that the cystine concentration in wool isolated from SFE was low [80].

4.6 Utilizing microwave irradiation to extract keratin

Microwave irradiation serves the primary purpose of expediting the processing time by heating the solution using this technology. Zoccola et al. achieved an extraction yield of approximately 60% by employing microwave irradiation within a power range of 150—570 W at a temperature of 180°C for 7 minutes. Notably, this microwave-based approach demonstrated greater efficiency than conventional steam processing [40]. However, a significant drawback of this method is the substantial loss of amino acids, particularly cysteine, in the final wool keratin sample. Zoccola et al. observed a decline in cysteine concentration from 9.4 mol% to around 0.5 mol% after 90 min of treatment using microwave irradiation [40]. Chen et al. highlighted that microwave heating significantly reduced the activation energy required for keratin extraction compared with conventional heating methods, which are often nonuniform. Despite the intricate structure of keratin, the interaction between electromagnetic radiation and the wool matrix remains poorly understood. Nevertheless, there is a hypothesis that the activation energy needed for the hydrolysis of ester groups is lower [81].

4.7 Techniques for keratin extraction using microbes and enzymes

The biotechnology and food industries use microbial and enzymatic keratin extraction processes, especially for breaking down keratin-rich materials like wool and feathers. Enzymes catalyze keratin hydrolysis commercially, providing a low-energy and ecologically benign substitute for conventional chemical techniques [82]. Numerous microorganisms, such as prokaryotes, keratinophilic fungi, and gram-positive bacteria, generate efficient keratinases in hydrolyzing keratin [83]. Keratinases are used in many sectors, such as sewage treatment, leather, textile, and wool [84].

Strains of Bacillus licheniformis are known to degrade feather proteins, while species like Chrysosporium and Dermatophytes exhibit keratinolytic fungal properties [85–88]. Kornillowicz-Kowalska et al. experimented with using a combination of 16 keratinophilic fungal strains to monitor keratin degradation [89]. After a 21-day cultivation period, the researchers observed a 50% solubilization of peptides. Furthermore, once Chrysosporium was cultivated for 21 days on a substrate made of feathers, around 75% of the nitrogen converted to ammonium. Similarly, almost 75% of the nitrogen in a wool-based substrate was converted to ammonia when Streptomyces fradiae bacteria were used as a breakdown source [90]. Employing feathers as a substrate converted around 20% of nitrogen into peptides and amino acids. The lysate protein composition included 10%–20% cystine/cysteine and 20%–30% serine [89]. Keratin degradation occurs through the breakdown of protein disulfide links into cysteine and S-sulfocysteine by sulfite material produced by bacteria. The oxidation of sulfur amino acids by oxygen leads to the formation of cysteic acid.

4.8 Applications of keratin in biomedicine

In-depth exploration of keratin's chemical, physical, and biological attributes has resulted in the development of biomaterials based on this substance. Inherently, keratin-based biomaterials exhibit self-assembly, biocompatibility, biodegradability, and the ability to support cell proliferation [18]. This inherent self-assembly characteristic, extensively explored at both the nanoscale and macroscale, enables polymerization into porous scaffolds. Cell-binding motifs like glutamic acid-aspartic acid-serine (EDS) and leucine-aspartic acid-valine (LDV) binding residues are present in biomaterials from keratin found in wool and hair, facilitating cellular attachment. Together, these characteristics improve cell adhesion and growth in a three-dimensional matrix structure [91,92]. In the last 30 years, many experiments have been carried out to develop novel keratin-based biomaterials, such as films, sponges, fibers, gels, and scaffolds. For several biological uses, including bone tissue engineering [93–95], ocular regeneration [96], wound healing [97,98], nerve regeneration [99,100], skin replacement [101], and controlled drug administration, keratin has been well studied [102–104].

4.9 Keratin films serve as a carrier for bone morphogenic protein 2 and contribute to the reconstruction of the ocular surface

Commonly, methods like solvent casting, compress molding, thermal pressing, electrospinning, and layer-by-layer (LbL) deposition are employed in the production of keratin films. Numerous studies in recent decades have aimed to investigate the biological and physicochemical properties of keratin films [105–108]. Yamauchi et al. researched keratin derived from wool, focusing on the breakdown biodegradation and physical and chemical aspects of solvent-cast keratin films [37]. Their study also delved into the cellular attachment and proliferation of these keratin films, revealing that, when compared to collagen, these films acted as a more adhesive substrate for cells [109]. Fujii et al. demonstrated a rapid casting technique, showcasing that keratin films derived from hair could incorporate bioactive molecules like alkaline phosphatase. Furthermore, these films were identified as suitable substrates for the controlled release of these molecules despite their relatively poor mechanical strength. Collectively, these preliminary studies underscore the potential medical applications of keratin films [110].

4.9.1 Different approaches for incorporating different organic and inorganic polymers

Several studies have been conducted to improve the physical properties of these films while maintaining their exceptional biological characteristics [71,111,112]. Yamauchi's group has used different strategies to incorporate natural and artificial polymers into pure keratin formulations, such as chitosan in 2002 [112]. The interactions between silk fibroin and keratin films have been extensively studied, with a reported change from a random coil to a beta-sheet structure in fibroin due to interactions with polar amino acids in keratin [113–116]. The antithrombogenic properties of these blended films were superior to those of pure keratin or SF films. Vasconcelos et al. investigated keratin-SF films' degradation and physical properties, observing distinct interactions between the two proteins' molecules [112].

4.9.2 Keratin-based scaffolds to carry Bone Morphogenic Protein 2

In vivo study, researchers investigated keratose, the water-soluble component of keratin, as a carrier for Bone Morphogenic Protein 2 (BMP2) in the healing of rat femoral bone defects. The study observed enhanced bone regeneration and a reduction in fat tissue [117].

5. Keratin-based scaffolds for advancing urinary tract tissue engineering

In 2001, Tachibana et al. pioneered the development of wool-derived keratin scaffolds for extended cell culture, harnessing their unique ability to polymerize and self-assemble into a three-dimensional porous structure [118]. Through a controlled freeze-drying process, they successfully produced a uniform, porous, and heat-stable structure [119]. Subsequently, in 2005, Tachibana et al. advanced the technology by hybridizing keratin sponges with calcium phosphate [120]. The hybridization process involved chemically bonding calcium and phosphate ions within the sponges or integrating hydroxyapatite particles into the keratin carboxy-sponge structure. Both types of hybridized sponges exhibited positive promotion of osteoblastic cultivation. However, achieving optimal cellular penetration and ensuring appropriate nutritional supply necessitated careful adjustment of the pore diameter in the porous scaffold. Addressing the challenge of managing pore size and porosity during lyophilization, Katoh et al. introduced an alternative approach. They employed compression molding to precisely control the pore size of keratin scaffolds, providing a valuable method for enhancing scaffold customization [121].

Peplow et al. conducted a study to examine the in vivo degradation of reconstituted keratin rectangular bars and establish a connection between physical strength and mass. They subcutaneously implanted these bars into rats and measured both the elastic modulus and dry weight over 18 weeks. The results indicated a significant 22% weight decrease at 18 weeks, with a marked reduction in elastic modulus observed between Weeks 3 and 6. Consequently, the researchers concluded that keratin in this form could serve as an implant material in non-load-bearing locations due to its rapid loss of mechanical integrity and progressive disintegration [122].

In response to the inherent brittleness and low mechanical characteristics of keratin composites, various researchers have incorporated synthetic polymers such as PVA, PCL, PLLA, and PEO to enhance mechanical properties [93,123–126]. Electrospinning, known for its efficacy in producing fibers with high porosity and surface area, has been employed to destabilize the beta-sheet structure simultaneously. Aluigi et al. utilized electrospinning to create a 50:50 ratio mixture of keratin/PEO, while Edwards et al. electrospun PCL/keratin fibers at different ratios [127]. Zhao et al. improved the biocompatibility and mechanical properties of PCL/keratin by introducing hydroxyapatite particles [128]. This comprehensive approach aims to address the brittleness and low mechanical characteristics associated with keratin composites, presenting promising advancements in the realm of implant materials [124].

5.1 The application of keratin-based scaffolds in tissue engineering for the urinary tract

In recent years, tissue engineering techniques have shown promise in addressing urinary tract strictures or abnormalities resulting from cancer, congenital disorders, trauma, and inflammation [129]. Biomaterials play a crucial role in this context by providing a three-dimensional framework for seeded cells [130]. Researchers have extensively studied various matrices, including synthetic polyesters, protein, and collagen-based matrices. However, addressing challenges related to the survival of seeded cells and the antibacterial properties of implanted biomaterials requires the development of an optimal technique [131]. To overcome these limitations, researchers have developed biomaterials capable of generating oxygen. This innovation facilitates the adequate diffusion of oxygen and prevents necrosis in cell-seeded implants. Observations indicate that these biomaterials preserve cell viability under hypoxic conditions and actively inhibit necrosis. This advancement holds significant promise for improving the effectiveness of tissue engineering in addressing urinary tract complications [130,131].

Recently, keratin from human hair, gelatin, silk, and calcium peroxide were used by researchers to create a novel biomaterial (CPO). In vitro tests revealed that this film, primarily made of 2% gelatin, silk/keratin (60:40), and 20% calcium peroxide, can reliably release oxygen for 2 weeks. The resultant film was examined using various techniques by the researchers, including confocal laser scanning microscopy, Fourier Transform Infrared (FTIR) spectroscopy, scanning electron microscopy, and tensile testing. Aside from that, they evaluated other attributes like cellular growth, antibacterial activity, cytotoxicity, breakdown, and oxygen-release behavior—dogs with urethral abnormalities healed more quickly after watching films that included CPO. Comparatively speaking, animals treated with CPO-containing films showed a more ordered pattern in the epithelial layer and muscle bundles than those treated with non-CPO films [131].

5.2 Keratin hydrogels as a flexible matrix for medication administration and wound healing

Utilizing a variety of natural and synthetic materials, such as films, gels, scaffolds, or nanoparticles, for the targeted delivery of therapeutic drugs to prevent infection and enhance healing is a common practice [132−135]. In drug delivery, researchers extensively investigated numerous synthetic and natural polymers, such as alginates, polyphosphazene, polyanhydrides, polyorthoesters, chitosan, collagen, and keratin. Proteins-based biomaterials are gaining attention in drug administration due to their abundant availability, low toxicity, emulsifying capability, and water retention ability [136]. Researchers frequently use keratose, keratin's water-soluble component, to produce keratin hydrogel [97,137]. By incorporating Ciprofloxacin into a keratin hydrogel, researchers gradually released 60% of the antibiotic over 10 days [138]. Keratin hydrogel demonstrated effectiveness in preventing postoperative adhesion following abdominal or peritoneal surgery. Peyton et al. employed keratose hydrogel as a physical barrier and Halofuginone (HF) as the medication, revealing that HF-keratin hydrogel reduced adhesion density in a rodent cecal abrasion model. This hydrogel exhibits versatility, serving as a gel with multiple applications and facilitating targeted drug delivery. However, challenges associated with using these hydrogels for drug release applications include a high degradation rate and drug instability in the keratin matrix [139].

The biological process of wound healing is intricate and involves many cellular components to restore damaged or destroyed tissue integrity [140]. Because it is widely available and has great biocompatibility [92,141,142], researchers extensively studied keratin hydrogel derived from human hair as a matrix for enhanced wound healing [141]. Recently, keratin-based in situ researchers created cross-linkable hydrogels made from human hair to serve as a matrix for better wound healing. These hydrogels were reported to accelerate the reepithelization process in animal models with full-thickness wounds. Researchers observed numerous biological interactions between human skin keratinocytes and hair-derived keratin, encompassing proliferation, morphological changes, and alterations in gene and protein expression profiles. Using an animal model with a full-thickness skin defect, researchers assessed the hydrogel's capacity to repair wounds [141].

5.2.1 Keratin hydrogel actively contributes to nerve regeneration

Addressing peripheral nerve abnormalities and restoring autonomic and sensory systems presents a significant clinical challenge, especially as nerve fiber degeneration begins. Treatment options include tubular conduits, end-to-end repair, and autologous grafts. When conduits are chosen as a therapeutic alternative, commonly used biomaterials like chitosan, fibrin, and hyaluronic acid are employed to fill the deficiency [100,142]. According to Sierpinski and Apel, the use of keratin hydrogel in this situation may increase nerve cell activity and proliferation via chemotactic mechanisms [99,142]. Subsequent in vivo studies demonstrated axon regrowth. The identical study team conducted a histological analysis to examine the nerve regeneration process over time precisely with a conduit filled with keratin hydrogel [99,102,143].

6. Conclusions

This chapter introduces keratin as a dependable bioactive material with a variety of manipulable forms, including films, sponges, fibers, and hydrogels, which are ideal for repairing damaged and diseased tissues. Keratin is based on nanocomposites for tissue engineering used in the field of biomedical and regenerative medicine. Keratin differs from conventional biomaterials due to its distinct mechanical and biological characteristics, which include its chemical structure, innate capacity for self-assembly, presence of cell-binding domains, and bacteriostatic effects. Over the past few decades, keratin-based biomaterials, including hydrogels, films, fibers, sponges, scaffolds, and wound patches, have been thoroughly investigated and created by researchers. This research highlights the potential of combining several natural and synthetic polymers with keratin to improve its mechanical and biological properties for a range of technical applications. The antibacterial capabilities of keratin have been significantly enhanced by the addition of antimicrobial agents to provide a bacteriostatic effect. Furthermore, the review highlights continuing research efforts to gain a thorough understanding of keratin's involvement in maintaining cell attachment and proliferation as well as cellular interactions with it. For keratin to be used in the biomedical area, it is essential to improve the mechanical-physical properties of sponges, films, and composites made of keratin and to carry out molecular-level research on how keratin interacts with other natural or synthetic polymers.

Acknowledgments

The authors appreciate the Short Term Grant (304/PKIMIA/6315580) by Universiti Sains Malaysia.

References

[1] O'brien FJ. Biomaterials and scaffolds for tissue engineering. Mater Today March 1, 2011;14(3):88–95.

[2] Tallawi M, Rosellini E, Barbani N, Cascone MG, Rai R, Saint-Pierre G, Boccaccini AR. Strategies for the chemical and biological functionalization of scaffolds for cardiac tissue engineering: a review. J R Soc Interface July 6, 2015;12(108).

[3] Wang G, Zreiqat H. Functional coatings or films for hard-tissue applications. Materials July 2010;3(7):3994–4050.

[4] Zujur D, Moret J, Rodriguez D, Cruz L, Lira J, Gil L, Dominguez E, Alvarez-Barreto J. A novel photocrosslinkable and cytocompatible chitosan coating for Ti6Al4V surfaces. J Appl Biomater Funct Mater July 2015;13(3):210–9.

[5] Ben Cao Gang Mu SL. Volume IX: fowls, domestic and wild animals, human substances. Univ of California Press; February 2, 2021.

[6] Noishiki Y, Ito H, Miyamoto T, Inagaki H. Application of denatured wool keratin derivatives to an antithrombogenic biomaterial-vascular graft coated with a heparinized keratin derivative. Kobunshi Ronbunshu January 1, 1982;39(4):221–7.

[7] Schweizer J, Bowden PE, Coulombe PA, Langbein L, Lane EB, Magin TM, Maltais L, Omary MB, Parry DA, Rogers MA, Wright MW. New consensus nomenclature for mammalian keratins. J Cell Biol July 17, 2006;174(2):169–74.

[8] Fraser RD, MacRae TP, Parry DA, Suzuki E. Intermediate filaments in alpha-keratins. Proc Natl Acad Sci USA March 1986;83(5):1179–83.

[9] Moll R, Divo M, Langbein L. The human keratins: biology and pathology. Histochem Cell Biol June 2008;129:705–33.

[10] Yu J, Yu DW, Checkla DM, Freedberg IM, Bertolino AP. Human hair keratins. J Invest Dermatol July 1, 1993;101(1):S56–9.

[11] Pracella M, Haque MM, Paci M, Alvarez V. Property tuning of poly (lactic acid)/cellulose bio-composites through blending with modified ethylene-vinyl acetate copolymer. Carbohydrate Polymers February 10, 2016;137:515–24.

[12] Dogu B, Kaynak C. Behavior of polylactide/microcrystalline cellulose biocomposites: effects of filler content and interfacial compatibilization. Cellulose February 2016;23:611–22.

[13] Song K, Gao A, Cheng X, Xie K. Preparation of the superhydrophobic nano-hybrid membrane containing carbon nanotube based on chitosan and its antibacterial activity. Carbohydrate Polymers October 5, 2015;130:381–7.

[14] Tran CD, Mututuvari TM. Cellulose, chitosan and keratin composite materials: facile and recyclable synthesis, conformation and properties. ACS Sustainable Chem Eng March 7, 2016;4(3):1850–61.

[15] Xu X, Wang Z, Li M, Su Y, Zhang Q, Zhang S, Hu J. Reconstructed hierarchically structured keratin fibers with shape-memory features based on reversible secondary-structure transformation. Adv Mater October 2023;35(41).

[16] Mu B, Xu L, Yang Y. Rational fabrication of completely amorphous chitosan-formyl-sucrose sorbents with excellent durability and regenerability for high-throughput dye removal. Chem Eng J April 1, 2023;461.

[17] Ramadoss P, Arul KT, Ramya JR, Begam MR, Chandra VS, Manikandan E. Enhanced mechanical strength and sustained drug release of gelatin/keratin scaffolds. Mater Lett January 1, 2017;186:109–12.

[18] McLellan J, Thornhill SG, Shelton S, Kumar M. Keratin-based biofilms, hydrogels, and biofibers. Keratin as a protein biopolymer: extraction from waste biomass and applications. 2019. p. 187–200.

[19] Zhen LS, Mu BC. The time literature and art press. Jilin, China: Changchun; 2005.

[20] Rouse JG, Van Dyke ME. A review of keratin-based biomaterials for biomedical applications. Materials February 3, 2010;3(2):999–1014.
[21] Hofmeier J. Horn-lime plastic masses from keratin substances. German Pat. DE184915 December 18, 1905;18.
[22] Anker CA, Inventor; General Mills Inc, assignee. Method of preparing keratin-containing films and coatings. United States patent US 1972 Feb 15;3(642):498.
[23] Kawano Y, Okamoto S. Film and gel of keratins. Kagaku to Seibutsu 1975;13(5):291–2.
[24] Okamoto S. On the formation of films from some proteins. Nippon Shokuhin Kogyo Gakkaishi January 15, 1977;24(1):40–50.
[25] Miyamoto T, Takahashi SI, Ito H, Inagaki H, Noishiki Y. Tissue biocompatibility of cellulose and its derivatives. J Biomed Mater Res January 1989;23(1):125–33.
[26] Fraser RD, MacRae TP, Rogers GE. Keratins: their composition, structure and biosynthesis. Food Cosmet Toxicol 1973;11(5):892.
[27] Donato RK, Mija A. Keratin associations with synthetic, biosynthetic and natural polymers: an extensive review. Polymers December 23, 2019;12(1):32.
[28] Jones LN, Simon M, Watts NR, Booy FP, Steven AC, Parry DA. Intermediate filament structure: hard α-keratin. Biophys Chem October 1, 1997;68(1–3):83–93.
[29] Squire J, Vibert PJ, Elliott A. Fibrous protein structure: a volume dedicated to Dr Arthur Elliott. London; San Diego, Calif.: Academic Press; 1987.
[30] Fraser RB, Parry DA. The structural basis of the filament-matrix texture in the avian/reptilian group of hard β-keratins. J Struct Biol February 1, 2011;173(2):391–405.
[31] Isarankura Na Ayutthaya S, Tanpichai S, Wootthikanokkhan J. Keratin extracted from chicken feather waste: extraction, preparation, and structural characterization of the keratin and keratin/biopolymer films and electrospuns. J Polym Environ December 2015;23:506–16.
[32] Aluigi A, Tonetti C, Rombaldoni F, Puglia D, Fortunati E, Armentano I, Santulli C, Torre L, Kenny JM. Keratins extracted from Merino wool and Brown Alpaca fibres as potential fillers for PLLA-based biocomposites. J Mater Sci September 2014;49:6257–69.
[33] Park M, Kim BS, Shin HK, Park SJ, Kim HY. Preparation and characterization of keratin-based biocomposite hydrogels prepared by electron beam irradiation. Mater Sci Eng C December 1, 2013;33(8):5051–7.
[34] Poole AJ, Lyons RE, Church JS. Dissolving feather keratin using sodium sulfide for bio-polymer applications. J Polym Environ December 2011;19:995–1004.
[35] Tonin C, Aluigi A, Varesano A, Vineis C. Keratin-based nanofibres. Nanofibers February 2010;1:139–58.
[36] Gunnarsson M, Larsson S, Malak M, Ericson MB, Topgaard D, Sparr E. Molecular mobility in keratin-rich materials monitored by nuclear magnetic resonance: a tool for the evaluation of structure-giving properties. Biomacromolecules May 18, 2023;24:2661–73.
[37] Yamauchi K, Yamauchi A, Kusunoki T, Kohda A, Konishi Y. Preparation of stable aqueous solution of keratins, and physiochemical and biodegradational properties of films. J Biomed Mater Res August 1996;31(4):439–44.
[38] Buchanan JH. A cystine-rich protein fraction from oxidized alpha-keratin. Biochem J November 11, 1977;167(2):489.
[39] Tsuda Y, Nomura Y. Properties of alkaline-hydrolyzed waterfowl feather keratin. Animal Sci J February 2014;85(2):180–5.
[40] Zoccola M, Aluigi A, Patrucco A, Vineis C, Forlini F, Locatelli P, Sacchi MC, Tonin C. Microwave-assisted chemical-free hydrolysis of wool keratin. Textil Res J November 2012;82(19):2006–18.

[41] Tonin C, Zoccola M, Aluigi A, Varesano A, Montarsolo A, Vineis C, Zimbardi F. Study on the conversion of wool keratin by steam explosion. Biomacromolecules December 11, 2006;7(12):3499–504.
[42] Xie H, Li S, Zhang S. Ionic liquids as novel solvents for the dissolution and blending of wool keratin fibers. Green Chem 2005;7(8):606–8.
[43] Savige WE. The dispersion of wool protein by thiols in acid solution. Textil Res J January 1960;30(1):1.
[44] O'donnell IJ, Thompson EO. Studies on reduced wool. Aust J Biol Sci 1964;17(4):973–8.
[45] Smith AL, Harris M. Oxidation of wool: photochemical oxidation. J Res Natl Bur Stand (US) July 1936;17:97–100.
[46] Arai KM, Takahashi R, Yokote Y, Akahane K. Amino-acid sequence of feather keratin from fowl. Eur J Biochem May 1983;132(3):501–7.
[47] Gortner RA, Sinclair WB. Sulfur in proteins: IV. The effect of alkalies upon cystine. J Biol Chem September 1, 1929;83(3):681–96.
[48] Nagai Y, Nishikawa T. Alkali solubilization of chicken feather keratin. Agricult Biol Chem January 1, 1970;34(1):16–22.
[49] Jiang-Tao XU, Ping ZH, Lin ZH, Shu-ying SU, Zhao-hong DO, Yi ZU. Study of keratin extraction from human hair. Wool Text J May 1, 2015;43(5).
[50] Earland C, Knight CS. Studies on the structure of keratin: I. The analysis of fractions isolated from wool oxidized with peracetic acid. Biochim Biophys Acta January 1, 1955;17:457–61.
[51] Strasheim A, Buijs K. An infra-red study of the oxidation of the disulphide bond in wool. Biochim Biophys Acta March 4, 1961;47(3):538–41.
[52] Robbins CR, Robbins CR. Chemical and physical behavior of human hair. Berlin: Springer; February 23, 2012.
[53] de Guzman RC, Merrill MR, Richter JR, Hamzi RI, Greengauz-Roberts OK, Van Dyke ME. Mechanical and biological properties of keratose biomaterials. Biomaterials November 1, 2011;32(32):8205–17.
[54] Toennies G, Homiller RP. The oxidation of amino acids by hydrogen peroxide in formic acid. J Am Chem Soc December 1942;64(12):3054–6.
[55] Yoo CG, Pu Y, Ragauskas AJ. Ionic liquids: promising green solvents for lignocellulosic biomass utilization. Curr Opin Green Sustainable Chem June 1, 2017;5:5–11.
[56] Ji Y, Chen J, Lv J, Li Z, Xing L, Ding S. Extraction of keratin with ionic liquids from poultry feather. Separat Purificat Technol August 20, 2014;132:577–83.
[57] Ghosh A, Clerens S, Deb-Choudhury S, Dyer JM. Thermal effects of ionic liquid dissolution on the structures and properties of regenerated wool keratin. Polym Degrad Stabil October 1, 2014;108:108–15.
[58] Zheng S, Nie Y, Zhang S, Zhang X, Wang L. Highly efficient dissolution of wool keratin by dimethylphosphate ionic liquids. ACS Sustainable Chem Eng November 2, 2015;3(11):2925–32.
[59] Zhang H, Wu J, Zhang J, He J. 1-Allyl-3-methylimidazolium chloride room temperature ionic liquid: a new and powerful nonderivatizing solvent for cellulose. Macromolecules October 4, 2005;38(20):8272–7.
[60] Feng L, Chen ZL. Research progress on dissolution and functional modification of cellulose in ionic liquids. J Mol Liq August 20, 2008;142(1–3):1–5.
[61] Li R, Wang D. Preparation of regenerated wool keratin films from wool keratin–ionic liquid solutions. J Appl Polym Sci February 15, 2013;127(4):2648–53.
[62] Idris A, Vijayaraghavan R, Rana UA, Fredericks D, Patti AF, Macfarlane DR. Dissolution of feather keratin in ionic liquids. Green Chem 2013;15(2):525–34.
[63] Wang YX, Cao XJ. Extracting keratin from chicken feathers by using a hydrophobic ionic liquid. Process Biochem May 1, 2012;47(5):896–9.

[64] Fernández JF, Waterkamp D, Thöming J. Recovery of ionic liquids from wastewater: aggregation control for intensified membrane filtration. Desalination April 15, 2008;224(1−3):52−6.
[65] Hameed N, Guo Q. Blend films of natural wool and cellulose prepared from an ionic liquid. Cellulose August 2010;17:803−13.
[66] Tran CD, Mututuvari TM. Cellulose, chitosan, and keratin composite materials. Controlled drug release. Langmuir February 3, 2015;31(4):1516−26.
[67] Sun P, Liu ZT, Liu ZW. Particles from bird feather: a novel application of an ionic liquid and waste resource. J Hazard Mater October 30, 2009;170(2−3):786−90.
[68] Idris A, Vijayaraghavan R, Rana UA, Patti AF, Macfarlane DR. Dissolution and regeneration of wool keratin in ionic liquids. Green Chem 2014;16(5):2857−64.
[69] Phillips DM, Drummy LF, Conrady DG, Fox DM, Naik RR, Stone MO, Trulove PC, De Long HC, Mantz RA. Dissolution and regeneration of Bombyx mori silk fibroin using ionic liquids. J Am Chem Soc November 10, 2004;126(44):14350−1.
[70] Jin HJ, Fridrikh SV, Rutledge GC, Kaplan DL. Electrospinning Bombyx mori silk with poly (ethylene oxide). Biomacromolecules November 11, 2002;3(6):1233−9.
[71] Shavandi A, Silva TH, Bekhit AA, Bekhit AE. Keratin: dissolution, extraction and biomedical application. Biomater Sci 2017;5(9):1699−735.
[72] Sanchez OJ, Cardona CA. Trends in biotechnological production of fuel ethanol from different feedstocks. Bioresour Technol September 1, 2008;99(13):5270−95.
[73] Sun XF, Xu F, Sun RC, Fowler P, Baird MS. Characteristics of degraded cellulose obtained from steam-exploded wheat straw. Carbohydr Res January 17, 2005;340(1):97−106.
[74] Khan MA, Ahmad A, Umar K, Nabi SA. Synthesis, characterization, and biological applications of nanocomposites for the removal of heavy metals and dyes. Ind Eng Chem Res January 14, 2015;54(1):76−82.
[75] Zhang L, Wang T, Jiao S, Hao C, Mao Z. Effect of steam-explosion on biodegradation of lignin in wheat straw. In: 2007 ASAE annual meeting. American Society of Agricultural and biological Engineers; 2007. p. 1.
[76] Young RA, Akhtar M, editors. Environmentally friendly technologies for the pulp and paper industry. John Wiley and Sons; November 19, 1997.
[77] McKendry P. Energy production from biomass (part 2): conversion technologies. Bioresour Technol May 1, 2002;83(1):47−54.
[78] Miyamoto T, Amiya T, Inagaki H. Preparation of wool powder by explosive-puffing treatment. Kobunshi Ronbunshu January 1, 1982;39(11):679−85.
[79] Xu W, Ke G, Wu J, Wang X. Modification of wool fiber using steam explosion. Eur Polym J September 1, 2006;42(9):2168−73.
[80] Zhao W, Yang R, Zhang Y, Wu L. Sustainable and practical utilization of feather keratin by an innovative physicochemical pretreatment: high density steam flash-explosion. Green Chem 2012;14(12):3352−60.
[81] Chen J, Ding S, Ji Y, Ding J, Yang X, Zou M, Li Z. Microwave-enhanced hydrolysis of poultry feather to produce amino acid. Chem Eng Process: Process Intensif January 1, 2015;87:104−9.
[82] Brandelli A. Bacterial keratinases: useful enzymes for bioprocessing agroindustrial wastes and beyond. Food Bioprocess Technol June 2008;1:105−16.
[83] Saleem M, Rehman A, Yasmin R, Munir B. Biochemical analysis and investigation on the prospective applications of alkaline protease from a Bacillus cereus strain. Mol Biol Rep June 2012;39:6399−408.
[84] Chaturvedi V, Bhange K, Bhatt R, Verma P. Production of kertinases using chicken feathers as substrate by a novel multifunctional strain of Pseudomonas stutzeri and its dehairing application. Biocatal Agric Biotechnol April 1, 2014;3(2):167−74.

[85] Burtt JEH, Ichida JM. Occurrence of feather-degrading bacilli in the plumage of birds. The Auk April 1, 1999;116(2):364–72.
[86] Goldstein G, Flory KR, Browne BA, Majid S, Ichida JM, Burtt JEH. Bacterial degradation of black and white feathers. The Auk July 1, 2004;121(3):656–9.
[87] Abdullah A, Abdullah AZ, Ahmed M, Khan J, Shahadat M, Umar K, Alim MA. A review on recent developments and progress in sustainable acrolein production through catalytic dehydration of bio-renewable glycerol. J Clean Prod March 20, 2022;341.
[88] Gunderson AR, Forsyth MH, Swaddle JP. Evidence that plumage bacteria influence feather coloration and body condition of eastern bluebirds Sialia sialis. J Avian Biol July 2009;40(4):440–7.
[89] Korniłłowicz-Kowalska T, Bohacz J. Biodegradation of keratin waste: theory and practical aspects. Waste Manage August 1, 2011;31(8):1689–701.
[90] Noval JJ, Nickerson WJ. Decomposition of native keratin by Streptomyces fradiae. J Bacteriol March 1959;77(3):251–63.
[91] Costa F, Silva R, Boccaccini AR. Fibrous protein-based biomaterials (silk, keratin, elastin, and resilin proteins) for tissue regeneration and repair. Peptid Protein Biomat Tissue Regener Repair January 2018;1:175–204.
[92] Patrucco A, Visai L, Fassina L, Magenes G, Tonin C. Keratin-based matrices from wool fibers and human hair. Material Biomed Eng January 1, 2019:375–403.
[93] Li JS, Li Y, Liu X, Zhang J, Zhang Y. Strategy to introduce an hydroxyapatite–keratin nanocomposite into a fibrous membrane for bone tissue engineering. J Mater Chem B 2013;1(4):432–7.
[94] Tachibana A, Nishikawa Y, Nishino M, Kaneko S, Tanabe T, Yamauchi K. Modified keratin sponge: binding of bone morphogenetic protein-2 and osteoblast differentiation. J Biosci Bioeng November 1, 2006;102(5):425–9.
[95] Mir NA, Haque MM, Khan A, Umar K, Muneer M, Vijayalakshmi S. Semiconductor mediated photocatalysed reaction of two selected organic compounds in aqueous suspensions of Titanium dioxide. J Adv Oxid Technol July 1, 2012;15(2):380–91.
[96] Borrelli M, Joepen N, Reichl S, Finis D, Schoppe M, Geerling G, Schrader S. Keratin films for ocular surface reconstruction: evaluation of biocompatibility in an in-vivo model. Biomaterials February 1, 2015;42:112–20.
[97] Ham TR, Lee RT, Han S, Haque S, Vodovotz Y, Gu J, Burnett LR, Tomblyn S, Saul JM. Tunable keratin hydrogels for controlled erosion and growth factor delivery. Biomacromolecules January 11, 2016;17(1):225–36.
[98] Nakata R, Tachibana A, Tanabe T. Preparation of keratin hydrogel/hydroxyapatite composite and its evaluation as a controlled drug release carrier. Mater Sci Eng C August 1, 2014;41:59–64.
[99] Apel PJ, Garrett JP, Sierpinski P, Ma J, Atala A, Smith TL, Koman LA, Van Dyke ME. Peripheral nerve regeneration using a keratin-based scaffold: long-term functional and histological outcomes in a mouse model. J Hand Surg November 1, 2008;33(9):1541–7.
[100] Lin YC, Ramadan M, Van Dyke M, Kokai LE, Philips BJ, Rubin JP, Marra KG. Keratin gel filler for peripheral nerve repair in a rodent sciatic nerve injury model. Plast Reconstr Surg January 1, 2012;129(1):67–78.
[101] Xu S, Sang L, Zhang Y, Wang X, Li X. Biological evaluation of human hair keratin scaffolds for skin wound repair and regeneration. Mater Sci Eng C March 1, 2013;33(2):648–55.
[102] Yin XC, Li FY, He YF, Wang Y, Wang RM. Study on effective extraction of chicken feather keratins and their films for controlling drug release. Biomater Sci 2013;1(5):528–36.

[103] Guo J, Pan S, Yin X, He YF, Li T, Wang RM. H-sensitive keratin-based polymer hydrogel and its controllable drug-release behavior. J Appl Polym Sci March 5, 2015;132(9).
[104] Umar K, Mfarrej MF, Rahman QI, Zuhaib M, Khan A, Zia Q, Banawas S, Nadeem H, Khan MF, Ahmad F. ZnO Nano-swirlings for Azo Dye AR183 photocatalytic degradation and antimycotic activity. Sci Rep August 18, 2022;12(1):14023.
[105] Borrelli M, Witt J, Roth M, Reichl S, Bradenbrink P, Schoppe M, Schrader S, Geerling G. Keratin films for ocular surface reconstruction: wound healing in an in-vivo model. Exp Eye Res February 1, 2023;227:109356.
[106] Sharma S, Kumar A, Adelere IA, Latee A. Keratin as a protein biopolymer. Springer series on polymer and composite materials. 2019.
[107] Umar K. Water contamination by organic-pollutants: TiO 2 photocatalysis. Modern age environmental problems and their remediation. 2018. p. 95—109.
[108] Fortunato GM, Da Ros F, Bisconti S, De Acutis A, Biagini F, Lapomarda A, Magliaro C, De Maria C, Montemurro F, Bizzotto D, Braghetta P. Electrospun structures made of a hydrolyzed keratin-based biomaterial for development of in vitro tissue models. Front Bioeng Biotechnol July 17, 2019;7:174.
[109] Yamauchi K, Maniwa M, Mori T. Cultivation of fibroblast cells on keratin-coated substrata. J Biomater Sci Polym Ed January 1, 1998;9(3):259—70.
[110] Fujii T, Ogiwara D, Arimoto M. Convenient procedures for human hair protein films and properties of alkaline phosphatase incorporated in the film. Biol Pharm Bull 2004;27(1):89—93.
[111] Vasconcelos A, Freddi G, Cavaco-Paulo A. Biodegradable materials based on silk fibroin and keratin. Biomacromolecules April 14, 2008;9(4):1299—305.
[112] Fujii T, Ide Y. Preparation of translucent and flexible human hair protein films and their properties. Biol Pharm Bull 2004;27(9):1433—6.
[113] Tanabe T, Okitsu N, Tachibana A, Yamauchi K. Preparation and characterization of keratin—chitosan composite film. Biomaterials February 1, 2002;23(3):817—25.
[114] Umar K, Dar AA, Haque MM, Mir NA, Muneer M. Photocatalysed decolourization of two textile dye derivatives, Martius Yellow and Acid Blue 129, in UV-irradiated aqueous suspensions of Titania. Desal Water Treat August 1, 2012;46(1—3):205—14.
[115] Lee KY, Ha WS. DSC studies on bound water in silk fibroin/S-carboxymethyl kerateine blend films. Polymer June 1, 1999;40(14):4131—4.
[116] Lee KY, Kong SJ, Park WH, Ha WS, Kwon IC. Effect of surface properties on the antithrombogenicity of silk fibroin/S-carboxymethyl kerateine blend films. J Biomater Sci Polym Ed January 1, 1998;9(9):905—14.
[117] de Guzman RC, Saul JM, Ellenburg MD, Merrill MR, Coan HB, Smith TL, Van Dyke ME. Bone regeneration with BMP-2 delivered from keratose scaffolds. Biomaterials February 1, 2013;34(6):1644—56.
[118] Tachibana A, Furuta Y, Takeshima H, Tanabe T, Yamauchi K. Fabrication of wool keratin sponge scaffolds for long-term cell cultivation. J Biotechnol February 14, 2002;93(2):165—70.
[119] Rahmani Del Bakhshayesh A, Annabi N, Khalilov R, Akbarzadeh A, Samiei M, Alizadeh E, Alizadeh-Ghodsi M, Davaran S, Montaseri A. Recent advances on biomedical applications of scaffolds in wound healing and dermal tissue engineering. Artific Cell Nanomed Biotechnol May 19, 2018;46(4):691—705.
[120] Tachibana A, Kaneko S, Tanabe T, Yamauchi K. Rapid fabrication of keratin—hydroxyapatite hybrid sponges toward osteoblast cultivation and differentiation. Biomaterials January 1, 2005;26(3):297—302.

[121] Katoh K, Tanabe T, Yamauchi K. Novel approach to fabricate keratin sponge scaffolds with controlled pore size and porosity. Biomaterials August 1, 2004;25(18):4255–62.
[122] Peplow PV, Dias GJ. A study of the relationship between mass and physical strength of keratin bars in vivo. J Mater Sci Mater Med November 2004;15:1217–20.
[123] El-Kheir AA, Popescu C, Mowafi S, Salama M, El-Sayed H. Physico-chemical properties of keratin-polyvinyl alcohol composite. Fibers Polym March 2015;16:537–42.
[124] Zhao X, Lui YS, Choo CK, Sow WT, Huang CL, Ng KW, Tan LP, Loo JS. Calcium phosphate coated Keratin–PCL scaffolds for potential bone tissue regeneration. Mater Sci Eng C April 1, 2015;49:746–53.
[125] Safian MT, Umar K, Ibrahim MN. Synthesis and scalability of graphene and its derivatives: a journey towards sustainable and commercial material. J Clean Prod October 10, 2021;318:128603.
[126] Aluigi A, Vineis C, Varesano A, Mazzuchetti G, Ferrero F, Tonin C. Structure and properties of keratin/PEO blend nanofibres. Eur Polym J August 1, 2008;44(8):2465–75.
[127] Aluigi A, Varesano A, Montarsolo A, Vineis C, Ferrero F, Mazzuchetti G, Tonin C. Electrospinning of keratin/poly (ethylene oxide) blend nanofibers. J Appl Polym Sci April 15, 2007;104(2):863–70.
[128] Edwards A, Jarvis D, Hopkins T, Pixley S, Bhattarai N. Poly (ε-caprolactone)/keratin-based composite nanofibers for biomedical applications. J Biomed Mater Res B Appl Biomater January 2015;103(1):21–30.
[129] Horst M, Madduri S, Milleret V, Sulser T, Gobet R, Eberli D. A bilayered hybrid microfibrous PLGA–acellular matrix scaffold for hollow organ tissue engineering. Biomaterials February 1, 2013;34(5):1537–45.
[130] Gholipourmalekabadi M, Zhao S, Harrison BS, Mozafari M, Seifalian AM. Oxygen-generating biomaterials: a new, viable paradigm for tissue engineering? Trends Biotechnol December 1, 2016;34(12):1010–21.
[131] Lv X, Li Z, Chen S, Xie M, Huang J, Peng X, Yang R, Wang H, Xu Y, Feng C. Structural and functional evaluation of oxygenating keratin/silk fibroin scaffold and initial assessment of their potential for urethral tissue engineering. Biomaterials April 1, 2016;84:99–110.
[132] Kumar D, Babu G, Krishnan S. Study on mechanical and thermal properties of PCL blended graphene biocomposites. Polímeros July 4, 2019;29.
[133] Lee K, Kaplan D, editors. Tissue engineering I: scaffold systems for tissue engineering. Springer; October 6, 2006.
[134] Umar K, Adnan R. Biomass mediated green synthesis of ZnO/TiO2 nanocomposite and enhanced photocatalytic activity for the decolorization of rhodamine B under visible light. Key Eng Mater June 16, 2022;920:36–42.
[135] Mano JF, Silva GA, Azevedo HS, Malafaya PB, Sousa RA, Silva SS, Boesel LF, Oliveira JM, Santos TC, Marques AP, Neves NM. Natural origin biodegradable systems in tissue engineering and regenerative medicine: present status and some moving trends. J R Soc Interface December 22, 2007;4(17):999–1030.
[136] Curcio M, Blanco-Fernandez B, Diaz-Gomez L, Concheiro A, Alvarez-Lorenzo C. Hydrophobically modified keratin vesicles for GSH-responsive intracellular drug release. Bioconjugate Chem September 16, 2015;26(9):1900–7.
[137] Tomblyn S, Pettit Kneller EL, Walker SJ, Ellenburg MD, Kowalczewski CJ, Van Dyke M, Burnett L, Saul JM. Keratin hydrogel carrier system for simultaneous delivery of exogenous growth factors and muscle progenitor cells. J Biomed Mater Res B Appl Biomater July 2016;104(5):864–79.

[138] Saul JM, Ellenburg MD, de Guzman RC, Dyke MV. Keratin hydrogels support the sustained release of bioactive ciprofloxacin. J Biomed Mater Res September 15, 2011;98(4):544–53.
[139] Peyton CC, Keys T, Tomblyn S, Burmeister D, Beumer JH, Holleran JL, Sirintrapun J, Washburn S, Hodges SJ. Halofuginone infused keratin hydrogel attenuates adhesions in a rodent cecal abrasion model. J Surg Res December 1, 2012;178(2):545–52.
[140] Pastar I, Stojadinovic O, Yin NC, Ramirez H, Nusbaum AG, Sawaya A, Patel SB, Khalid L, Isseroff RR, Tomic-Canic M. Epithelialization in wound healing: a comprehensive review. Adv Wound Care July 1, 2014;3(7):445–64.
[141] Kim SY, Park BJ, Lee Y, Park NJ, Park KM, Hwang YS, Park KD. Human hair keratin-based hydrogels as dynamic matrices for facilitating wound healing. J Ind Eng Chem May 25, 2019;73:142–51.
[142] Gao F, Li W, Deng J, Kan J, Guo T, Wang B, Hao S. Recombinant human hair keratin nanoparticles accelerate dermal wound healing. ACS Appl Mater Interfaces April 30, 2019;11(20):18681–90.
[143] Sierpinski P, Garrett J, Ma J, Apel P, Klorig D, Smith T, Koman LA, Atala A, Van Dyke M. The use of keratin biomaterials derived from human hair for the promotion of rapid regeneration of peripheral nerves. Biomaterials January 1, 2008;29(1):118–28.

CHAPTER 9

Zein-based nanocomposites for tissue engineering

Mohammad Mushaf[1], Khalid Umar[2], Tabassum Parveen[3], Noor Haida Mohd Kaus[2] and Mohd Jameel[4]

[1]Institute of Eminence Teaching Fellow, Talent Development Center, Indian Institute of Science, Challakere, Karnataka, India; [2]School of Chemical Sciences, Universiti Sains Malaysia, Penang, Malaysia; [3]Department of Botany, Aligarh Muslim University, Aligarh, Uttar Pradesh, India; [4]Molecular Cancer Genetics & Translational Research Laboratory, Section of Genetics, Department of Zoology, Aligarh Muslim University, Aligarh, Uttar Pradesh, India

1. Introduction

Nanotechnology has introduced innovative ideas to enhance diverse fields, including tissue engineering (TE). The primary goal of TE is to regenerate damaged tissue using a ceramic or polymeric scaffold positioned at a specific anatomical site. However, these scaffolds face numerous challenges in replicating the cellular environment, such as establishing a vascular network, achieving the correct pore size to handle mechanical stress, and maintaining structural integrity, with the vascular network being a major obstacle [1,2]. To address the vascular network issue, it is essential to preload the scaffold with cells before placing it at the desired anatomical location [3]. Moreover, for the proliferation of preloaded cells, the scaffold must meet criteria for anatomical structure, functionality, esthetic requirements, mechanical properties, histocompatibility, degradation capacity, growth factors, minerals (e.g., iron as a bone TE cofactor), and even magnetic forces [1,4–7].

In the context of bone TE, the scaffold's material matrix should be derived from natural sources to capitalize on potential advantages in cell recognition near the damaged site without triggering rejection. Scaffolds are essential for cellular growth and proliferation in TE and provide chances to encapsulate extra characteristics. The synergistic combinations of synthetic, natural, and inorganic components have markedly improved the mechanical characteristics of zein-based scaffolds and extracellular matrices. For example, bovine collagen is a natural and promising scaffold matrix source,

Protein-Based Nanocomposites for Tissue Engineering
ISBN 978-0-323-99357-9
https://doi.org/10.1016/B978-0-323-99357-9.00013-2

exhibiting high biocompatibility. Unfortunately, its application in supporting body structures is limited due to its poor mechanical properties [8]. The advent of biopolymers has spurred the exploration and utilization of various techniques and monomer materials, creating versatile materials with diverse properties applicable across various uses. Notably, the biomaterial sector has experienced significant progress, as these developed materials with varied attributes contribute to advancements in medical and healthcare fields [9]. Spun fiber-derived polymers offer a versatile platform for fabricating filaments, sheets, and coaxial scaffolds, presenting favorable attributes for biomedical applications. These materials exhibit porosity, flexibility, and a substantial surface area, making them particularly advantageous for various medical purposes [10].

Zein is a useful tool in the biomedical field because of its malleability and chemical manipulability. Zein, particularly in micro- and nanoparticle form, exhibits promise as a metal particle substitute in medicinal and diagnostic applications. The remarkable physicochemical characteristics of the protein support its use as a substitute for current synthetic polymers, especially in applications involving the intracellular transport of genetic elements and therapeutic peptides. Biomedical applications have extensively utilized a diverse range of both natural and artificial polymers. These applications include heart valves, hard contact lenses, enteric pharmaceutical coatings, drug encapsulation, wound dressings, surgical meshes, nerve regeneration, and bone tissue regeneration. In these contexts, the unique properties of spun fiber-derived polymers contribute to developing biomedical devices and interventions that capitalize on their porous nature, flexibility, and ample surface area [11,12]. Naturally occurring polymers can be obtained from both plant and animal sources, and they are deemed environmentally friendly and sustainable alternatives to their synthetic counterparts. Some examples of naturally derived protein compounds that can be utilized in producing polymers are fibroin, which is the primary element of silk, collagen, keratin, gelatin, and zein [13,14].

Zein-based nanocomposites, which combine nanotechnology with biocompatibility, biodegradability, and customizable characteristics, are a ground-breaking approach to TE. These materials can significantly improve the development of scaffolds for regenerative medicine by resolving issues with the controlled release of bioactive compounds and the construction of vascular networks [15]. More than 80% of the total protein content in maize comes from the protein complex called zein, which is kept in the endosperm tissue of corn [16,17]. Zein-based compounds demonstrate the properties seen in intriguing natural materials, with exceptional resistance to heat, moisture, abrasion, and water. Moreover, the maize-derived zein protein may increase the longevity of biomolecules [15,16]. Zinc has exceptional mechanical qualities in addition to its structural stability, which makes it appropriate for use in film production [18].

Zein has found diverse applications, including its use in food packaging [19], delivery systems for medicine [20,21], wound dressing [22], and serving as a scaffold in TE [23–25]. In their study, Lin et al. [26] developed nanofiber scaffolds using Zein and collagen for wound healing applications. They incorporated berberine into the nanofiber membrane for its antibiotic properties. Another study by Lin et al. [27] utilized "green" food proteins as electrospun scaffolds for skin revitalization engineering. The findings indicated that green proteins like Soy and Zein created a conducive environment for skin cell cultures. Due to the inherent limitations, such as low tensile strength and poor stability in aqueous media in electrospun fibers of Zein and other protein biomaterials [28], considerable efforts have been directed toward enhancing the stability of these fibers. Unnithan et al. [29] addressed this by manufacturing composite scaffolds from Zein, polyurethane, and cellulose acetate designed for wound dressing. Consequently, current scientific endeavors are concentrated on exploring its innovative applications in biomedicine, particularly in areas such as the controlled delivery of biologically active compounds or for promoting tissue regeneration [30–32].

2. Zein protein

Zein is a protein frequently found in corn (Zea mays), between 44 and 79% of the endosperm's protein content. Using a solvent, Zein is extracted from maize gluten meal, a protein-rich residue of wet milling corn [17]. Usually, it is offered as a yellow fine powder [33]. The abundance of low-polar and nonpolar amino acid residues increases Zein's solubility [34,35]. Its hydrophobic component makes it soluble in solutions with ethanol concentrations ranging from 60% to 95% or in pH 11 aqueous alkaline solutions, giving it an isoelectric point of 6.2 [36]. Leucine and alanine are responsible for zein's hydrophobic properties. Zein is also greaseproof and has a low permeability to water vapor. Zein comes in four different varieties: α-, β-, γ-, and δ-Zein. 80% of total zein comprises α-zein, while the proportion of β and γ-zein is usually between 10 and 15% [37]. The remaining is δ-zein; α-zein ranges in molecular weight from 18 to 27 kDa, β-zein is roughly

Table 9.1 Lists a few of the Zein protein's significant characteristics.

Property	Value	References
Denaturation temperature	80.32–87.1°C	[40]
The α-zein glass transition temperature	165°C	[18]
The point at which α-zein thermally degrades	280°C	[18]
The molecular weight of α-zein	22–24 kDa	[38]
The molecular weight of β-zein	17 kDa	[38]
The molecular weight of δ-zein	10 kDa	[38]
The molecular mass of γ-zein	18–27 kDa	[38]
Degree of polymerization of α-zein	210–245	[18]
The isoelectric point of α-zein pH	6.2	[18,41]
Partial specific volume of α-zein	0.771	[18]
Zein flavor	Flavorless	[40]
Zein color	Yellowish	[40]
Zein odor	Odorless	[40]
Zein composition	Glutamine, 21%–26% Leucine 20% Proline 10% Alanine	[42]

17 kDa, and δ-zein is between 22 and 24 kDa [38,39]. Table 9.1 shows some Zein protein's significant characteristics.

3. Methods of extraction of zein protein

The literature reports several techniques for zein extraction. Here are a few of them.

1. The first method involves extracting zein using an alcohol-water solvent system for commercial zein production at a constant temperature. The concentration of aqueous alcohol is varied from 2% to 60% to attain the maximum solubility of zein. Higher temperatures are required when more than 65% of zein is needed. The denaturation of zein protein was also reduced by using acetone, dioxane, and dioxolane instead of aqueous alcohol [43].
2. The aqueous solvent method, which involves using acidified or alkalized water with a pH greater than 1 or 12, has converted insoluble amines into soluble salts. Although this approach has proven to be effective, it has some drawbacks. For instance, alkaline solutions can lead to significant degradation of zein protein and require substantial quantities

of solvents. In addition, the formation of a zein/phosphatidate complex with lecithin, which exhibits emulsifying properties across a range of pH levels, has been reported [44].

3. Some studies have reported successful production of water-soluble zein through enzymatic hydrolysis using alkalase, while other enzymes have demonstrated limited success in achieving this outcome [45].
4. Gelation qualities serve as a guide for selecting a solvent for zein extraction. Several parameters, including solvent type, concentration, temperature, pH, and agitation, can affect the length of the gelation process. Achieving high solution stability for commercial purposes involves using an organic solvent, such as a combination of acetone and water with 5% formaldehyde [46].
5. A hybrid strategy combining solvent and enzymatic extraction techniques was used in a recent study. A commercial approach employing 88% aqueous 2-propanol was compared with an alternative method that used either 70% aqueous ethanol (v/v) or 70% aqueous 2-propanol (w/w) in the study. Notably, in this experiment, the pretreatment of samples with a combination of cellulose and pectinase enzymes did not affect the amount of zein produced [47].

3.1 Characterization of zein

The complete understanding of the zein protein structure remains elusive despite the application of various methods in the past. However, distinct molecular weight fractions of zein have been identified using extraction, electrophoresis, and chromatography techniques. These findings suggest the existence of two major protein structures ($M = 19$ and 22 kDa) indicative of zein's heterogeneity [48].

Zein's stability is attributed to hydrogen bonds, and its structure exhibits a helical wheel shape with nine homologous repeating units arranged antiparallelly. Subsequent research employing the small-angle X-ray scattering technique (SAXS) has revealed that the monomer structure of zein consists of 10 folded helical segments. Contrarily, a recent study contends that the zein structure comprises nine α-helices organized into superhelical structures, each consisting of three helices stacked end to end [49].

4. Zein as a biopolymer

The heightened production of petroleum-derived polymers in recent years has resulted in environmental harm, primarily because of their resistance to decomposition. Microplastics, anticipated to reach an estimated 12,000 million tons by 2050, have become the ocean's predominant pollutants. In response to this issue, bioplastics have emerged as a promising alternative. They stand out due to their nontoxic nature, renewable origin, compatibility with living organisms, and ability to undergo biodegradation [50]. Zein has found extensive applications as a biopolymer across various industrial and scientific domains, with the electrospinning method being employed to produce zein films and fibers. The electrospinning protocol includes utilizing a 70% concentrated ethanol-water solution, applying a 15–20 kV voltage, and positioning a plate at a 10–12 cm distance to collect the resulting fibers. A syringe pump achieves a pressure of about 1.244 KPa and an outlet stream of approximately 0.9 mL/h (less than 3 g/h). Subsequently, the fibers undergo further drying in a desiccator [18].

The nanofibers generated through this process offer numerous advantages, such as a high surface area-to-volume ratio, making them highly attractive for various applications. These fibers are easily functionalized, allow for straightforward material combination, entail relatively low startup costs, and facilitate deposition onto other substrates [51].

Characterizing zein-based fibers commonly involves scanning electron microscopy (SEM) and Fourier transform infrared spectroscopy (FTIR). SEM aids in visualizing the fiber diameter, ranging from as small as 237 nm to as large as 830 nm. The morphology of zein varies with its content, exhibiting ribbon-like structures or, in the case of cylindrical structures, experiencing flat structures due to the impact of a magnetic field. When using FTIR to characterize zein-based films, specific peaks are observed at 3294–3350/cm, corresponding to –OH functional groups. In addition, peaks at 2968–2922/cm represent C–H groups, 1538–1546/cm signify N–H, 1649–1653/cm denote C=O, and 1428–1451/cm indicate C–N functional groups [52,53] (Fig. 9.1).

4.1 The significance of zeins in tissue engineering

Various biomolecules, including proteins, polysaccharides, and proteoglycans, constitute the extracellular matrix (ECM), supporting cell attachment, proliferation, differentiation, and migration. Cells must execute similar functions in novel and artificial environments, such as reconstructing lost tissue or repairing injured tissue. Due to its cost-effectiveness and versatile fiber production technique, the electrospinning method proves helpful in generating the ECM matrix. A synergistic effect can be achieved

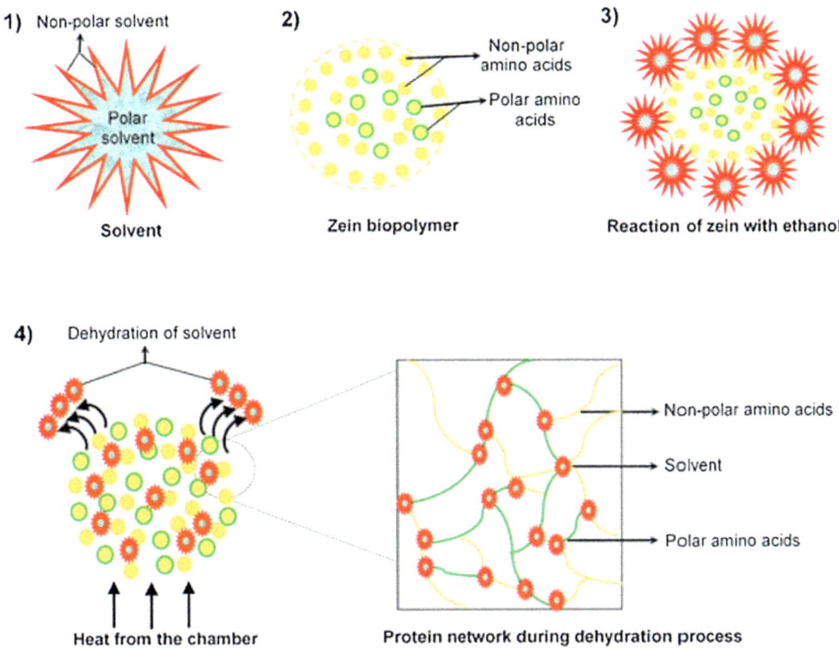

Figure 9.1 Zein biopolymer components and dehydration reaction [53].

by blending nanofibers from natural and synthetic sources [23]. In contrast, synthetic materials maintain suitable mechanical stability without cell binding and acid generation. Throughout the biodegradation process, natural-based fibers may experience a reduction in mechanical strength. Conversely, nanofibers derived from animal sources in the ECM may indicate immune response or disease transmission. Consequently, researchers have scrutinized plant-based nanofibers, revealing that they offer more advantages than their animal-based counterparts [54]. In TE, zein was selected due to its resistance to microorganisms, flexibility, compatibility with the human body, and biodegradability. Electrospun zein has demonstrated antibacterial activity along with these characteristics. Scaffolds can be created using other fibers such as cellulose acetate, polyurethane, and gum arabic. To address the fragility issue in skin regeneration, polycaprolactone (PCL) has been suggested. Furthermore, PCL offers biocompatibility, nontoxicity, and high mechanical strength. For instance, Pedram Rad and colleagues developed and thoroughly characterized a nanocomposite scaffold for skin TE, incorporating polycaprolactone (PCL), zein, and gum arabic [55,56]. In conjunction with zein and gum arabic, polycaprolactone is a promising solution for developing skin regeneration and support scaffolds. According to a study by Pedram Rad, the porosity of these scaffolds is greater than 77%, which is advantageous for cell infiltration. In addition, including cyanogenic glycosides in gum arabic imparts antimicrobial properties and increases the hydrophilicity of composite scaffolds. The hydrophilicity of scaffolds is essential for improving cell survival and proliferation. Synthetic polymers have a low affinity for cells because of their low hydrophilicity and lack of cell recognition sites. In contrast, polymers derived from natural sources exhibit better cell affinities because of their interactions with membrane receptors. Blending zein with poly (glycerol sebacate) for producing fibers via electrospinning technology suggests that zein may be suitable for cardiac tissue-engineering applications [57,58]. Researchers have suggested using composites made from graphene oxide, TiO_2, carbon nanotubes, and hydroxyapatite to enhance the mechanical strength of scaffolds [59—61]. The addition of nanoparticles such as hydroxyapatite has also been shown to increase the regeneration rate of the scaffold and reduce its breakdown rate. Furthermore, the combination of zein and hydroxyapatite has been found to improve osteoblast function [25]. Hydroxyapatite (HA), a component of this combination, contains vancomycin, an antibiotic with a negative charge that the release of HA can control. Osteoblast differentiation and proliferation are improved when growth factors are incorporated into nanofibers. Dexamethasone (DEX) and recombinant human bone morphogenetic protein 2 (rhBMP-2) enhance the differentiation efficacy of TE cells. Maintaining a stable release of these factors [62]. The creation of scaffolds can be achieved through various means, one of which is electrospinning, which offers the utmost versatility. Other methods, such as melt-drawing, centrifugal spinning, freeze-drying, and 3D extrusion, can also customize scaffold properties. Centrifugal spinning is a technique for producing gelatin-based scaffolds, where gelatin, a natural polymer derived from the hydrolysis of collagen, is employed. Gelatin is prone to rapid degradation due to its poor water resistance. Still, the hydrophobicity of zein can enhance its properties, resulting in a material that can be utilized for various purposes, including drug delivery, hernia repair, and TE. Studies have shown that a homogeneous blend of gelatin and zein (at a ratio of 1:4) can effectively improve the tensile and hydrophobic properties of materials, as demonstrated by a water contact angle of 115 degrees. The study used human fibroblasts to evaluate cell viability, revealing a slight toxic effect. The scaffolds were also tested for their ability to release the medication berberine, showing a sustained release

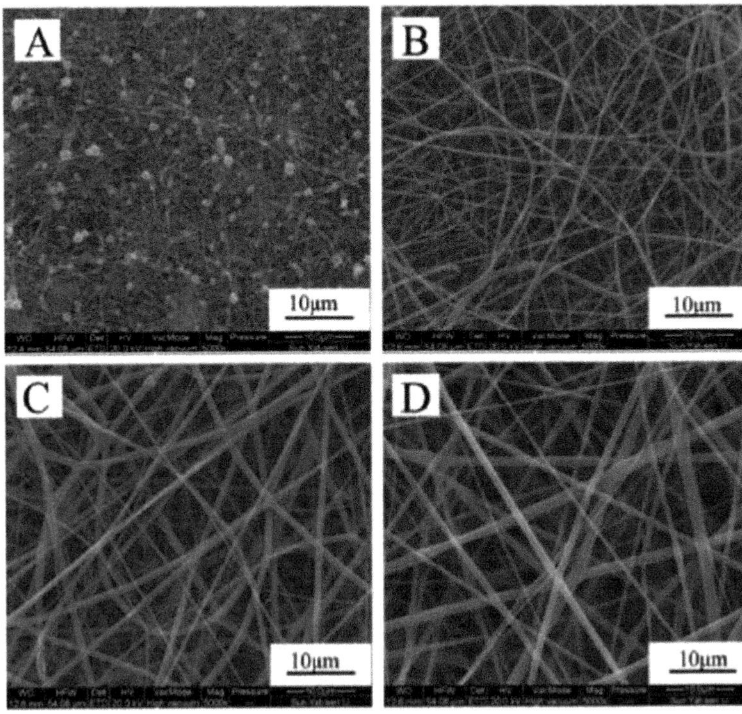

Figure 9.2 Displays the morphological analysis of electrospun nanofibers, including zein (A), zein/gelatin-1 (B), zein/gelatin-2 (C), and zein/gelatin-3 (D) [63].

rate over 15 days [35]. The coelectrospinning process can also create scaffolds based on a zein/gelatin complex, which offers several advantages. For instance, adding gelatin increased the elastic modulus and hydrophilicity of the resulting nanofibers. However, high concentrations of gelatin can lead to the formation of weak membranes. Electrospinning regulates various properties, such as porosity, surface, cytocompatibility, mechanical strength, fiber form, and cellular adherence [42]. The results indicated that the scaffolds exhibited a smooth and homogeneous appearance, except for A, which displayed a beaded structure, as depicted in Fig. 9.2 [63].

Poly(hydroxybutyrate) (PHB), a biodegradable thermoplastic produced by bacteria and compatible with the human body, finds applications in packaging and orthopedic wound treatment. To manufacture fibers, a blend of poly(3-hydroxybutyrate-co-4-hydroxybutyrate) (P(3HB-co-4HB)) and zein was electrospun in N, N-dimethylformamide. Achieving ultrathin fibers ranging from 60 to 650 nm, the tensile strength increased from 4.8 to 7.1 MPa, and elongation at break improved from 15% to 69% with varying P(3HB-co-4HB) content (20%–80%) [64]. In recent studies, zein-based electrospun fibers incorporating bioactive glass with antibacterial properties were developed. Addressing zein's inherent mechanical limitations, the researchers combined inorganic substances, such as bioactive Cu-based glasses, to create composite materials with enhanced mechanical characteristics. Testing these materials in TE applications revealed positive outcomes in cell culture experiments with MG-63 and C2C12 cells [65]. The fiber mats containing both forms of bioactive glass promoted cell proliferation and growth. In addition, the inorganic composite scaffolds exhibited antibacterial properties when tested against *Staphylococcus* aureus and *Escherichia coli* bacteria. Despite Cu's antibacterial characteristics, it had minimal impact on cell behavior [65–67].

Natural composites can also be incorporated into zein scaffolds. Aloe vera, for instance, has a long history of application in healing skin problems and burns. Aloe vera facilitates collagen synthesis and enhances cellular adhesion and proliferation. Moreover, it exhibits antibiotic and antifungal activities against *Streptococcus pyogenes*, *Enterococcus faecalis*, *Candida albicans*, and *Staphylococcus aureus* [68]. Consequently, a deeper understanding of zein's role as a carrier could pave the way for introducing new bioactive molecules, contributing to better comprehension of their action processes. Zein has found utility as a wall material in nanoencapsulation within the pharmaceutical, food, and pesticide industries [69].

5. Zein-based drug delivery systems

Drugs are organic compounds utilized for treating, managing, and preventing various diseases. The demand for drugs with enhanced therapeutic efficacy has increased significantly, and bioinformatics has proven helpful in addressing this issue. However, challenges such as solubility, stability, and toxicity, persist. To mitigate these challenges, scientists have sought to improve the efficiency of drugs by developing a carrier that releases the compound at a controlled rate with low toxicity. This can be achieved through protein-based biopolymers, which possess advantages such as ease of manufacture and a high loading capacity. Common proteins used for this purpose include albumin, casein, gelatin, keratin, silk protein, and zein. Despite these advantages, biopolymers can undergo structural changes, leading to loss of protein function and rapid degradation [70].

Breast cancer is the most commonly occurring form of cancer in women. In its early stages, the cancer remains confined to the local area, but once it metastasizes, it spreads throughout the body. Sadly, 90% of breast cancer deaths are caused by the metastasis process. Fortunately, there have been advancements in treating this disease by using new drug delivery systems containing zein and hyaluronic acid. The combination of zein with hyaluronic acid has successfully delivered honokiol, a compound with anticarcinogenic, antiinflammatory, antioxidant, and neuroprotective properties. Honokiol acts on CD44 receptors, which are overexpressed on cancer cells. The success of the hyaluronic acid-zein-honokiol complex has been shown to reduce tumor growth by 77.3%, depending on the size of the tumor, which is three times more effective than free honokiol alone, with only 25.8% tumor inhibition [71]. Zein is commonly used as a natural excipient in drug delivery systems due to its biocompatibility, safety, affordability, adhesive properties, ease of molding, and flexibility. For example, mixing zein with the biologically active compound curcumin enhances its antioxidant and antiinflammatory properties. Curcumin's poor bioavailability, caused by low water solubility, chemical instability, and poor pharmacokinetics, has been addressed through various packing methods such as microcapsules, micelles, and inorganic nanoparticles. When combined with zein-poly (sulfobetaine methacrylate), curcumin showed increased stability, cytotoxicity against cancer cells, and improved pharmacokinetics. However, the resulting micelles had low macrophage activation and prolonged circulation time (over 72 h in mice). Still, they were sensitive to pH changes, making nanoencapsulation a potential alternative due to its pH stability [72]. To improve the stability of zein-based nanoparticles coated with curcumin, their dimensions have been reported to be around 65.17 ± 0.32 nm. However, it is possible to recoat these nanoparticles with sodium caseinate and sodium alginate to enhance their stability and increase their size to approximately 200.67 ± 0.65 nm [73]. Resveratrol, similar to curcumin, is utilized to prevent and treat gastrointestinal tract cancer; however, it has low solubility and bioavailability [74]. To overcome this issue, nanoencapsulation can be used to improve oral intake. Zein and pectin-based shells prevent aggregation caused by pH concentration, high salt concentration, and high temperatures. Zein-pectin core/shell nanoparticles loaded with resveratrol were produced through antisolvent precipitation and electrostatic deposition techniques. In addition, the encapsulation of resveratrol in biopolymer-based nanoparticles significantly enhanced its antioxidant activity [75].

5.1 Utilizing zein-based nanoparticles in the food industry

Nanomaterials in food products, known as nanofoods, may offer elevated nutritional value compared with conventional foods, but it also poses the risk of potential toxicity. Notably, zein, a protein derived from corn, has been deemed safe by the FDA as a GRAS (Generally Recognized as Safe) additive and is not associated with toxicity. As a result, zein-based nanoparticles are being utilized to deliver flavor compounds, food colors, and bioactive compounds [69]. Among these compounds, cinnamaldehyde, a flavor compound of interest in the food industry, displays antioxidant properties; however, it is susceptible to moisture, oxygen, light, and high temperatures [76]. Karim et al. employed zein as a wall material to encapsulate cinnamaldehyde within hydrophobic nanofibers created using a needleless electrospinning method to address this issue. Incorporating cinnamaldehyde nanocapsules into sausages has decreased the use of nitrite while concurrently enhancing the hardness of the sausages from 9.76 to 15.2 N during storage and reducing humidity. In addition, the nanoencapsulated cinnamaldehyde has exhibited antibacterial activity against *E. coli* O157:H7 and *S. aureus* PTCC 1337 [77]. Developing edible packaging using zein-starch films in a two-layer configuration, as demonstrated by Chen et al. can replace traditional plastic packaging materials. The improved mechanical and barrier properties of zein-starch films are attributed to the hydrogen bonds formed between the hydroxyl groups of starch and amino (carboxyl) zein molecules. This innovative edible film has significant potential for food packaging applications [78].

5.2 Application of zein as a carrier for pesticides

Zein has found a variety of applications, particularly in the packaging of pesticides and fertilizers. As the demand for agri-food products grows due to population expansion, there is an increased need for pesticides to protect crops. To minimize harmful side effects, there is a pressing need for pesticides that can be delivered in a controlled manner. Zein-based pesticide nanocarriers offer a solution by facilitating delivery through the root system and foliage, thereby reducing water and soil pollution [78]. A group of 16-membered macrocyclic lactones called avermectins, which are effective against nematodes, mites, and insects, are encapsulated in nanocarriers through a multistep process [79]. First, zein is phosphorylated with sodium caseinate to enhance its hydrophilicity. Then, avermectin is loaded onto the phosphorylated zein by mixing it with ethanol. Adding a modified carboxymethyl cellulose (CMC) solution via diallyldimethylammonium chloride (DMDAAC) improves the stability, UV resistance, and adhesion of avermectin-loaded phosphorylated zein [80]. DMDAAC is used to modify CMC because it cannot be directly used with phosphorylated zein [80]. Natamycin, a bacterial molecule that inhibits mycotoxin generation and is produced by a soil bacterium, is used in small amounts to control yeast and mold, even after fruit harvest. However, its main drawback is low photostability, making it expensive and limiting its availability and applicability. The stability of the zein core encapsulating natamycin is enhanced by the shell of carboxymethylchitosan, which provides photostability. The coated natamycin has a pH range of 2.0–8.0, and its photostability increases by 3.12 times [81].

5.3 Potential use of zein in bandages

Zein is also modified to make a zein/chitosan composite bandage that includes ellagic acid. Ellagic acid confers antiinflammatory, antioxidant, and anticarcinogenic qualities to the bandage [82]. The chitosan was diluted in a solution of 3.25% glycerol and 3% acetic acid as part of a synthetic technique developed by Tavares and associates. The zein was then submerged in a mixture of 1.2% ellagic acid and 70% ethanol. After 5 days of stirring the resultant solution, the solvent evaporated at 25°C. This procedure successfully created an antibacterial bandage resistant to *Staphylococcus aureus* and *Pseudomonas aeruginosa*. It was discovered as a result that zein was essential to the release of ellagic acid [83].

5.4 Zein's role as a coating material

Zein is a simple, quick coating solution that shows improved heat, humidity, and abrasion resistance when applied as a coating material. Zein has shown itself to be a flexible protective coating material. It was first used to improve the visual appeal of quickly released tablets or to disguise their taste while remaining economical [84]. The coating technique did not affect the core hardness in comparative research comparing the hardness of five common film-coating materials. Notably, tablets coated with zein film were more durable than those with hydroxypropyl methyl cellulose or cellulose acetate phthalate. A surfactant-free aqueous pseudolatex of zein coating for tablets and pellets was also developed as part of the innovation. The preservation effect of methyl or propyl paraben increased film coat flexibility. Metoprolol, a water-soluble drug, was included using an aqueous dispersion and an 80% ethanol solution for tablets coated with plasticized zein film. The resulting coated tablets performed similarly to PEG 400-glycerol plasticized film tablets regarding moisture sorption, erosion, and water vapor permeability [85,86].

6. Conclusions

This review covered the investigation of nanocomposites based on zein and its many roles in TE and nanotechnology applications. Zein is a biopolymer that is considered flexible. Its primary uses are as a scaffold for cellular support and as a wall material for encasing substances sensitive to the environment. In TE applications, scaffolds provide the ability to encapsulate extra characteristics in addition to promoting cellular development and proliferation. It has proven possible to improve the mechanical properties of scaffolds or extracellular matrices (ECM) by carefully combining synthetic, natural, or inorganic components. These improved scaffolds, first made to support cells, can now be filled with biological substances to promote cell development. Plant-derived proteins—especially zein—are perfect for biomedical applications because of their biocompatibility, safety, and adjustable characteristics.

Zein protein was first used in medicines, mainly for edible coatings, but due to its many uses, including its solubility and capacity to create films, its uses have greatly expanded. Zein has received significant validation in various fields, including drug administration, targeted therapy, imaging, theranostics, and tissue regeneration. It is an entirely natural, biodegradable, and reasonably priced material.

Zein is a beneficial tool in the biomedical area because of its ability to shape and manipulate chemicals. Zein can potentially replace metal particles used in many therapeutic and diagnostic applications, especially in micro- and nanoparticles. Zein protein has remarkable physical and chemical characteristics that make it a prospective candidate to replace synthetic polymers already in use for the intracellular delivery of genetic elements and therapeutic peptides.

Acknowledgments

The authors appreciate the Research Supporting Project (304/PKIMIA/6315580) by Universiti Sains Malaysia.

References

[1] Goranov V, Shelyakova T, De Santis R, Haranava Y, Makhaniok A, Gloria A, Tampieri A, Russo A, Kon E, Marcacci M, Ambrosio L. 3D patterning of cells in magnetic scaffolds for tissue engineering. Sci Rep February 10, 2020;10(1):2289.

[2] Oladapo BI, Obisesan OB, Oluwole B, Adebiyi VA, Usman H, Khan A. Mechanical characterization of a polymeric scaffold for bone implant. J Mater Sci July, 2020;55:9057−69.

[3] Bhatia S. Natural polymer drug delivery systems: nanoparticles, plants, and algae. Springer; September 23, 2016.

[4] Mehrian M, Lambrechts T, Papantoniou I, Geris L. Computational modeling of human mesenchymal stromal cell proliferation and extra-cellular matrix production in 3d porous scaffolds in a perfusion bioreactor: the effect of growth factors. Front Bioeng Biotechnol April 29, 2020;8:376.

[5] Li H, Pan S, Xia P, Chang Y, Fu C, Kong W, Yu Z, Wang K, Yang X, Qi Z. Advances in the application of gold nanoparticles in bone tissue engineering. J Biol Eng December, 2020;14:1−5.

[6] Dhivya S, Keshav Narayan A, Logith Kumar R, Viji Chandran S, Vairamani M, Selvamurugan N. Proliferation and differentiation of mesenchymal stem cells on scaffolds containing chitosan, calcium polyphosphate and pigeonite for bone tissue engineering. Cell Prolif February, 2018;51(1):e12408.

[7] Zhu Y, Yang Q, Yang M, Zhan X, Lan F, He J, Gu Z, Wu Y. Protein corona of magnetic hydroxyapatite scaffold improves cell proliferation via activation of mitogen-activated protein kinase signaling pathway. ACS Nano April 25, 2017;11(4):3690−704.

[8] A.M. Cícero, J.P. Issa, S. Feldman. Third generation matrices in bone tissue engineering.

[9] Rahman M, Dip TM, Haase T, Truong YB, Le TC, Houshyar S. Fabrication of zein-based fibrous scaffolds for biomedical applications—areview. Macromol Mater Eng 2023:2300175.

[10] Dos Santos DM, Correa DS, Medeiros ES, Oliveira JE, Mattoso LH. Advances in functional polymer nanofibers: from spinning fabrication techniques to recent biomedical applications. ACS Appl Mater Interf September 16, 2020;12(41): 45673−701.

[11] Madhumanchi S, Srichana T, Domb AJ. Polymeric biomaterials. Biomed Mater 2021:49−100.

[12] Angra V, Sehgal R, Kaur M, Gupta R. Commercialization of bionanocomposites. In: Bionanocomposites in tissue engineering and regenerative medicine. Woodhead Publishing; January 1, 2021. p. 587−610.

[13] DeFrates K, Markiewicz T, Gallo P, Rack A, Weyhmiller A, Jarmusik B, Hu X. Protein polymer-based nanoparticles: fabrication and medical applications. Int J Mol Sci June 9, 2018;19(6):1717.

[14] Song R, Murphy M, Li C, Ting K, Soo C, Zheng Z. Current development of biodegradable polymeric materials for biomedical applications. Drug Des Dev Ther September, 2018;24:3117−45.

[15] Tortorella S, Maturi M, Buratti VV, Vozzolo G, Locatelli E, Sambri L, Franchini MC. Zein as a versatile biopolymer: different shapes for different biomedical applications. RSC Adv 2021;11(62):39004−26.

[16] Li C, Song R. The regulation of zein biosynthesis in maize endosperm. Theor Appl Genet May, 2020;133(5):1443−53.

[17] Jaski AC, Schmitz F, Horta RP, Cadorin L, da Silva BJ, Andreaus J, Paes MC, Riegel-Vidotti IC, Zimmermann LM. Zein-a plant-based material of growing importance: new perspectives for innovative uses. Ind Crop Prod October 15, 2022;186:115250.

[18] Corradini E, Curti PS, Meniqueti AB, Martins AF, Rubira AF, Muniz EC. Recent advances in food-packing, pharmaceutical and biomedical applications of zein and zein-based materials. Int J Mol Sci December 4, 2014;15(12):22438–70.
[19] Kashiri M, Cerisuelo JP, Domínguez I, López-Carballo G, Muriel-Gallet V, Gavara R, Hernández-Muñoz P. Zein films and coatings as carriers and release systems of *Zataria multiflora Boiss* essential oil for antimicrobial food packaging. Food Hydrocoll September 1, 2017;70:260–8.
[20] Fereshteh Z, Fathi M, Bagri A, Boccaccini AR. Preparation and characterization of aligned porous PCL/zein scaffolds as drug delivery systems via improved unidirectional freeze-drying method. Mater Sci Eng C November 1, 2016;68:613–22.
[21] Yang JM, Zha LS, Yu DG, Liu J. Coaxial electrospinning with acetic acid for preparing ferulic acid/zein composite fibers with improved drug release profiles. Colloids Surf B Biointerfaces February 1, 2013;102:737–43.
[22] Dashdorj U, Reyes MK, Unnithan AR, Tiwari AP, Tumurbaatar B, Park CH, Kim CS. Fabrication and characterization of electrospun zein/Ag nanocomposite mats for wound dressing applications. Int J Biol Macromol September 1, 2015;80:1–7.
[23] Paliwal R, Palakurthi S. Zein in controlled drug delivery and tissue engineering. J Contr Release September 10, 2014;189:108–22.
[24] He M, Jiang H, Wang R, Xie Y, Zhao C. Fabrication of metronidazole loaded poly (ε-caprolactone)/zein core/shell nanofiber membranes via coaxial electrospinning for guided tissue regeneration. J Colloid Interface Sci March 15, 2017;490:270–8.
[25] Shahbazarab Z, Teimouri A, Chermahini AN, Azadi M. Fabrication and characterization of nanobiocomposite scaffold of zein/chitosan/nanohydroxyapatite prepared by freeze-drying method for bone tissue engineering. Int J Biol Macromol March 1, 2018;108:1017–27.
[26] Lin J, Li C, Zhao Y, Hu J, Zhang LM. Co-electrospun nanofibrous membranes of collagen and zein for wound healing. ACS Appl Mater Interface February 22, 2012;4(2):1050–7.
[27] Lin L, Perets A, Har-el YE, Varma D, Li M, Lazarovici P, Woerdeman DL, Lelkes PI. Alimentary 'green'proteins as electrospun scaffolds for skin regenerative engineering. J Tiss Eng Regenerat Med December, 2013;7(12):994–1008.
[28] Jiang Q, Yang Y. Water-stable electrospun zein fibers for potential drug delivery. J Biomater Sci January 1, 2011;22(10):1393–408.
[29] Unnithan AR, Gnanasekaran G, Sathishkumar Y, Lee YS, Kim CS. Electrospun antibacterial polyurethane–cellulose acetate–zein composite mats for wound dressing. Carbohydr Polym February 15, 2014;102:884–92.
[30] Kurakula M, Naveen NR. Electrospraying: a facile technology unfolding the chitosan based drug delivery and biomedical applications. Eur Polym J March 15, 2021;147:110326.
[31] Rial-Hermida MI, Rey-Rico A, Blanco-Fernandez B, Carballo-Pedrares N, Byrne EM, Mano JF. Recent progress on polysaccharide-based hydrogels for controlled delivery of therapeutic biomolecules. ACS Biomater Sci Eng June 17, 2021;7(9):4102–27.
[32] Lawton JW. Zein: a history of processing and use. Cereal Chem January, 2002;79(1):1–8.
[33] Laelorspoen N, Wongsasulak S, Yoovidhya T, Devahastin S. Microencapsulation of Lactobacillus acidophilus in zein–alginate core–shell microcapsules via electrospraying. J Funct Food March 1, 2014;7:342–9.
[34] Li M, Zheng H, Lin M, Zhu W, Zhang J. Characterization of the protein and peptide of excipient zein by the multi-enzyme digestion coupled with nano-LC-MS/MS. Food Chem August 15, 2020;321:126712.

[35] Mamidi N, Romo IL, Gutiérrez HM, Barrera EV, Elías-Zúñiga A. Development of forcespun fiber-aligned scaffolds from gelatin–zein composites for potential use in tissue engineering and drug release. MRS Communicat September, 2018;8(3):885–92.
[36] Moradkhannejhad L, Abdouss M, Nikfarjam N, Mazinani S, Heydari V. Electrospinning of zein/propolis nanofibers; antimicrobial properties and morphology investigation. J Mater Sci Mater Med November, 2018;29:1.
[37] Coleman CE, Herman EM, Takasaki K, Larkins BA. The maize gamma-zein sequesters alpha-zein and stabilizes its accumulation in protein bodies of transgenic tobacco endosperm. Plant Cell December 1, 1996;8(12):2335–45.
[38] Raza A, Hayat U, Bilal M, Iqbal HM, Wang JY. Zein-based micro-and nanoconstructs and biologically therapeutic cues with multi-functionalities for oral drug delivery systems. J Drug Deliv Sci Technol August 1, 2020;58:101818.
[39] Pérez-Guzmán CJ, Castro-Muñoz R. A review of zein as a potential biopolymer for tissue engineering and nanotechnological applications. Processes October 29, 2020;8(11):1376.
[40] Chen Y, Ye R, Xu H. Physicochemical properties of zein-based films by electrophoretic deposition using indium tin oxide electrodes: vertical and horizontal electric fields. Int J Food Prop May 3, 2016;19(5):945–57.
[41] Gu J, Xin Z, Meng X, Sun S, Qiao Q, Deng H. Recovering high value-added substances from corn distillers dried grains with solubles: a semi-continuous countercurrent downstream processing method. J Chem Technol Biotechnol 2016;91:1327–38.
[42] Demir M, Ramos Rivera L, Silva R, Nazhat SN, Boccaccini AR. Zein-based composites in biomedical applications. J Biomed Mater Res June, 2017;105(6):1656–65.
[43] Conroy JM, Esen A. An enzyme-linked immunosorbent assay for zein and other proteins using unconventional solvents for antigen adsorption. Anal Biochem February 15, 1984;137(1):182–7.
[44] Esen A, Conroy JM, Wang SZ. A simple and rapid dot-immunobinding assay for zein and other prolamins. Anal Biochem July 15, 1983;132(2):462–7.
[45] Landry J. Heterogenetics of corn grain glutelins, elective extraction and amino acid composition of the three isolated fractions. Bull Soc Chem Biol 1970;52:1021–37.
[46] Esen A. Separation of alcohol-soluble proteins (zeins) from maize into three fractions by differential solubility. Plant Physiol March 1, 1986;80(3):623–7.
[47] Mertz ET, Bates LS, Nelson OE. Mutant gene that changes protein composition and increases lysine content of maize endosperm. Science July 17, 1964;145(3629):279–80.
[48] Wang G, Han J, Meng X, Kang SS, Liu X, Sun YE, Luo Q, Ye K. Zein-based nanoparticles improve the therapeutic efficacy of a TrkB agonist toward Alzheimer's disease. ACS Chem Neurosci August 16, 2023;14(17):3249–64.
[49] Matsushima N, Danno GI, Takezawa H, Izumi Y. Three-dimensional structure of maize α-zein proteins studied by small-angle X-ray scattering. Biochim Biophys Acta Protein Struct Mol Enzymol April 25, 1997;1339(1):14–22.
[50] Tsung KL, Ilavsky J, Padua GW. Formation and characterization of zein-based oleogels. J Agric Food Chem October 13, 2020;68(46):13276–81.
[51] Fathi-Achachelouei M, Knopf-Marques H, Ribeiro da Silva CE, Barthès J, Bat E, Tezcaner A, Vrana NE. Use of nanoparticles in tissue engineering and regenerative medicine. Front Bioeng Biotechnol May 24, 2019;7:113.
[52] Wu Z, Li J, Zhang X, Li Y, Wei D, Tang L, Deng S, Liu G. Rational fabrication of folate-conjugated zein/soy lecithin/carboxymethyl chitosan core–shell nanoparticles for delivery of docetaxel. ACS Omega April 7, 2022;7(15):13371–81.
[53] Babatunde QO, Byun YH. Soil stabilization using zein biopolymer. Sustainability January 21, 2023;15(3):2075.

[54] Wu Y, Luo Y, Wang Q. Antioxidant and antimicrobial properties of essential oils encapsulated in zein nanoparticles prepared by liquid–liquid dispersion method. LWT-food Sci Technol October 1, 2012;48(2):283–90.
[55] Kale A, Zhu F, Cheryan M. Separation of high-value products from ethanol extracts of corn by chromatography. Ind Crop Prod June 1, 2007;26(1):44–53.
[56] Khan MA, Ahmad A, Umar K, Nabi SA. Synthesis, characterization, and biological applications of nanocomposites for the removal of heavy metals and dyes. Ind Eng Chem Res January 14, 2015;54(1):76–82.
[57] Abdullah A, Abdullah AZ, Ahmed M, Khan J, Shahadat M, Umar K, Alim MA. A review on recent developments and progress in sustainable acrolein production through catalytic dehydration of bio-renewable glycerol. J Clean Prod March 20, 2022;341:130876.
[58] Vogt L, Liverani L, Roether JA, Boccaccini AR. Electrospun zein fibers incorporating poly (glycerol sebacate) for soft tissue engineering. Nanomaterials March 8, 2018;8(3):150.
[59] Babaei M, Ghaee A, Nourmohammadi J. Poly (sodium 4-styrene sulfonate)-modified hydroxyapatite nanoparticles in zein-based scaffold as a drug carrier for vancomycin. Mater Sci Eng C July 1, 2019;100:874–85.
[60] Mir NA, Haque MM, Khan A, Umar K, Muneer M, Vijayalakshmi S. Semiconductor mediated photocatalysed reaction of two selected organic compounds in aqueous suspensions of Titanium dioxide. J Adv Oxid Technol July 1, 2012;15(2):380–91.
[61] Umar K, Mfarrej MF, Rahman QI, Zuhaib M, Khan A, Zia Q, Banawas S, Nadeem H, Khan MF, Ahmad F. ZnO Nano-swirlings for Azo Dye AR183 photocatalytic degradation and antimycotic activity. Sci Rep August 18, 2022;12(1):14023.
[62] Zhao H, Ma Y, Sun D, Ma W, Yao J, Zhang M. Preparation and characterization of coaxial electrospinning rhBMP2-loaded nanofiber membranes. J Nanomater August 2019;29(2019).
[63] Yang F, Miao Y, Wang Y, Zhang LM, Lin X. Electrospun zein/gelatin scaffold-enhanced cell attachment and growth of human periodontal ligament stem cells. Materials October 12, 2017;10(10):1168.
[64] Zhijiang C, Qin Z, Xianyou S, Yuanpei L. Zein/Poly (3-hydroxybutyrate-co-4-hydroxybutyrate) electrospun blend fiber scaffolds: preparation, characterization and cytocompatibility. Mater Sci Eng C February 1, 2017;71:797–806.
[65] Mariotti CE, Ramos-Rivera L, Conti B, Boccaccini AR. Zein-based electrospun fibers containing bioactive glass with antibacterial capabilities. Macromol Biosci July 2020;20(7):2000059.
[66] Wang GW, Yang H, Wu WF, Zhang P, Wang JY. Design and optimization of a biodegradable porous zein conduit using microtubes as a guide for rat sciatic nerve defect repair. Biomaterials July 1, 2017;131:145–59.
[67] Umar K. Water contamination by organic-pollutants: TiO_2 photocatalysis. Mod Age Environ Prob Remediat 2018:95–109.
[68] Ghorbani M, Nezhad-Mokhtari P, Ramazani S. Aloe vera-loaded nanofibrous scaffold based on Zein/Polycaprolactone/Collagen for wound healing. Int J Biol Macromol June 15, 2020;153:921–30.
[69] Kasaai MR. Zein and zein-based nano-materials for food and nutrition applications: a review. Trend Food Sci Technol September 1, 2018;79:184–97.
[70] Singh BG, Das RP, Kunwar A. Protein: a versatile biopolymer for the fabrication of smart materials for drug delivery. J Chem Sci September, 2019;131:1–4.
[71] Zhang Q, Wang J, Liu D, Zhu W, Guan S, Fan L, Cai D. Targeted delivery of honokiol by zein/hyaluronic acid core-shell nanoparticles to suppress breast cancer growth and metastasis. Carbohydr Polym July 15, 2020;240:116325.

[72] Chen S, Li Q, Li H, Yang L, Yi JZ, Xie M, Zhang LM. Long-circulating zein-polysulfobetaine conjugate-based nanocarriers for enhancing the stability and pharmacokinetics of curcumin. Mater Sci Eng C April 1, 2020;109:110636.
[73] Liu Q, Han C, Tian Y, Liu T. Fabrication of curcumin-loaded zein nanoparticles stabilized by sodium caseinate/sodium alginate: curcumin solubility, thermal properties, rheology, and stability. Process Biochem July 1, 2020;94:30−8.
[74] Leena MM, Yoha KS, Moses JA, Anandharamakrishnan C. Edible coating with resveratrol loaded electrospun zein nanofibers with enhanced bioaccessibility. Food Biosci August 1, 2020;36:100669.
[75] Huang X, Liu Y, Zou Y, Liang X, Peng Y, McClements DJ, Hu K. Encapsulation of resveratrol in zein/pectin core-shell nanoparticles: stability, bioaccessibility, and antioxidant capacity after simulated gastrointestinal digestion. Food Hydrocoll August 1, 2019;93:261−9.
[76] Balaguer MP, Borne M, Chalier P, Gontard N, Morel MH, Peyron S, Gavara R, Hernandez-Munoz P. Retention and release of cinnamaldehyde from wheat protein matrices. Biomacromolecules May 13, 2013;14(5):1493−502.
[77] Karim M, Fathi M, Soleimanian-Zad S. Nanoencapsulation of cinnamic aldehyde using zein nanofibers by novel needle-less electrospinning: production, characterization and their application to reduce nitrite in sausages. J Food Eng January 1, 2021;288:110140.
[78] Kacsó T, Neaga IO, Erincz A, Astete CE, Sabliov CM, Oprean R, Bodoki E. Perspectives in the design of zein-based polymeric delivery systems with programmed wear down for sustainable agricultural applications. Polym Degrad Stabil September 1, 2018;155:130−5.
[79] Cui B, Gao F, Zeng Z, Wang C, Wang Y, Sun C, Zhao X, Guo L, Shen Y, Liu G, Cui H. Construction and characterization of avermectin B2 solid nanodispersion. Sci Rep June 4, 2020;10(1):9096.
[80] Hao L, Lin G, Lian J, Chen L, Zhou H, Chen H, Xu H, Zhou X. Carboxymethyl cellulose capsulated zein as pesticide nano-delivery system for improving adhesion and anti-UV properties. Carbohydr Polym March 1, 2020;231:115725.
[81] Lin M, Fang S, Zhao X, Liang X, Wu D. Natamycin-loaded zein nanoparticles stabilized by carboxymethyl chitosan: evaluation of colloidal/chemical performance and application in postharvest treatments. Food Hydrocoll September 1, 2020;106:105871.
[82] Falahieh KH, Sarkaki A, Edalatmanesh M, Naseri MK, Farbood Y. Ellagic acid attenuates post-cerebral ischemia and reperfusion behavioral deficits by decreasing brain tissue inflammation in rats. Iran J Bas Med Sci May, 2020;23(5):645.
[83] Tavares WS, Tavares-Júnior AG, Otero-Espinar FJ, Martín-Pastor M, Sousa FF. Design of ellagic acid-loaded chitosan/zein films for wound bandaging. J Drug Deliv Sci Technol October 1, 2020;59:101903.
[84] Zhang Y, Cui L, Che X, Zhang H, Shi N, Li C, Chen Y, Kong W. Zein-based films and their usage for controlled delivery: origin, classes and current landscape. J Contr Release May 28, 2015;206:206−19.
[85] Tsai MJ, Weng YM. Novel edible composite films fabricated with whey protein isolate and zein: preparation and physicochemical property evaluation. Lwt March 1, 2019;101:567−74.
[86] Dubey NK, Dubey R. Edible films and coatings: an update on recent advances. In: Biopolymer-based formulations. Elsevier; January 1, 2020. p. 675−95.

CHAPTER 10

Collagen/gelatin-based hydrogels for tissue engineering

Sadiq Umar[1], Khalid Umar[2], Rani Rahat[1] and Showkat Ahmad Bhawani[3]

[1]College of Dentistry, University of Illinois, Chicago, IL, United States; [2]School of Chemical Sciences, Universiti Sains Malaysia, Penang, Malaysia; [3]Faculty of Resource Science and Technology, Universiti Malaysia Sarawak (UNIMAS), Kota Samarahan, Sarawak, Malaysia

1. Introduction

The aim of bone engineering is to develop innovative bone substitutes to replace damaged bone tissue and restore bone integrity. Bone is a naturally occurring, solid biological composite material with high strength, fracture toughness, and a distinctive multiscale hierarchical structure. Extracellular substances released by cells form the extracellular matrix (ECM) in natural tissues. These molecules give cells mechanical and spatial signals and physical support for the tissues. It plays a dynamic and adaptable role in determining cell behavior and tissue function and acting as a benign framework for the arrangement of cells in connective tissue. As a result, it makes sense to create a transplant that mimics the injured tissue or organ extracellular matrix and then gradually restores it [1].

Molecular chains immersed in water-rich environments create hydrogels, which are three-dimensional (3D) networks. Hydrogels have adjustable physical-chemical characteristics, high biomimicry of the extracellular matrix of natural tissues, and may be generated by various cross-linking methods. Furthermore, stimuli-responsive molecules and growth factors (GFs), which are physiologically and chemically active recognition cues, can be added to hydrogels to modify them further and improve their biofunctionality. Therefore, hydrogels can offer an environment that allows cells to proliferate, differentiate, and create structures resembling tissues [2].

Natural materials have become more popular over the last 10 years thanks to the development of a new generation of hydrogels designed to

Protein-Based Nanocomposites for Tissue Engineering
ISBN 978-0-323-99357-9
https://doi.org/10.1016/B978-0-323-99357-9.00010-7

fulfill the unique needs of various tissues and the use of cutting-edge methods. The many natural polymer cross-linking methods will be covered in this overview, followed by a discussion of pertinent examples of hydrogels made using these polymers, with a particular emphasis on—but not limited to—3D bioprinting applications. Next, it will address how to create biomimetic and bioinstructive natural hydrogels using blood derivatives and decellularized tissues. The last section provides an overview of the engineering of sophisticated hydrogels using nanotechnology and supramolecular chemistry [3].

Collagen makes up approximately one-third of the body's protein tissue mass and is the primary constituent of both soft and hard tissues in mammals. Teeth, tendons, skin, and bones are just a few tissues with a large amount of collagen. There are now 28 different forms of collagen known to exist, with type I collagen being the most prevalent in the extracellular matrix (ECM), particularly in tendons and bones. The architecture of the different collagens is similar; three interwoven chains, or a-polypeptide chains comprising homotrimers or heterotrimers, are present. Collagen type determines these structures, with each chain having a shape resembling polyalanine II. The repeating Gly-X-Y triplet, in which X is often proline (or any other amino acid) and Y is frequently hydroxyproline, gives rise to the impenetrable triple helix composition. Due to its tiny volume and ability to fill the restricted area in the triple helix center, glycine is necessary for every third position [4].

Gelatin has amphoteric behavior, is nonimmunogenic, and is readily soluble in water at 37°C. Due to these characteristics, gelatin-based hydrogels are utilized in the production of contact lenses, tissue engineering matrices, and drug delivery systems. Exploring novel applications for hydrogels based on gelatin is a significant field of academic study. Furthermore, various cross-linking agents, including as glutaraldehyde, genipin, and dextran dialdehyde, can be used to alter gelatin's mechanical and chemical characteristics. Using transglutaminase-catalyzed cross-linking, for instance, Crescenzi et al. created novel gelatin-based hydrogels from high-bloom pure gelatin A with or without hyaluronan to create more densely linked networks that promote cell regeneration [5].

Mechanical characteristics of chemically altered gelatin can be adjusted. Bulcke et al.'s study of the rheological characteristics of methacrylamide-modified gelatin-based hydrogels, for instance, revealed that the degree of modification, polymer concentration, photoinitiator concentration, and UV exposure time can all affect the rheological characteristics of gelatin-based hydrogels. Higher-degree modified gelatin-based hydrogels can form more acrylate bonds, produce denser networks and have higher elastic modulus values. The methacrylamide-modified gelatin undergoes photo-initiated chemical cross-linking, which creates a regulated chemical network that allows for predictable modulation of the hydrogels' strength [6]. This review will describe synthesis and fabrication techniques for preparing gelatin- and collagen-based hydrogels.

2. Tissue engineering

The creation, restoration, or substitution of damaged or absent tissue in humans and other animals is known as tissue engineering. In a bioreactor, tissue constructions for grafting into the animal later on may be created, or this engineering may occur inside the animal's body. The right kinds of cells are the bare minimum of ingredients needed. However, in most cases, inanimate substrates are also employed. These substrata could be no more than fillers for any spaces left by injured tissue, giving it the mechanical strength it has lost due to removal or injury. They could have two comparable roles in the bioreactor. When it comes to creating patterns, they are far more capable. The interactions between various cell types, the orientations and shape of the cells, and the arrangement of intercellular material as it is put down are all significant factors in the mending or building of tissue since they should closely mimic the appropriate normal tissue. Pattern creation is required for the majority of these needs.

From its beginnings a little over a decade ago, tissue engineering has attracted enormous interest. A recurring theme in this work is the idea that the application and control of cells, materials, and chemoactive proteins can guide the repair and regeneration of biological tissues despite the fact that the number of researchers in this field has grown significantly over the years and the potential applications have become more widespread. Therefore, the study of tissue engineering is fundamentally an interdisciplinary area that necessitates collaboration between scientists, engineers, and doctors.

The field of tissue engineering uses live cells in several methods to maintain, improve, or restore tissues and organs. Images of organs created from scratch in a laboratory and prepared for transplantation into terminally sick patients come to mind when one hears of tissue engineering. Yet, the field's potential effects are far-reaching: engineered tissues may 1 day significantly speed up the discovery of novel medications that may treat patients and eliminate the need for organ transplants by reducing the requirement for replacement organs.

In vitro cultured cells are cultivated on biodegradable scaffolds that provide chemical and physical cues to promote their differentiation and assembly into three-dimensional (3D) structures, enabling the creation of biological tissues [7]. Cell assembly into tissues is a carefully orchestrated series of activities requiring dimensions varying from 0.0001 to 10 cm and time frames ranging from seconds to weeks. The traditional engineering design challenge of guiding cells to build tissues dependably must be solved within the restrictions of government regulation, cost, society acceptability, and dependability.

2.1 Overview/background

These days, tissue engineering is considered a viable substitute for organ or tissue transplantation. This technique allows for the treatment of tissue loss or organ failure through the use of ex vivo perfusion devices or the implantation of a biological replacement that has been developed. Tissue-engineered products (like liver assist devices and encapsulated islets) may be completely functional during therapy or integrate and produce the intended functional tissue after implantation (like chondrocytes implanted in a matrix carrier). Biomaterials can occasionally be altered to promote the migration and adhesion of particular cell populations that replace or repair damaged tissue [8].

Tissue engineering originates in the science of biomaterials, which studies the materials found in the body and their impact on both the host and the material's biological environment. In many circumstances, using materials that were as inert as possible—that is, not damaged or detrimental to the host—was the goal. The application of bioactive materials—that is, materials made to interact with the body to promote tissue repair—was, in a way, the origin of tissue engineering. Three publications by Yannas and associates provide a significant early example and detail the creation of an artificial skin equivalent using collagen and glycosaminoglycan (GAG) [9].

Although regenerative medicine was formerly thought to be an unreachable goal, it is now becoming a reality due to recent technical developments and scientific efforts to produce cures for various illnesses. To achieve the goals of this discipline of medicine, sophisticated cell treatment, genetic engineering, and tissue engineering are among the primary domains in which this medical science collaborates [10]. "The science of designing and manufacturing new tissues for the functional restoration of altered organs and the replacement of structures damaged by trauma or disease" is the definition of tissue engineering [11]. As a result, it is a rapidly expanding interdisciplinary field encompassing several disciplines, including biology, chemistry, engineering, and medicine. The growth of this field of study led to the development of a brand-new class of materials known as biomaterials. The word "biomaterials" has been defined in various ways. Still, the most often used definition describes the substance as "a material designed to repair or restore the functionalities of a defective biological system" [12].

Regarding a historical overview, these items were originally covered in papers in the late 1960s and early 1970s [13,14]. Because of the adaptability of these materials, the examination of these materials has been one of the most researched areas over the years. Biomaterials have, therefore, improved throughout time as a result of their evolution. Target attributes include nontoxicity, biocompatibility, and a macroscopic structure that resembles the material to be replaced in terms of biomechanical, biofunctional, and biomimetic requirements. They also need to remain stable throughout insertion, storage, and sterilization. Depending on the application, they might be either temporary or permanent [15,16].

2.2 The importance of tissue engineering

Tissue engineering aims to replace or repair organs and tissues during surgery using scaffolds, DNA, proteins, and/or pieces of protein and transplanted cells. Biomaterials (new and creative delivery vehicles), cell and molecular biology (e.g., the isolation and manipulation of cells, genes, and growth factors), and the integration of biology and materials to deliver viable cells in compatible support structures are some of the major advancements that have contributed to the rapid advancements in tissue engineering. Numerous organs and tissues that need to be replaced have vital biomechanical roles. Indeed, these tissues' biomechanical characteristics are essential to their appropriate in vivo functioning [17].

A novel approach offering an alternate tissue and organ reconstruction strategy first surfaced about 30 years ago. Tissue engineering is that. Regenerating a patient's organs and tissues completely free of severe immunological rejection, limited biofunctionality, and poor biocompatibility is one of the unique characteristics of tissue engineering. Tissue engineering is frequently regarded as the perfect medical treatment because of its many benefits. Three fundamental techniques are used in biomedical engineering to regenerate new tissues: Cells, scaffolds, and growth factors. Not all three are utilized at the same time. For instance, bone morphogenetic protein (BMP) alone is adequate in some bone tissue engineering applications. In contrast, dermal tissue may be regenerated with only a porous collagen sheet applied over a full-thickness skin incision, obviating the need for cell seeding and growth factor administration. In this instance, the body absorbs the sheet simultaneously. Fibroblasts are drawn from the surrounding healthy skin tissue, move into the sheet's pores, and release proteins and glycosaminoglycans to create dermal tissue [18].

Human cells may have been used in tissue engineering for the first time in clinical settings to treat skin tissue utilizing fibroblasts, keratinocytes, or scaffolds (templates). It all began in the year 1980. A short while later, guided tissue regeneration (GTR) and guided bone regeneration (GBR)—two methods that guarantee the preservation of the site for tissue regeneration by blocking fibroblast invasion—were tried to repair the periodontal and alveolar bone tissues. While Wakitani et al. (1989) reported repairing rabbit articular surfaces with transplanted chondrocytes embedded in collagen gel, Vacanti et al. (1988) investigated cell transplantation utilizing bioabsorbable synthetic polymers as matrix. The review paper "Tissue Engineering," published by Langer and Vacanti in 1993, has made a significant contribution to the global advancement of tissue engineering research [19].

3. Collagen and gelatin as biomaterials

3.1 Structure and properties

Collagen, an essential protein constituting a significant portion of the human body's structural framework, is renowned for its intricate hierarchical structure. At the molecular level, collagen manifests as a triple-helical configuration formed by three polypeptide chains, commonly called α chains [20]. This unique structure arises from a distinct amino acid sequence, dominated by glycine, proline, and hydroxyproline. This triple helix is the foundation of collagen's flexible strength and resilience, providing tissues with the ability to withstand mechanical stresses.

The diversity in collagen types, ranging from Type I to Type XXVIII, plays a crucial role in tailoring the material to specific tissue environments [21]. Type I collagen, found predominantly in skin, tendons, and bones, is known for its high tensile strength. In contrast, Type II collagen, abundant in cartilage, imparts resilience to this load-bearing tissue. The self-assembly of collagen molecules into fibrils, followed by their organization into fibers, contributes to the structural integrity of tissues across a spectrum of physiological contexts.

Gelatin, a derivative of collagen obtained through partial hydrolysis, retains essential characteristics of its parent protein while introducing properties advantageous for various applications [22]. Hydrolysis involves the enzymatic or acidic cleavage of peptide bonds within the collagen structure, yielding a soluble mixture of polypeptides and amino acids. This partial degradation results in the solubility of gelatin in water, setting it apart from the insoluble nature of native collagen.

Structural alterations during the hydrolysis process influence the type of gelatin obtained, such as Type A (acidic) and Type B (basic). Extraction of gelatine as shown in Fig. 10.1. Despite the partial disruption of the triple-helical conformation, gelatin maintains crucial cell-adhesive motifs, ensuring its utility as a biomaterial for tissue engineering applications. The solubility and ease of processing further enhance the versatility of gelatin in the design of biomimetic scaffolds.

One of the distinctive features contributing to the effectiveness of collagen and gelatin in tissue engineering is their structural mimicry of the natural ECM [24]. The molecular architecture of collagen closely resembles that of native tissues, providing a biomimetic scaffold that supports

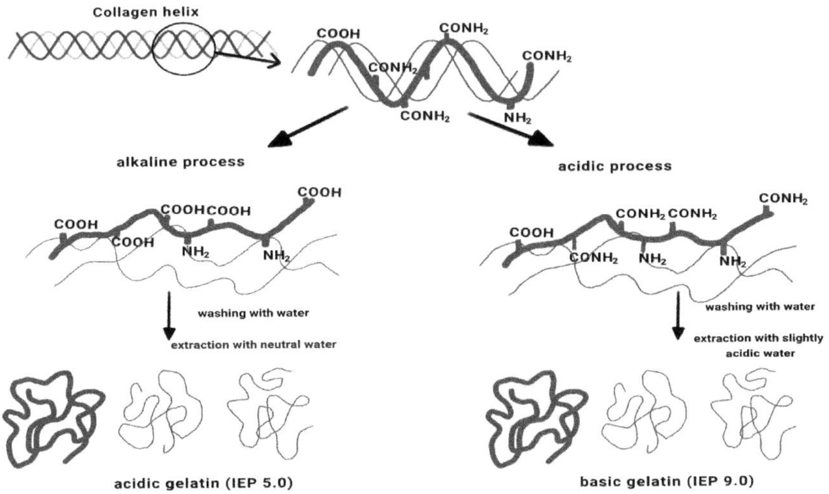

Figure 10.1 Two techniques are available for extracting gelatin from collagen-containing tissues [23].

biochemical signaling and cellular differentiation. This mimicry extends to the triple-helical structure of collagen, which shows mechanical strength and serves as a signaling cue for cells, influencing their behavior and fate. Gelatin, derived from collagen, retains critical cell-adhesive motifs, further ensuring effective cellular interactions within the biomaterial.

Besides that, collagen and gelatin-based hydrogels offer a unique advantage in their tunable mechanical properties. The mechanical characteristics of these biomaterials can be tailored to match the specific requirements of different tissues. By adjusting factors such as protein concentration and employing various cross-linking techniques, researchers can modulate the hydrogels' stiffness, elasticity, and overall mechanical behavior. This tunability is crucial for creating biomimetic environments that provide structural support and mimic the dynamic mechanical cues experienced by cells in their native microenvironments.

Collagen and gelatin-based biomaterials also serve as effective carriers for controlled drug delivery. Their porous structures and the ability to encapsulate bioactive molecules make them suitable for delivering therapeutic agents in a controlled and sustained manner. This property is particularly advantageous in tissue engineering applications where localized and targeted drug delivery is desired. By incorporating growth factors, cytokines, or other therapeutic compounds into the biomaterial matrix, collagen and gelatin hydrogels can enhance tissue regeneration and modulate the cellular response [24,25].

3.2 Biocompatibility and biodegradability

Collagen and gelatin stand out in biomaterials due to their exceptional biocompatibility, a property that plays a critical role in their successful integration into biological systems; as natural components of the extracellular matrix (ECM), collagen and gelatin provide a microenvironment that closely mimics the body's native tissue. This fundamental biocompatibility fosters favorable interactions with living cells, promoting adhesion, migration, and proliferation processes.

The molecular structure of collagen, with its characteristic triple-helical conformation and cell-binding domains, enables strong interactions with cell surface receptors [26]. This interaction is adhesive and instructive, influencing cellular behavior and responses. Integrin-binding sites in collagen allow for specific cell recognition, encouraging a seamless interface between the biomaterial and surrounding tissues. As a result, collagen and gelatin serve as substrates that support cellular activities, creating a conducive environment for tissue regeneration.

In tissue engineering, the biocompatibility of collagen and gelatin is particularly crucial. It ensures the implanted biomaterial does not cause adverse immune responses or chronic inflammation. This property is fundamental for the success of regenerative strategies, as the biomaterial needs to seamlessly integrate with host tissues, facilitating the restoration of normal physiological functions.

Another key property of collagen and gelatin is their biodegradability, which aligns with the dynamic nature of tissue regeneration. Biodegradation is the process by which a material is broken down into smaller components by enzymatic or cellular activity, eventually metabolizing and clearing from the body [27]. Controlled biodegradation is crucial for several reasons in the context of collagen and gelatin.

First, the biomaterial's gradual degradation matches the pace of tissue regeneration. As new tissue forms, the scaffold provided by collagen and gelatin progressively breaks down, allowing the emerging tissue to assume the structural and functional roles previously held by the biomaterial [28]. This controlled degradation prevents the persistence of foreign materials, reducing the risk of chronic inflammation and promoting a natural transition from the implanted scaffold to functional tissue.

Second, the breakdown products of collagen and gelatin are metabolically manageable by the body. The hydrolysis of peptide bonds during biodegradation yields amino acids and small peptides that can be readily incorporated into cellular processes or excreted. This metabolic compatibility ensures that the by-products of biodegradation do not impose unnecessary stress on the host organism.

In practical terms, the biodegradability of collagen and gelatin allows for the design of temporary scaffolds. These scaffolds provide temporary support during the critical phases of tissue regeneration and gradually disappear as the regenerated tissue matures. This property is particularly advantageous in applications where a permanent implant may not be desirable or necessary.

3.3 Advantages

First, collagen and gelatin exhibit unparalleled biocompatibility, naturally derived proteins that closely resemble the components of the extracellular matrix (ECM). Their biological origin reduces the risk of immune rejection or adverse reactions, fostering a favorable microenvironment for cellular interactions. The biocompatibility of these biomaterials promotes cell adhesion, migration, and proliferation, critical aspects for tissue regeneration in various medical applications [29]. The structural mimicry of collagen and gelatin to the native ECM is a distinct advantage. Their molecular architecture, especially the triple-helical structure in collagen, provides a biomimetic scaffold that supports biochemical signaling. This allows for complex signaling interactions between the biomaterial and cells, influencing cellular behavior, differentiation, and tissue-specific functions. The biomimicry enhances the ability of collagen and gelatin to guide and organize the regeneration of functional tissues.

Next, the versatility of collagen and gelatin is a significant asset in tissue engineering. Their adaptability enables the design of scaffolds that can mimic the unique properties of various tissues, including skin, bone, cartilage, and vascular tissues. This versatility makes collagen and gelatin valuable tools in creating customized biomimetic environments tailored to the specific needs of different tissue regeneration strategies. The biodegradability of collagen and gelatin aligns seamlessly with the dynamic tissue regeneration process. These biomaterials undergo controlled degradation over time, ensuring the scaffold gradually gives way to newly formed tissue. The controlled degradation prevents the persistence of foreign materials, reducing the risk of chronic inflammation and enabling a natural transition from the biomaterial to functional tissue.

Collagen and gelatin-based hydrogels also offer a unique advantage in their tunable mechanical properties. Researchers can manipulate the mechanical characteristics of these biomaterials by adjusting factors such as protein concentration and employing various cross-linking techniques [30,31]. This tunability allows for the creation of biomimetic environments that provide not only structural support but also mimic the dynamic mechanical cues experienced by cells in their native microenvironments. Other than that, collagen and gelatin serve as effective carriers for controlled drug delivery [32]. Their porous structures and ability to encapsulate bioactive molecules make them suitable for delivering therapeutic agents in a controlled and sustained manner. This property is particularly advantageous in tissue engineering applications where localized and targeted drug delivery is desired, enhancing tissue regeneration and modulating the cellular response in a spatiotemporal manner.

The advantages of collagen and gelatin as biomaterials make them prominent players in the field of tissue engineering and regenerative medicine. Their biocompatibility, structural mimicry, versatility, biodegradability, mechanical tunability and drug delivery capabilities collectively position them as versatile and effective tools for creating biomimetic environments conducive to tissue repair and regeneration. The ongoing research in this area holds promise for the development of advanced therapeutic strategies that leverage the unique advantages offered by collagen and gelatin.

4. Material (collagen/gelatin) modifications and fabrication method

4.1 Collagen and gelatin types used

Gelatin is an organic biopolymer that is formed from animal collagen found in skins, bones, and tendons by partial acid hydrolysis (gelatin type A) or alkaline hydrolysis (gelatin type B). Gelatin has a structure with varied physical characteristics and chemical heterogeneity due to variations in collagen sources and fabrication methods [33]. Gelatin is a naturally occurring biopolymer that is highly valued for its abundance of benefits, despite variations in its manufacturing process.

It has been observed that 19 amino acids are somewhat orderedly linked together in gelatin [26]. The majority of the amino acid groups in the gelatin molecule are four. Of the amino acid residues found in gelatin, 330 are glycine, 132 are proline, 112 are alanine, and 93 are hydroxyproline per 1000 residues. The remaining ones are leftovers. The triple helical structure of gelatin is a result of the representation (GlycineX-Proline)n, where X stands for the amino acids lysine, arginine, methionine, and valine in most cases. Gelatin has a polyampholyte as one of its surface properties.

On the contrary, the gelatin has a positive charge at a lower pH and a negative charge at a higher pH. Around pH 9 (gelatin type A) and pH 5 (gelatin type B), gelatin becomes polyampholyte [34,35]. The charge distribution pattern of type A and type B gelatins in aqueous solutions with varying pH values is shown in Fig. 10.2 [36].

As a basis for both cell-based and cell-free tissue healing, collagen offers several benefits. When implanted into subcutaneous pockets in normal rats, porous collagen sponges manufactured from pepsin-digested (i.e., telopeptide-free) bovine skin collagen were shown to be biocompatible, unlike sponges prepared in the same way from acid-soluble bovine skin collagen. Sponge formed from collagens containing telopeptides caused a slight inflammatory reaction; thus, to prevent issues with cell compatibility

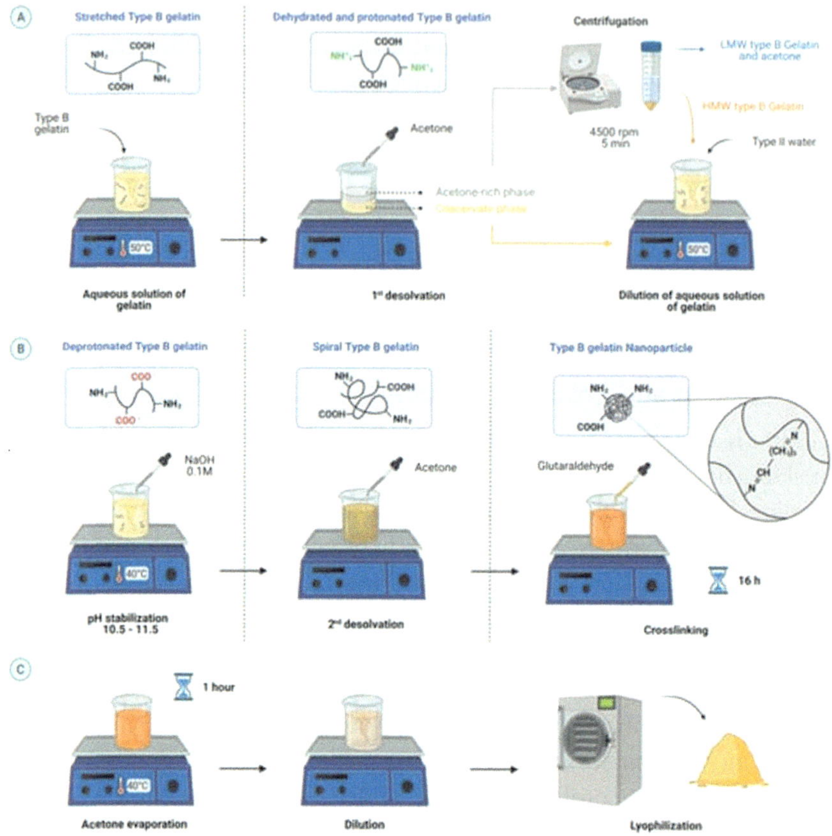

Figure 10.2 A schematic detailing the synthesis of type B gelatin nanoparticles (GNPs) is presented, employing a two-step desolvation method utilizing acetone. In the initial step (A), type B gelatin is dissolved, dehydrated, and protonated. Subsequently, in step (B), high molecular weight (HMW) type B gelatin undergoes deprotonation, facilitating controlled gelatin coiling and cross-linking. Finally, in step (C), the recovery of GNPs takes place [36].

and regeneration processes, they were not employed in future in vitro and in vivo research [34].

The interconnected holes in collagen sponges produced from 0.5 weight percent solutions, lyophilized to preserve a porous surface, and cross-linked by UV light are ideal for cellular in-growth and histogenesis. They include 120–200 μm pore sizes and are more than 95% porous. When rehydrated without cross-linking, they turned into amorphous hydrogels that prevented cell migration. The first application of the porous collagen sponges was in vitro cartilage formation. An abundant supply of cells for evaluating the impact of growth hormones, mechanical forces, and other matrix components on chondrogenesis was the bovine articular chondrocyte (bAC).2. It is possible that for the best in vitro histogenesis, various tissue types need distinct circumstances. We have identified many factors that augment chondrogenesis induced by beta-adrenergic acids [34].

4.2 Physical and chemical modifications of collagen and gelatin

Physical and chemical alterations are essential to customize collagen and gelatin's characteristics for various biomaterials and tissue engineering applications. Collagen may be physically altered by applying techniques like cross-linking, which strengthens the connections that hold collagen molecules together and makes them more resistant to enzymatic breakdown. Collagen-based materials' mechanical strength and rate of deterioration can be controlled using cross-linking techniques, such as chemicals or radiation. Chemical alterations include changing the chemical structure of collagen or gelatin, a derivative of it, to impart certain qualities [37].

To increase collagen's resistance to enzymatic degradation, thermal stability, and biocompatibility, it can be acetylated, phosphorylated, or methacrylated. Partially hydrolyzed collagen is the source of gelatin, which may also be chemically modified to improve its mechanical qualities and other functionalities. One such alteration is greater cross-linking. Through these changes, scientists may better tailor gelatin and collagen's properties, resulting in flexible and adaptable biomaterials for various biological uses [26].

4.3 Fabrication techniques

The diagram below illustrates the process of forming hydrogels based on collagen and gelatin, using the manufacture of collagen hydrogels as an example. By freezing the solutions containing collagen/gelatin and cross-linkers at a somewhat negative temperature, ice crystals develop throughout the preparation process and function as porogens. Thus, the produced crystals primarily regulate the size and shape of the pores in cryogels. Meanwhile, gelation processes occur when cross-linkers and collagen/gelatin are compressed into an unfrozen phase between ice crystals [26]. Gelatin-based hydrogels and collagen-based hydrogels with interconnecting macropores are created once the freezing system is thawed at ambient temperature.

4.4 Cross-linking methods

Cross-linkers are ideal for toughening collagen-based hydrogels and gelatin-based hydrogels. These will be briefly covered in the following. CBCs and GBCs may be classified into two categories based on the cross-linking mechanisms: physically cross-linked and chemically (covalently) cross-linked [38].

4.4.1 Physical/noncovalent cross-linking

Only physical interactions, such as hydrogen bonds, hydrophobic interactions, chain entanglement, etc., may produce physically cross-linked CBCs and GBCs [26]. These types of hydrogels often have limited mechanical strength, a quick rate of disintegration, and poor thermal stability, which restricts their usefulness.

4.4.2 Covalent/chemical cross-linking

Regarding covalent cross-linking, the $-NH_2$, $-COOH$, and $-OH$ active groups on the side chains of collagen and gelatin offer favorable cross-linking sites. When collagen-based hydrogels and gelatin-based hydrogels are covalently cross-linked instead of physically cross-linked, they often exhibit better mechanical and thermal stability. In addition, four types of cross-linkers may be used to categorize collagen-based hydrogels and gelatin-based hydrogels: those that use small-molecule cross-linkers, those that use macromolecular cross-linkers, and hydrogels made by enzymatic cross-linking or free-radical polymerization.

4.4.3 Cross-linking via small-molecule cross-linkers

Presently, 1-ethyl-3-(3-dimethyl aminopropyl) carbodiimide/N-hydroxysuccinimide (EDC/NHS), genipin, and aldehydes [39] are the most often employed small-molecule cross-linkers in the production of collagen and gelatin-based products. Due to its lower toxicity than formaldehyde, glutaraldehyde is the most commonly employed aldehyde-type cross-linker for collagen and gelatin [40,41]. Furthermore, earlier research has shown that under somewhat cold conditions, Schiff's base reaction between collagen/gelatin and glutaraldehyde can still occur [29,30]. Using gelatin as an example, the chemical process between collagen and glutaraldehyde occurred and the development of aldimine linkage ($CH{=}N$) enhances the mechanical strength of collagen and gelatin-based hydrogels. Research indicates that when the content of glutaraldehyde rises, so does the compressive strength of gelatin-based hydrogels. It is important to remember that the remaining glutaraldehyde in these hydrogels may be poisonous, affecting the hydrogels' biocompatibility and restricting their use in biomedical applications.

5. Properties of collagen/gelatin hydrogels

5.1 Mechanical properties

Collagen and gelatin hydrogels play a pivotal role in tissue engineering due to their unique mechanical properties, which can be finely tuned to mimic the structural characteristics of native tissues. Understanding and manipulating the mechanical aspects of these hydrogels are crucial for designing biomimetic scaffolds that provide the necessary support for cellular activities, guide tissue regeneration, and integrate seamlessly with host tissues. First, collagen and gelatin hydrogels are naturally viscoelastic, exhibiting both solid-like and fluid-like behavior. This property is crucial in replicating the softness of many natural tissues, such as skin or cartilage. The viscoelastic nature allows the hydrogel to deform under applied stress and recover when the stress is removed, mimicking the dynamic mechanical environment experienced by cells in vivo.

One of the standout features of collagen and gelatin hydrogels is their tunable mechanical properties. These hydrogels' mechanical strength, stiffness, and elasticity can be adjusted by varying factors such as protein concentration, cross-linking density, and fabrication methods [42]. This tunability is invaluable for modifying hydrogels to match the specific mechanical requirements of different tissues and organs. The mechanical stability of collagen and gelatin hydrogels is often achieved through cross-linking, a process that forms covalent bonds between polymer chains, reinforcing the three-dimensional network of the hydrogel [43]. Cross-linking methods, including chemical, physical, or enzymatic approaches, allow researchers to control the degree of connectivity within the hydrogel, influencing its mechanical strength and resilience.

Tissues in the human body exhibit a wide range of mechanical properties, from the softness of brain tissue to the stiffness of bone. Collagen and gelatin hydrogels can be tailored to closely mimic specific tissues' mechanics. For instance, hydrogels with low stiffness may be suitable for applications in brain tissue engineering, while those with higher stiffness can replicate the mechanical properties of bone. Collagen and gelatin hydrogels also can exhibit dynamic responses to environmental stimuli, such as changes in pH, temperature, or the presence of ions. This property is particularly advantageous for applications like drug delivery, where the hydrogel can undergo controlled changes in mechanical properties in response to specific indications, enabling on-demand release of therapeutic agents [43–45].

Lastly, collagen and gelatin hydrogels often exhibit time-dependent mechanical behavior, a feature known as viscoelasticity over time. This dynamic response is crucial in applications where the hydrogel must accommodate mechanical stresses and strains over extended periods, such as in load-bearing tissues or long-term tissue regeneration processes. Their viscoelasticity, tunability, cross-linking capabilities, ability to mimic native tissue mechanics and dynamic responsiveness collectively contribute to creating biomimetic scaffolds that provide the mechanical cues necessary for successful tissue regeneration [45]. Hydrogel is used in biomedical applications, as shown in Fig. 10.3.

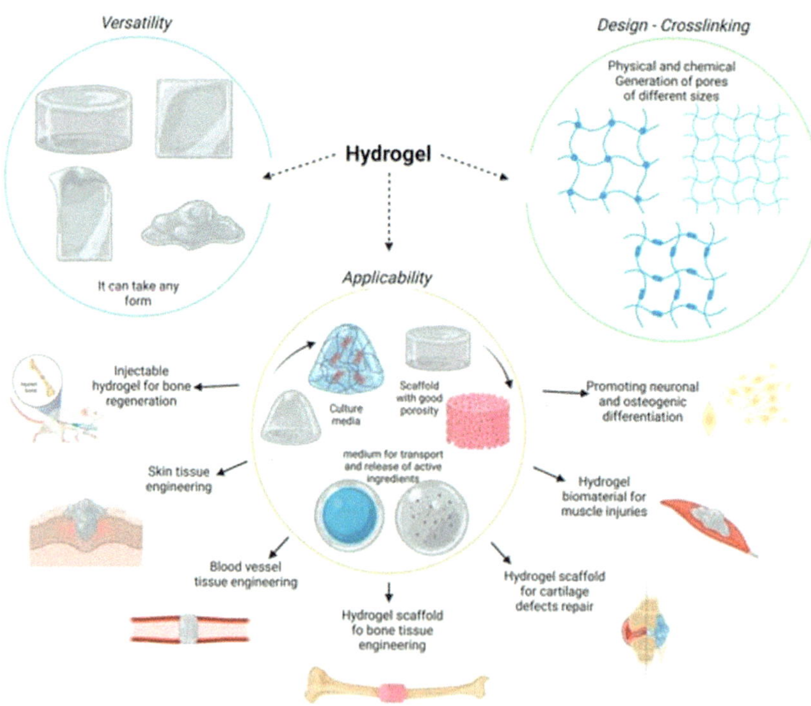

Figure 10.3 Versatile and pliable biomaterials, hydrogels find numerous medical applications [45].

5.2 Pore properties

The pore properties of collagen and gelatin hydrogels play a crucial role in determining their suitability for tissue engineering applications. These properties influence cell infiltration, nutrient transport, waste removal, and tissue regeneration within the three-dimensional scaffold. Understanding and manipulating the pore architecture of these hydrogels are essential for creating biomimetic environments that support cellular activities and promote successful tissue regeneration. Collagen and gelatin hydrogels are inherently porous due to their hydrophilic nature and the water content within the gel matrix. This porosity allows the hydrogels to mimic the porous structure of the extracellular matrix (ECM) in natural tissues, facilitating cell infiltration and promoting the exchange of nutrients and signaling molecules.

One of the advantages of collagen and gelatin hydrogels is the ability to control the pore size. The pore size directly impacts cell behavior, with smaller pores offering increased surface area for cell attachment and larger pores facilitating cell migration and tissue ingrowth. Researchers can tailor the pore size of these hydrogels through adjustments in the gelation process, biomaterial concentration, or using porogens during fabrication [43]. The interconnectedness of pores is critical for effective cell migration and nutrient diffusion throughout the hydrogel scaffold. Collagen and gelatin hydrogels can be designed to form a well-connected network of pores, ensuring that cells can penetrate the entire depth of the scaffold and receive the necessary cues for proliferation and differentiation.

The three-dimensional architecture of collagen and gelatin hydrogels allows for a porous structure beneficial to cell infiltration. Cells can navigate through the interconnected pores, enabling even distribution and colonization within the hydrogel. This property is particularly important for promoting homogeneous tissue regeneration and avoiding issues like cellular necrosis at the scaffold's core. The pore properties of collagen and gelatin hydrogels will significantly impact cellular activities within the scaffold. Cells interact with the surrounding microenvironment, and the pore structure influences cell adhesion, migration, and proliferation. Properly tuned pore properties create a microenvironment that closely mimics the natural tissue, enhancing cell functionality and supporting tissue-specific functions [45].

Other than that, the pore properties of hydrogels are directly linked to nutrient and oxygen transport within the scaffold [30]. Adequate pore size and interconnectedness facilitate efficient diffusion of nutrients and oxygen to cells within the hydrogel, ensuring their metabolic needs are met. This is crucial for maintaining cell viability and promoting tissue regeneration. Tailoring the pore properties of collagen and gelatin hydrogels allows researchers to create environments that are conducive to tissue-specific regeneration. Different tissues have varying requirements for pore size and structure, and the ability to customize these properties enables the development of scaffolds that closely mimic the target tissue, promoting more accurate and successful regeneration.

5.3 Swelling

The swelling properties of collagen and gelatin hydrogels represent a critical aspect of their behavior, influencing their performance in various biomedical applications. Swelling is an inherent characteristic of hydrogels, and it is particularly pronounced in collagen and gelatin-based matrices due to their hydrophilic nature. Understanding the swelling behavior is crucial for tailoring these hydrogels to specific applications in tissue engineering, drug delivery, and wound healing.

Collagen and gelatin hydrogels are inherently hydrophilic, meaning they have a strong affinity for water. This hydrophilicity arises from polar functional groups, such as hydroxyl and amino groups, in the molecular structure of collagen and gelatin [46,47]. As a result, when these hydrogels come into contact with water, they exhibit a rapid and extensive uptake of water molecules, leading to significant swelling. The degree of swelling in collagen and gelatin hydrogels can be modulated by adjusting the biomaterial composition. Factors such as protein concentration, cross-linking density, and the degree of hydrolysis in the case of gelatin influence the swelling behavior. Higher concentrations and increased cross-linking generally reduce swelling due to restricted water absorption.

The swelling properties of collagen and gelatin hydrogels are interconnected with their mechanical behavior. As these hydrogels absorb water, they undergo volumetric expansion, leading to mechanical properties such as stiffness and elasticity changes. The extent of swelling can be tuned to achieve desired mechanical characteristics, which is critical for matching the mechanical environment of the target tissue. The kinetics of swelling in collagen and gelatin hydrogels are influenced by pH, temperature, and ionic strength [48]. Environmental conditions can alter the hydrogel's swelling behavior, making it responsive to external cues. pH-sensitive hydrogels, for instance, may exhibit differential swelling in response to variations in the local pH, allowing for controlled drug release or modulation of mechanical properties.

The swelling properties of collagen and gelatin hydrogels are exploited in drug delivery applications. These hydrogels can capture therapeutic agents, and as they swell in the presence of water, the loaded drugs are released gradually. The controlled release of drugs from the swollen hydrogel matrix provides a sustained and localized therapeutic effect, making collagen and gelatin hydrogels promising candidates for drug delivery systems. In tissue engineering, the swelling properties of collagen and gelatin hydrogels are significant for achieving tissue compatibility. The hydrogels' ability to swell and absorb water mimics the hydration state of natural tissues, promoting a microenvironment that supports cell viability, proliferation, and tissue regeneration.

6. Applications for tissue engineering

6.1 Skin and muscle tissue regeneration

Collagen and gelatin-based hydrogels have emerged as valuable tools in skin tissue regeneration, addressing clinical needs ranging from wound healing to treating extensive burns. The unique properties of these biomaterials make them well-suited for creating scaffolds that closely mimic the native extracellular matrix of the skin. Collagen and gelatin hydrogels accelerate wound healing by providing a supportive environment for cell migration, proliferation, and tissue repair [48]. These hydrogels create a temporary matrix that promotes hemostasis, prevents infection, and facilitates the regeneration of skin layers. Their biocompatibility ensures minimal harmful reactions, making them suitable for various dermatological applications.

In the context of burn injuries, collagen and gelatin hydrogels contribute significantly to the regeneration of damaged skin. By providing a biomimetic scaffold, these hydrogels support the growth of keratinocytes and fibroblasts, which are critical for forming new skin tissue [49]. The controlled degradation of the hydrogel aligns with the dynamic nature of the healing process, ensuring seamless integration with the regenerated skin. Collagen-based hydrogels also find applications in cosmetic and esthetic medicine for soft tissue augmentation and rejuvenation. Injectable collagen fillers, derived from hydrogels, are used to enhance facial contours, reduce wrinkles, and restore volume, providing a nonsurgical approach to cosmetic procedures.

Collagen and gelatin hydrogels repair musculoskeletal injuries, providing a scaffold supporting muscle cells' growth and alignment. These hydrogels can be modified to mimic the mechanical properties of specific muscles, promoting the regeneration of functional tissue in cases of injuries or degenerative conditions. Volumetric muscle loss, resulting from trauma or surgery, presents a significant challenge in tissue regeneration. Collagen and gelatin hydrogels offer a potential solution by providing a three-dimensional framework for muscle cell growth. The hydrogels' tunable mechanical properties enable the recreation of muscle tissue's dynamic and contractile nature, facilitating functional recovery. Successful muscle tissue regeneration requires the formation of muscle fibers and the integration of neurovascular networks. Collagen and gelatin hydrogels can support the co-culture of muscle cells with neurons and blood vessel cells, promoting the development of functional neuromuscular junctions and ensuring proper nutrient and oxygen supply to the regenerating muscle tissue [49,50].

6.2 Bone tissue engineering

Bone tissue engineering represents a dynamic and evolving field that seeks to address bone defects, fractures, and degenerative conditions by developing biomimetic scaffolds. Collagen and gelatin-based hydrogels play a crucial role in bone tissue engineering, offering versatile platforms for the regeneration of functional and structurally sound bone tissue.

For fracture healing, the hydrogels contribute to the natural healing process by providing a scaffold that mimics the extracellular matrix of bone. These hydrogels support cell adhesion, proliferation, and differentiation, enabling the recruitment of osteoblasts and the formation of new bone tissue [30,51]. The controlled degradation of the hydrogel aligns with the timeline of bone healing, ensuring seamless integration with the regenerated bone. In bone defects resulting from trauma, tumors, or congenital abnormalities, collagen and gelatin-based hydrogels can be customized to fill the void and guide the regeneration of missing bone. The tunable mechanical properties of these hydrogels enable the creation of scaffolds that match the specific mechanical requirements of the target bone tissue.

Collagen and gelatin hydrogels are also utilized to develop orthopedic implants and prosthetics [51,52]. These implants aim to mimic bone tissue's

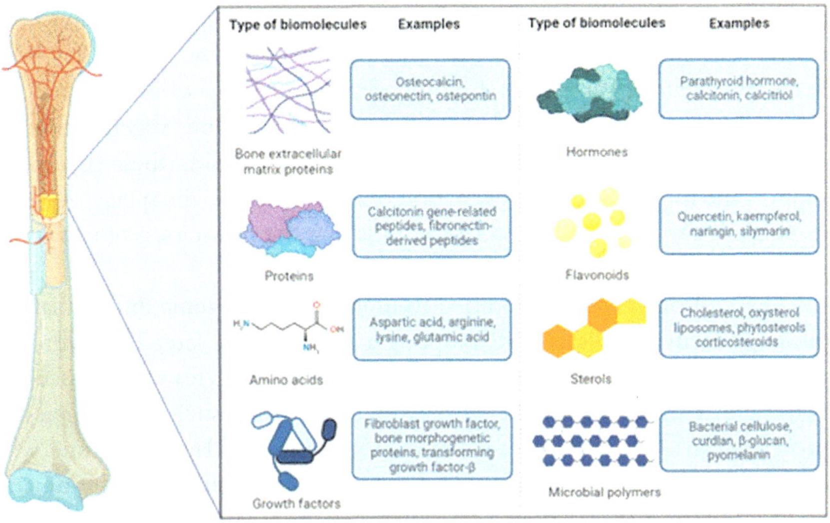

Figure 10.4 Application of bone tissue engineering [53].

natural architecture and support damaged or weakened skeletal structures. The biocompatibility of collagen and gelatin ensures that the implants seamlessly integrate with the surrounding bone, promoting long-term stability [51,52]. The tunable mechanical properties of collagen and gelatin hydrogels are crucial for achieving biomechanical stability in bone tissue engineering. By adjusting factors such as protein concentration and cross-linking density, researchers can tailor the hydrogel scaffold's stiffness and elasticity to match the target bone's mechanical characteristics. This is particularly important in load-bearing applications where the scaffold must endure mechanical stresses similar to those experienced by natural bone. The application of bone tissue engineering is shown in Fig. 10.4 [53].

6.3 Cartilage tissue engineering

Cartilage tissue engineering is promising for addressing the challenges associated with cartilage injuries, degenerative conditions, and osteoarthritis. Collagen and gelatin-based hydrogels have emerged as key components in cartilage tissue engineering, offering versatile platforms to replicate the unique properties of articular cartilage and promote effective tissue regeneration.

Collagen and gelatin hydrogels are utilized to develop scaffolds aimed at intervening in the progression of osteoarthritis, a condition characterized by the deterioration of cartilage in joints. These hydrogels provide a supportive matrix that aids in cartilage repair, reduces inflammation, and offers relief from osteoarthritic symptoms. In joint injuries or trauma cases, collagen and gelatin-based hydrogels contribute to the repair and regeneration of damaged cartilage. By creating a biomimetic scaffold, these hydrogels support the infiltration and production of chondrocytes, the specialized cells responsible for cartilage maintenance, ensuring the restoration of functional joint tissue [49].

The hydrogels can be modified to induce chondrogenic differentiation, guiding precursor cells toward adopting a chondrocytic fate. The hydrogels provide a favorable microenvironment for chondrocytes to produce the extracellular matrix components specific to cartilage, such as collagen and proteoglycans [54]. This is essential for forming a cartilage-like tissue with biomechanical properties resembling native articular cartilage. The tunable mechanical properties of collagen and gelatin hydrogels are crucial for mimicking the load-bearing nature of cartilage. Researchers can customize these hydrogels to match the stiffness and elasticity required for specific joints, ensuring that the engineered cartilage can withstand mechanical stresses similar to natural cartilage. This is particularly relevant for applications in weight-bearing joints like the knee or hip.

Moreover, the biodegradability of collagen and gelatin hydrogels aligns with the dynamic nature of cartilage regeneration. These hydrogels undergo controlled degradation over time, ensuring the scaffold gradually gives way to newly formed cartilage tissue. The controlled degradation minimizes the risk of chronic inflammation and supports the seamless integration of the engineered cartilage with the surrounding joint environment.

6.4 Nerve tissue regeneration

Collagen and gelatin hydrogels are utilized to repair and regenerate peripheral nerve injuries. These hydrogels provide a supportive matrix that facilitates the growth of nerve cells, guiding axons to bridge the gap in injured nerves. The biocompatibility of these hydrogels ensures minimal harmful reactions, promoting the integration of the scaffold with the surrounding nerve tissue [55]. The three-dimensional architecture of collagen and gelatin hydrogels can be engineered to provide precise guidance for axonal outgrowth. The hydrogel scaffold serves as a conduit for regenerating nerve fibers, directing axons across the injury site, and promoting the reconnection of nerve pathways. This is crucial for restoring sensory and motor functions in cases of nerve injury.

While regeneration in the central nervous system poses greater challenges, collagen, and gelatin-based hydrogels are also explored for their potential in Central Nervous System (CNS) repair. These hydrogels can create progressive environments for neural cell growth and may contribute to the repair of spinal cord injuries or other CNS disorders [55] by employing the hydrogels in neural tissue engineering to create three-dimensional environments that mimic the extracellular matrix of neural tissue. These hydrogels support the differentiation of neural stem cells into specific neuronal and glial cell types, fostering the development of functional neural networks.

Furthermore, the biocompatibility of collagen and gelatin hydrogels is crucial for minimizing immune responses and inflammation during nerve regeneration. These hydrogels create a microenvironment that supports cell adhesion and growth without triggering adverse reactions. In addition, they can be engineered to modulate immune responses, reducing inflammation and promoting a favorable environment for nerve tissue regeneration. It also can be functionalized to deliver growth factors and neurotrophic molecules. Incorporating these bioactive agents into the hydrogel matrix enhances cell survival, promotes neurite outgrowth, and stimulates the expression of factors that support nerve regeneration. This targeted delivery is critical for creating an environment conducive to the intricate processes involved in nerve tissue regeneration.

6.5 Corneal reconstruction

Collagen and gelatin-based hydrogels have emerged as valuable tools in corneal tissue engineering, providing a biomimetic environment for regenerating the transparent and avascular cornea [55,56]. Collagen and gelatin hydrogels are well-suited for corneal tissue engineering due to their transparency and biocompatibility. These hydrogels create a scaffold that mimics the structure of the natural cornea, facilitating the regeneration of clear and optically functional tissue. In corneal injuries or diseases affecting the stromal layer, collagen and gelatin-based hydrogels contribute to the repair and regeneration of the corneal stroma [55]. These hydrogels provide a three-dimensional matrix that supports the infiltration and alignment of corneal stromal cells, promoting the restoration of tissue integrity.

Collagen and gelatin hydrogels also play a role in reconstructing the corneal epithelium, the cornea's outermost layer. These hydrogels can be engineered to support the adherence, proliferation, and differentiation of corneal epithelial cells, ensuring the reconstruction of a functional and protective epithelial layer [56,57]. They are also utilized in the development of keratoprostheses and artificial corneas. These prosthetic devices aim to replace damaged or diseased corneas, offering a transparent and biocompatible alternative. The hydrogel scaffold supports cell attachment and tissue integration, ensuring the success of the artificial cornea in restoring vision.

The precision and customization offered by collagen and gelatin-based hydrogels enable the development of patient-specific corneal grafts. These grafts can be tailored to match the dimensions and curvature of individual patients' corneas, providing a personalized approach to corneal transplantation. This is particularly relevant in cases where conventional grafts may not be ideal. The biodegradability of collagen and gelatin hydrogels aligns with the dynamic nature of corneal regeneration. These hydrogels undergo controlled degradation, ensuring the scaffold gradually gives way to the regenerated corneal tissue. The controlled degradation minimizes the risk of inflammation and promotes the seamless integration of the hydrogel with the host cornea.

7. Hydrogels in tissue engineering

In theory, hydrogels are networks of three-dimensional (3D) polymers saturated with water. The water content varies depending on the concentration of the polymer and can reach up to 90%–99%. This explains why hydrogels have high hydrophilicity and why adding living entities (cells and proteins) is safe without causing aggregation. Generally speaking, hydrogels exhibit viscoelastic mechanical behavior related to water and the flow of polymer networks in fluid. Natural polymers including collagen, gelatin, alginate, hyaluronic acid (HA), and chitosan, as well as synthetic polymers like polyethylene glycol (PEG), polyacrylamide (PAA), and polydimethylsiloxane (PDMS), are common components of hydrogels [58].

Cross-linking techniques, whether physical or chemical, facilitate the gelation of hydrogels. While chemical cross-links provide strong bindings between polymer chains, weak interactions across polymer networks allow for physical gelation. Chemically cross-linked hydrogels resist permanent deformation, but physically cross-linked hydrogels readily relax under stress. Chemical cross-link techniques, such as UV curing, are frequently added,

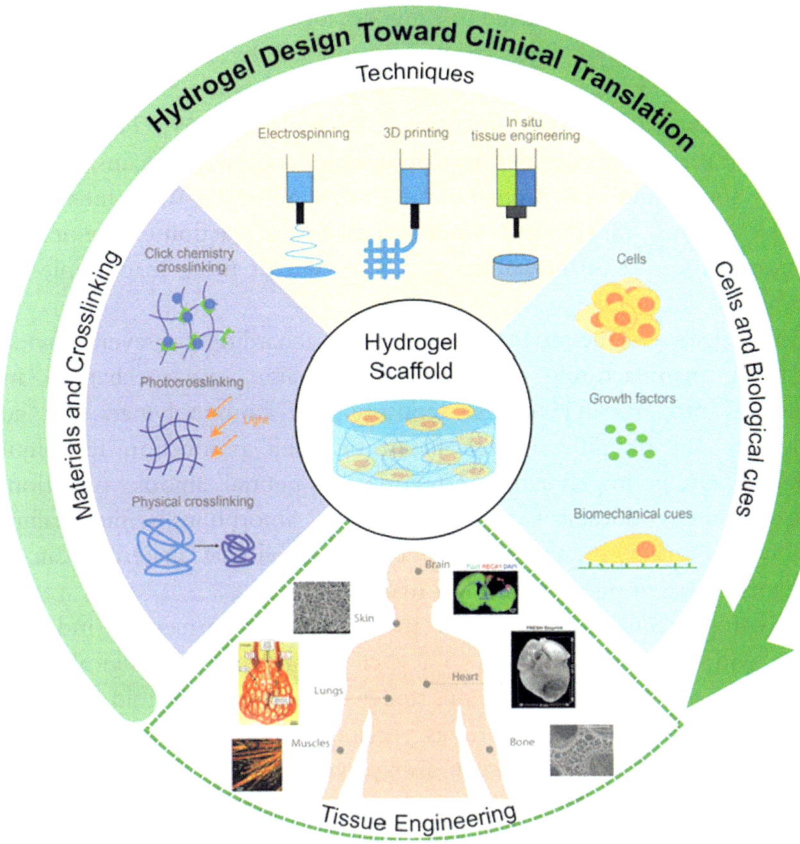

Figure 10.5 Illustrates the application of hydrogel in tissue engineering [59].

even though many natural polymers gel through physical interactions upon pH or temperature change. Readers are advised to consult the work of Caliari and Burdick for information on the types of hydrogels and their characteristics [58]. Fig. 10.5 illustrates the application of hydrogel in tissue engineering.

7.1 Role of hydrogels

The first implementation of hydrophilic networks of cross-linked poly(2-hydroxyethyl methacrylate) (pHEMA) as a soft contact lens material was developed by Wichterle and Lim in 1960, which is when hydrogels were first applied [60]. The growing number of publications on hydrogel-based materials from 1995 to the present suggests that hydrogels have attracted more attention throughout the past few decades. Hydrogels are defined in a wide range of ways. The definition provided by Peppas is the most commonly cited: Water-swollen, cross-linked polymeric structures with four different types of cross-links are called hydrogels [61]. These include (1) physical cross-links caused by entanglements between chains, (2) association bonds (such as hydrogen bonds or strong van der Waals interactions between chains), (3) covalent bonds created by the reaction of one or more comonomers, and (4) crystallites that join two or more macromolecular chains.

Hydrogels can be divided into groups according to several factors, including manufacturing technique, total charge, and mechanical and structural properties. Hydrogels consisting of homopolymers and copolymers can be differentiated based on their production technique. Alternatively, hydrogels can be categorized as neutral, anionic, or cationic based on the constituent parts' charges. Lastly, amorphous, semicrystalline, hydrogen-bonded, supramolecular, or hydrocolloidal materials can be categorized based on their physical makeup.

Hydrogels find great use in the medical and pharmaceutical industries for a wide range of purposes. They closely resemble biological tissues because of their soft, rubbery consistency and capacity to hold enormous amounts of water. Furthermore, as previously mentioned by Ovsianikov et al. their high water content also plays a role in their exceptional biocompatibility [22]. Porous gelatin-based hydrogels made by two-photon polymerization have already been shown to have the potential to be used as mesenchymal stem cell carriers.

In addition, the planted cells developed into the expected lineage when applying osteogenic stimulation. Because hydrogels have a low interfacial tension, they also exhibit less inclination to absorb proteins from bodily fluids [24]. Nevertheless, it should be mentioned that natural polymers, such as collagen, gelatin, glycosaminoglycans, and their derivatives, frequently have a strong affinity for serum proteins. Van Vlierberghe et al. for instance, have demonstrated that gelatin treated with methacrylamide has a strong affinity for fibronectin [62,63].

7.2 Importance of collagen and gelatin in hydrogel development

The primary natural protein that gives tissues their structural integrity is collagen, present in most soft, lax, semirigid, and rigid connective tissues (skin, bones, tendon, basal membranes, etc.). According to reports, collagen makes up over 80% of the dry, dermal substances near the skin's surface. High hydrophilicity, changeable ionic character, and various functionality are characteristics of the polymer collagen, which may be used in various interaction systems with other micro- and macromolecular components [64].

Hydrophobic segments produced from hydrophobic amino acids and polar groups coexist in the tight triple helix conformation of collagen, an amphoteric macromolecule. All forms of intramolecular electrostatic, dipole—dipole, hydrogen, and hydrophobic connections can thus be formed in the aqueous medium at pH values outside of the isoelectric range between the molecules, fibrils, and chain fragments of the nondenatured type I fibrillar collagen. Compared with denatured collagen (gelatin or collagen hydrolysates), which has molecules in the shape of statistical coils, this might be why aqueous systems of this kind of collagen gel at low concentrations [64].

The most popular collagen extracts, type I collagen gels and solutions, are fundamental resources for producing medical biomaterials. A gel is an arrangement of qualities halfway between a fluid and a solid. As a result, a gel might be an extremely dense solid or a less viscous liquid. Collagen gel disperses at isoelectric pH because the fibers and fibrils detach from the gel. Tropocollagen solutions are mono-dispersed, having only molecules with triple helix conformation; in contrast, collagen gels and solutions are poly-dispersed colloidal systems [64].

Conventional gelatin is formed from animal sources, including the bones, cartilage, tendons, ligaments, and skin of fish, poultry, pigs, and cattle. Gelatin, as previously indicated, is produced by partially hydrolyzing the collagen protein that was previously reported in sources. Because of this, when it has been hydrolyzed, it can also be referred to as hydrolyzed collagen, hydrolyzed gelatin, or collagen peptide. The finished substance is soluble and colorless after this treatment [65].

One of the most widely used nontoxic and biodegradable substances in the food and nonfood sectors, gelatin may be employed for various tasks, including film formation, gelation promotion, stabilization, thickening, and emulsification. Since every product must be sustainable, sanitary treatment is costly, and space delimitation is a major concern for governments and communities, biodegradability is becoming increasingly crucial. If it does n't, the product may have issues with its future usage. It has been proven that even when the gelatin or desired product is extracted from it, its biodegradable properties remain, and it may help create new materials with a high potential for biodegradability both within the human body and in the environment [65].

Gelatin is utilized to give hydrogels firmness and viscosity, and because it is renewable and biodegradable, it can be a valuable source of sustainable hydrogels. These days, gelatin's structure and texture properties determine how it is used to create hydrogels for various uses, from the biomedical or biotechnological fields to the most varied water and waste treatments. Consequently, gelatin-based hydrogels are very intriguing materials because of their versatility.

7.3 Advantages of hydrogels

The compositions and gel properties, including texture and structure that may be created in hydrogels, are the most varied. Research on various polymers has shown that these materials are highly valuable for various applications and are inventive, sustainable, and renewable [66]. These materials have also been researched in environmental and biological fields [67–69]. Their vast application and formulation possibilities with various polymers and compositions might improve their performance and make their usage both technically and financially feasible.

Pollutant emissions and environmental pollution have become major issues for humanity to address and lessen today. Hydrogels may be significant in this case because of their excellent contaminant adsorption capability and versatility in production methods and material modifications. For the manufacture of hydrogels, a variety of matrices have been utilized, including gelatin, poly(vinyl alcohol) (PVA), acrylamide, alginate dialdehyde-gelatin (ADA-GEL) [70], dialdehyde carboxymethyl cellulose-dextrin, and gelatin [71]. To increase their adsorbent capabilities, several additional ingredients have also been added, and they include graphene oxide/lapndonite/gelatin hydrogels, lignin, montmorillonite, and gelatin ionically modified by bacterial cellulose [22].

The biodegradable hydrogels with chelating groups and ion exchange have garnered significant interest because of their nontoxicity, biodegradability, swelling characteristics, and substantial water content. A variety of moieties on the hydrogel surface, such as amine (-NH2), hydroxyl (-OH), carboxyl (-COOH), and thiol (-SH), can serve as active binding sites. The 3D network structure can offer a diffusion pathway to demonstrate better adsorption kinetics and capacities for the contaminants found in water [24].

7.4 Limitations/challenges

One biomaterial frequently used in tissue engineering is collagen; however, when creating engineered tissues, there are several restrictions to consider. A major limitation is its intrinsic low mechanical strength, which makes it especially inappropriate for tissues that support weight, such as cartilage and bones. One further obstacle that might jeopardize the long-term stability of tissue constructions is the fast breakdown of collagen in vivo. Its immunogenicity also raises questions regarding collagen's universal biocompatibility by potentially causing negative responses in certain people [72].

Due to its animal origins, collagen has problems with batch-to-batch variability, potential for disease transmission, and ethical considerations. For example, exact manipulation of collagen's cross-linking is still difficult to do, which affects customized and reproducible tissue engineering. To overcome these constraints, current research investigates substitute origins, sophisticated production methodologies, and amalgamations with other biomaterials to augment the comprehensive efficacy and adaptability of collagen-derived tissue engineering strategies [72].

Although the protein gelatin is easily biodegradable in the environment, it is not as stable at high temperatures because prolonged exposure to temperatures above 40°C might cause denaturation of the protein after it has been dissolved. Furthermore, the water solubility of gelatin might be a challenge for creating tidy gelatin structures. Glycine-X-Y repeating units are typically used to make gelatin. What makes gelatin unique is the high concentration of the amino acids hydroxyproline (10%), proline (12%), and hydroxylysine (0.5%). Proline and hydroxyproline contents can vary depending on the source; fish gelatin is recognized to have fewer amino acids than gelatin derived from mammals. This has a detrimental effect on fish gelatin's ability to gel, which worsens the material's mechanical qualities and lowers the gelation and melting temperatures [72].

8. Conclusion

In conclusion, collagen and gelatin-based hydrogels in tissue engineering highlight these biomaterials' remarkable versatility and efficiency in advancing regenerative medicine. The unique combination of biocompatibility, tunable mechanical properties, and bioactive potential has positioned collagen and gelatin hydrogels as pivotal components in the quest for innovative solutions across various tissue engineering applications.

The structural and biochemical similarities between collagen/gelatin and the natural extracellular matrix make these hydrogels highly conducive to cell adhesion, proliferation, and differentiation. The ability to modulate their mechanical properties allows researchers to tailor hydrogels to match the specific requirements of diverse tissues, from load-bearing bone to flexible cartilage. Moreover, the controlled degradation of these hydrogels aligns seamlessly with the dynamic nature of tissue regeneration, promoting integration with the host environment. Across different tissues, collagen and gelatin hydrogels have demonstrated their function in advancing angiogenesis, supporting vascularization, and facilitating the formation of three-dimensional tissue constructs. Their applications span skin and muscle tissue regeneration, bone repair, cartilage engineering, nerve regeneration, and vascular reconstruction. The success in these diverse applications indicates the adaptability and effectiveness of collagen and gelatin hydrogels in replicating the microenvironment necessary for optimal tissue regeneration.

Some challenges persist, including achieving long-term stability, addressing immune responses, and optimizing mechanical properties for various tissues. Ongoing research industries aim to overcome these challenges by incorporating advanced technologies, growth factors, and enhanced fabrication techniques. The trajectory of collagen and gelatin-based hydrogels in tissue engineering promises continued innovation and transformative impacts on regenerative medicine. As interdisciplinary collaborations flourish and technological advancements unlock new possibilities, these hydrogels are poised to play an even more vital role in addressing complex challenges, ultimately translating into improved clinical outcomes and a brighter future for tissue engineering.

References

[1] Curtis A, Riehle M. Tissue engineering: the biophysical background. Phys Med Biol 2001;46(4):47–65.

[2] Bonassar LJ, Vacanti CA. Tissue engineering: the first decade and beyond. J Cell Biochem 1998;72(S30–31):297–303.

[3] Caló E, Khutoryanskiy VV. Biomedical applications of hydrogels: a review of patents and commercial products. Eur Polym J Apr. 2015;65(1):252–67.

[4] Li Y, et al. Collagen-based biomaterials for bone tissue engineering. Mater Des Nov. 2021;210:110049.

[5] Griffith LG, Gail N. Tissue engineering—current challenges and expanding opportunities. Science 2002;295(5557):1009–14.

[6] Aebischer P, Winn SR, Tresco PA, Greene LA, Jaeger CB. Transplantation of polymer encapsulated neurotransmitter secreting cells: effect of the encapsulation technique. J Biomech Eng 1991;113:178–83.

[7] Wang Y, et al. Advances in hydrogel-based vascularized tissues for tissue repair and drug screening. Bioact Mater Mar. 2022;9:198–220.
[8] Skalak R, Fox CF. Tissue engineering. In: Granlibakken, lake tahoe: Proc wrkshop. New York: Liss; 1988. p. 26–9.
[9] Chapekar MS. Tissue engineering: challenges and opportunities. J Biomed Mater Res 2000;53(6):617–20.
[10] Chen Q, et al. Elastomeric biomaterials for tissue engineering. Prog Polym Sci Mar. 2013;38(3–4):584–671.
[11] Mertz L. Tissue engineering and regenerative medicine: the promise, the challenges, the future. IEEE Pulse 2017;8:15–8.
[12] Reddi AH. Morphogenesis and tissue engineering of bone and cartilage: inductive signals, stem cells, and biomimetic biomaterials. Tissue Eng 2000;6:351–9.
[13] Teo WE, Ramakrishna S. A review on electrospinning design and nanofibre assemblies. Nanotechnology 2000;9:211–5.
[14] Lewin-Epstein J. Polyvinyl sponge (Ivalon) as a scaffold for bone. Br J Oral Surg 1964;2:115–9.
[15] Vracko R, Benditt EP. Basal lamina: the scaffold for orderly cell replacement. Observations on regeneration of injured skeletal muscle fibers and capillaries. J Cell Biol 1972;55:406–19.
[16] Li WJ, Cooper JA. In: Burdick JA, Mauck RL, editors. Biomaterials for tissue engineering applications. Vienna, Austria: Springer Vienna; 2011.
[17] Williams DF. On the nature of biomaterials. Biomaterials 2009;30:5897–909.
[18] Butler DL, et al. Functional tissue engineering: the role of biomechanics. J Biomech Eng 2000;122(6):570–5.
[19] Challenges in tissue engineering. J Royal Soc Interface 2019;62(11):141–53.
[20] Bhattacharjee A, Bansal M. Collagen structure: the Madras triple helix and the current scenario 2005;57(3):161–72.
[21] Salvatore L, et al. Marine collagen and its derivatives: versatile and sustainable bioresources for healthcare. Mater Sci Eng C Mater Biol Appl 2020;103:110963.
[22] Ahmed MA, Al-Kahtani HA, Jaswir I, AbuTarboush H, Ismail EA. Extraction and characterization of gelatin from camel skin (potential halal gelatin) and production of gelatin nanoparticles. Saudi J Biol Sci 2020;27:1596–601.
[23] Said NS, Sarbon NM. Physical and mechanical characteristics of gelatin-based films as a potential food packaging material: a review. Membranes April 19, 2022;12(5):442.
[24] Elango J, Hou C, Bao B, Wang S, Maté Sánchez de Val JE, Wenhui W. The molecular interaction of collagen with cell receptors for biological function. Polymers 2022;14(5):876.
[25] Abdullah A, Abdullah AZ, Ahmed M, Khan J, Shahadat M, Umar K, Alim MA. A review on recent developments and progress in sustainable acrolein production through catalytic dehydration of bio-renewable glycerol. J Clean Prod March 20, 2022;341:130876.
[26] Chiou BS, Avena-Bustillos RJ, Bechtel PJ, Jafri H, Narayan R, Imam SH, Glenn GM, Orts WJ. Cold water fish gelatin films: effects of cross-linking on thermal, mechanical, barrier, and biodegradation properties. Eur Polym J 2008;44:3748–53.
[27] Salgado CL, Grenho L, Fernandes MH, Colaço BJ, Monteiro FJ. Biodegradation, biocompatibility, and osteoconduction evaluation of collagen-nanohydroxyapatite cryogels for bone tissue regeneration. J Biomed Mater Res, Part A 2015;104:57–70.
[28] Kim H, Kumbar SG, Nukavarapu SP. Biomaterial-directed cell behavior for tissue engineering. Curr Opin Biomed Eng 2021;17:100–20.
[29] He Y, Wang C, Wang C, Xiao Y, Lin W. An overview on collagen and gelatin-based cryogels: fabrication, classification, properties and biomedical applications. Polymers 2021;13:2299.

[30] Li J, Wang Y, Zhang L, Xu Z, Dai H, Wu W. Nanocellulose/gelatin composite cryogels for controlled drug release. ACS Sustainable Chem Eng 2019;7:6381–9.
[31] Mir NA, Khan A, Umar K, Muneer M. Photocatalytic study of a xanthene dye derivative, phloxine B in aqueous suspension of TiO_2: adsorption isotherm and decolourization kinetics. Energy Environ Focus September 1, 2013;2(3):208–16.
[32] Naahidi S, Jafari M, Logan M, Wang Y, Yuan Y, Bae H, Dixon B, Chen P. Biocompatibility of hydrogel-based scaffolds for tissue engineering applications. Biotechnol Adv 2017;35(5):530–44.
[33] Wichterle O, Lim D. Hydrophilic gels for biological use. Nature 1960;185:117–8.
[34] Glowacki J, Mizuno S. Collagen scaffolds for tissue engineering. Biopolymers 2007;89(5):338–44.
[35] Mir NA, Haque MM, Khan A, Umar K, Muneer M, Vijayalakshmi S. Semiconductor mediated photocatalysed reaction of two selected organic compounds in aqueous suspensions of Titanium dioxide. J Adv Oxid Technol July 1, 2012;15(2):380–91.
[36] Gonzalez-Melo C, Garcia-Brand AJ, Quezada V, Reyes LH, Muñoz-Camargo C, Cruz JC. Highly efficient synthesis of type B gelatin and low molecular weight chitosan nanoparticles: potential applications as bioactive molecule carriers and cell-penetrating agents. Polymers November 24, 2021;13(23):4078.
[37] Zhao S, Wang D, Zhu S, Liu X, Zhang H. 3D cryogel composites as adsorbent for isolation of protein and small molecules. Talanta 2019;191:229–34.
[38] Mahmoud ME, Abouelanwar ME, Mahmoud SEM, Salam MA. Doping starch-gelatin mixed hydrogels with magnetic spinel Ferrite@biochar@molybdenum oxide as a highly efficient nanocomposite for removal of lead (II) ions. J Environ Chem Eng 2021;9:1066826.
[39] Maity J, Ray SK. Removal of Cu (II) ion from water using sugar cane bagasse cellulose and gelatin based composite hydrogels. Int J Biol Macromol 2017;97:238–48.
[40] Huang Y, Zhao W, Zhang X, Peng H, Gong Y. Thiol-ene synthesis of thioether/carboxyl-functionalized polymers for selective adsorption of silver (I) ions. Chem Eng J 2019;375:121935.
[41] Umar K, Mfarrej MF, Rahman QI, Zuhaib M, Khan A, Zia Q, Banawas S, Nadeem H, Khan MF, Ahmad F. ZnO Nano-swirlings for Azo Dye AR183 photocatalytic degradation and antimycotic activity. Sci Rep August 18, 2022;12(1):14023.
[42] Thang NH, Chien TB, Cuong DX. Polymer-based hydrogels applied in drug delivery: an overview. Gels 2023;9:523.
[43] Mu C, Liu F, Cheng Q, Li H, Wu B, Zhang G, Lin W. Collagen cryogel cross-linked by dialdehyde starch. Macromol Mater Eng 2010;295:100–7.
[44] Umar K. Water contamination by organic-pollutants: TiO 2 photocatalysis. Modern age environmental problems and their remediation. 2018. p. 95–109.
[45] Guillén-Carvajal K, Valdez-Salas B, Beltrán-Partida E, Salomón-Carlos J, Cheng N. Chitosan, gelatin, and collagen hydrogels for bone regeneration. Polymers June 21, 2023;15(13):2762.
[46] Allan IU, Tolhurst B, Shevchenko RV, Dainiak MB, Illsley M, Ivanov A, Jungvid H, Galaev IY, James SL, Mikhalovsky SV, et al. An in vitro evaluation of fibrinogen and gelatin containing cryogels as dermal regeneration scaffolds. Biomater Sci 2016;4:1007–14.
[47] Umar K, Dar AA, Haque MM, Mir NA, Muneer M. Photocatalysed decolourization of two textile dye derivatives, Martius Yellow and Acid Blue 129, in UV-irradiated aqueous suspensions of Titania. Desalination Water Treat August 1, 2012;46(1–3):205–14.
[48] Ferreira AM, Gentile P, Chiono V, Ciardelli G. Collagen for bone tissue regeneration. Acta Biomater 2012;8:3191–200.

[49] Dinescu S, et al. Collagen-based hydrogels and their applications for tissue engineering and regenerative medicine. Polym polym compos: a reference series. 2019. p. 978–83.
[50] Umar K, Adnan R. Biomass mediated green synthesis of ZnO/TiO_2 nanocomposite and enhanced photocatalytic activity for the decolorization of rhodamine B under visible light. Key Eng Mater June 16, 2022;920:36–42.
[51] Safian MT, Umar K, Ibrahim MN. Synthesis and scalability of graphene and its derivatives: a journey towards sustainable and commercial material. J Clean Prod October 10, 2021;318:128603.
[52] Kuo C-Y, Chen C-H, Hsiao C-Y, Chen J-P. Incorporation of chitosan in biomimetic gelatin/chondroitin-6-sulfate/hyaluronan cryogel for cartilage tissue engineering. Carbohydr Polym 2015;117:722–30.
[53] Szwed-Georgiou A, Płociński P, Kupikowska-Stobba B, Urbaniak MM, Rusek-Wala P, Szustakiewicz K, Piszko P, Krupa A, Biernat M, Gazińska M, Kasprzak M. Bioactive materials for bone regeneration: biomolecules and delivery systems. ACS Biomater Sci Eng August 16, 2023;9(9):5222–54.
[54] Liu W, Merrett K, Griffith M, Fagerholm P, Dravida S, Heyne B, Scaiano JC, Watsky MA, Shinozaki N, Lagali N, Munger R, Li F. Recombinant human collagen for tissue engineered corneal substitutes. Biomaterials 2008;29(9):1147–58.
[55] Lee J-H, Kim H-W. Emerging properties of hydrogels in tissue engineering. J Tissue Eng 2018;9.
[56] Khan MA, Ahmad A, Umar K, Nabi SA. Synthesis, characterization, and biological applications of nanocomposites for the removal of heavy metals and dyes. Ind Eng Chem Res January 14, 2015;54(1):76–82.
[57] Peppas NA, Bures P, Leobandung W, Ichikawa H. Hydrogels in pharmaceutical formulations. Eur J Pharm Biopharm 2000;50(1):27–46.
[58] Ovsianikov A, Deiwick A, Van Vlierberghe S, Dubruel P, Moller L, Drager G, Chichkov B. Laser fabrication of three-dimensional cad scaffolds from photosensitive gelatin for applications in tissue engineering. Biomacromolecules 2011;12(4):851–8.
[59] Xu F, Dawson C, Lamb M, Mueller E, Stefanek E, Akbari M, Hoare T. Hydrogels for tissue engineering: addressing key design needs toward clinical translation. Front Bioeng Biotechnol May 5, 2022;10:849831.
[60] Gupta P, Vermani K, Garg S. Hydrogels: from controlled release to pH-responsive drug delivery. Drug Discov Today 2002;7:569–79.
[61] Van Vlierberghe S, Vanderleyden E, Dubruel P, De Vos F, Schacht E. Affinity study of novel gelatin cell carriers for fibronectin. Macromol Biosci 2009;9:1105–15.
[62] Morales A, Labidi J, Gullón P. Effect of the formulation parameters on the absorption capacity of smart lignin-hydrogels. Eur Polym J 2020;129:109631.
[63] Khalid U, Tabassum P, Khan MA, Mohamad N, Akil A, Mohd R. Degradation of organic pollutants using metal-doped TiO2 photocatalysts under visible light: a comparative study. Desalination Water Treat 2019;161:275–82.
[64] Monavari M, Homaeigohar S, Fuentes-Chandía M, Nawaz Q, Monavari M, Venkatraman A, Boccaccini AR. 3D printing of alginate dialdehyde-gelatin (ADA-GEL) hydrogels incorporating phytotherapeutic icariin loaded mesoporous SiO2-CaO nanoparticles for bone tissue engineering. Mater Sci Eng C 2021;131:112470.
[65] Yang W, Wang J, Han Y, Luo X, Tang W, Yue T, Li Z. Robust MOF film of self-rearranged UiO-66-NO2 anchored on gelatin hydrogel via simple thermal-treatment for efficient Pb(II) removal in water and apple juice. Food Control 2021;130:108409.
[66] Marciano JS, Ferreira RR, de Souza AG, Barbosa RFS, de Moura Junior AJ, Rosa DS. Biodegradable gelatin composite hydrogels filled with cellulose for chromium (VI) adsorption from contaminated water. Int J Biol Macromol 2021;181:112–24.

[67] Manish V, Arockiarajan A, Tamadapu G. Influence of water content on the mechanical behavior of gelatin based hydrogels: synthesis, characterization, and modeling. Int J Solid Struct 2021;233:111219.

[68] Tahari N, de Hoyos-Martinez PL, Abderrabba M, Ayadi S, Labidi J. Lignin-montmorillonite hydrogels as toluene adsorbent. Colloids Surf A Physicochem Eng Asp 2020;602:125108.

[69] Haseen U, Umar K, Ahmad H, Parveen T, Mohamad Ibrahim MN. Graphene and its composites: applications in environmental remediation. Modern age waste water problems: solutions using applied nanotechnology. 2020. p. 85–91.

[70] Sharma AK, Kaith BS, Shree B. Borax mediated synthesis of a biocompatible self-healing hydrogel using dialdehyde carboxymethyl cellulose-dextrin and gelatin. React Funct Polym 2021;166:104977.

[71] Cheng YH, Cheng SJ, Chen HH, Hsu WC. Development of injectable graphene oxide/laponite/gelatin hydrogel containing wharton's jelly mesenchymal stem cells for treatment of oxidative stress-damaged cardiomyocytes. Colloids Surf B Biointerfaces 2022;209:112150.

[72] Lotz C, et al. Cross-linked collagen hydrogel matrix resisting contraction to facilitate full-thickness skin equivalents. ACS Appl Mater Interfaces 2017;9(24):20417–25.

CHAPTER 11

Fibrin-based hydrogels for tissue engineering

Abhishek Kumar[1,2], Rakesh Pandey[2], Anant Narayan Bhatt[2] and Mohd Saquib Ansari[1]
[1]Department of Biomedical Sciences, Shaheed Rajguru College of Applied Sciences for Women, University of Delhi, Delhi, New Delhi, India; [2]Institute of Nuclear Medicine and Allied Sciences, Defence Research and Development Organization, Delhi, New Delhi, India

1. Introduction

Tissue engineering aims to artificially construct biological substitutes for the reconstruction, regeneration, and repair of damaged tissues. Tissue engineering employs modified biocompatible hydrogel scaffolds that are mechanically stable and include embedded cells with bioactive factors that enhance cellular function and differentiation [1].

Hydrogels made from protein-based polymers like fibrin are highly biocompatible and bioactive. These proteins are derived from the extracellular matrix (ECM) and have an inherent ability to mimic vital biochemical properties that can regulate tissue repair and regeneration. Fibrin hydrogels form an ECM-like matrix at the injury site, providing multiple binding sites for cell adhesion and ultimately on-site cellular proliferation to heal wounds. Fibrin-based hydrogels are composed of fibrinogen, which is degraded by thrombin by the removal of fibrinopeptides. Finally, the fibrin monomers self-assemble into a fibrous fibrin gel, which can be further degraded by plasmin-mediated fibrinolysis, providing excellent degradability to the fibrin gels [2].

Fibrin-based hydrogels have a clinical implementation in surgical procedures as hemostatic aids with the ability to seal such surgical wounds acting as excellent bioadhesives [3]. Trauma-induced injury or related insult to a tissue or organ exposes the site to foreign contaminants and infectious agents. When applied to such sites, a fibrin hydrogel provides a scaffold for the recruitment and attachment of neutrophils and macrophages, which clears

Protein-Based Nanocomposites for Tissue Engineering
ISBN 978-0-323-99357-9
https://doi.org/10.1016/B978-0-323-99357-9.00003-X

the site of any dead or necrotic cells while disposing of any infectious agents that have breached the outer epidermal protection [4]. It also acts as a clotting agent by mimicking the endpoint of the blood coagulation cascade, resulting in the formation of a fibrin clot which, more importantly, remains bound to the site of injury, plugging the tear in tissue preventing further leakage of bodily fluids while providing cellular attachment platform for migration, differentiation, and proliferation of fibroblasts for tissue repair progression [5].

Many natural biopolymers such as alginate [6,7], chitosan [8,9], natural gums [10], and cellulose [11,12] have favorable biological and mechanical properties. Fibrin hydrogels cross-linked with such natural and other synthetic polymers provide enhanced mechanical and chemical properties in different In vivoenvironments. The use of naturally occurring polymers like alginate, chitosan, and collagen in combination with fibrin gels has been reported in various clinical applications like the construction of artificial arteries and veins and spinal cord and peripheral nerve regeneration [13–15]. Gelatin and albumin combined fibrin gels have an application in cartilage and bone tissue engineering, respectively [16,17]. In the case of synthetic polymers, fibrin hydrogels loaded with Polyethylene Glycol (PEG) and Poly (DL-lactic-co-glycolic acid) (PLGA) have been applied in peripheral nerve regeneration and spinal cord regeneration, respectively [18,19]. Scaffolds prepared with the addition of polypropylene fumarate (PPF) and poly(L-lactide) (PLLA) have shown exemplary implementation in bone and cartilage tissue engineering [20,21]. Melt spun polylactic acid (PLA) integrated fibrin fibers have also demonstrated potential in cardiovascular tissue engineering [22]. Once injected, these hydrogels conform to the shape of tissue defects. They can provide mechanical, growth, and repair support at the injury site by creating an integrative hydrogel-tissue interface. These fibrin hydrogels can be modified as cellular carriers that can be developed to protect the desired cells from preparation and delivery forces. These cell-carrying hydrogels are highly compatible with high cellular density and uniform cell distribution for minimally invasive cellular delivery to repair damaged tissue and organs [23]. This chapter aims to develop an understanding of the current uses, advances, and applications of fibrin-based hydrogel-mediated tissue engineering.

2. Structure and synthesis of fibrin hydrogels

Fibrinogen is a 340 KDa fibrous protein, and it was first characterized by its distinct α-helical coiled structure using X-ray diffraction [24]. It is an essential component of human blood plasma, mainly involved in hemostatic action. In case of trauma to the vessel walls, the fibrinogen is activated to fibrin by the enzymatic activity of thrombin circulating in the blood, causing highly regulated deposition of fibrin at the site of injury exposed tissue resulting in the formation of stable fibrin clots while also avoiding any persistent thromboembolic complications [25]. Fibrinogen is composed of a pair of three polypeptide chains, Aα, Bβ, and γ, forming three domains, two outer D-regions, each of which is connected to the middle E-region by an α-helical coiled segment held together by 29 disulfide bonds (Fig. 11.1A) [26]. The fibrinogen Aα and Bβ chains contain an N-terminal fibrinopeptide A (FpA) and fibrinopeptide B (FpB), respectively. Thrombin cleaves the FpA and FpB from the E-region, exposing polymerization sites to interact with the binding pockets on γ polypeptide present in the D-

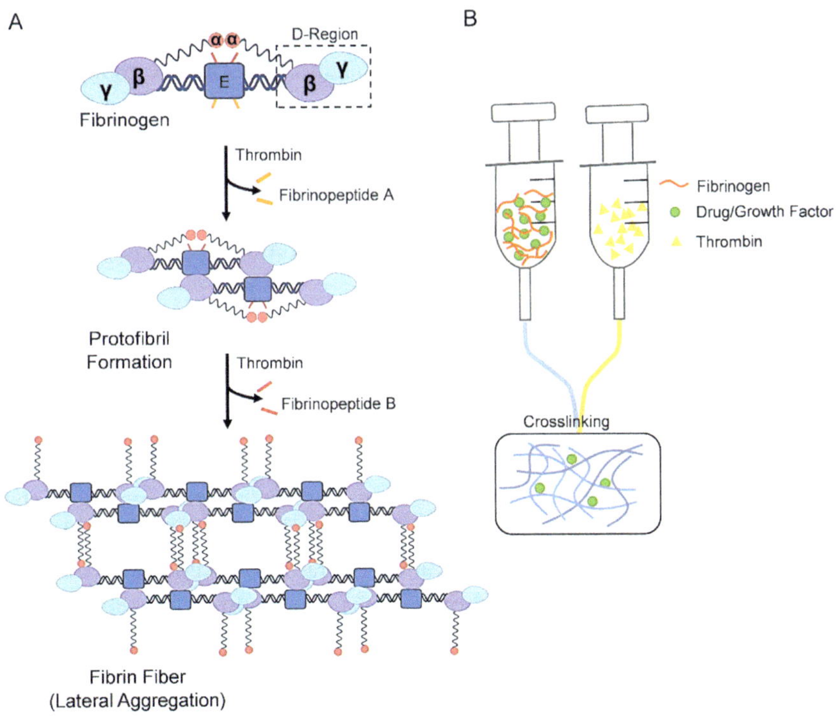

Figure 11.1 (A) Diagrammatic representation of the structure of fibrinogen and cleavage of FpA and FpB by thrombin resulting in the formation of fibrin mesh. (B) Schematic representation of injectable device carrying fibrinogen and thrombin (supplemented with growth factors, drug, or cells) in separate syringes for on-site application.

region [27]. This initial interaction causes staggered overlapping of the middle-end domains of fibrinogens, resulting in double-stranded fibrils. This formation is further strengthened by lateral interactions of fibrinogens, forming a mesh-like fibrin network (Fig. 11.1A) [28].

Hydrogels fabricated with fibrin as their polymer backbone are versatile for in-situ applications in tissue repair, targeted drug/cell delivery, and tissue engineering. These hydrogels support the addition and incorporation of desired natural/synthetic drugs and related growth factors securely enclosed inside the fibrin mesh for targeted delivery of the compounds. The fibrin mesh encompasses the cells/drugs securely and shields them from the physical forces of preparation and delivery [23]. Fibrin gels and other fibrin-based products are sourced from fibrinogen derived from human plasma to minimize the risks of any immunological reaction. Whereas thrombin is extracted from bovine plasma. Both the solutions are stored in separate injectable vessels, and the addition of natural/synthetic drugs and related growth factors to one or both of these syringes can be performed to obtain a self-assembling modified fibrin mesh on injection of both the syringes onto the site (Fig. 11.1B) [29]. The mechanical properties of the fibrin hydrogel prepared using this methodology can be modulated by changing the thrombin concentration. Increasing the thrombin concentration in the hydrogel causes the formation of densely packed fibrin mesh with thinner fibers, whereas decreasing the thrombin concentration leads to highly porous gels [30].

3. Clinical applications in tissue repair and bioengineering

3.1 Fibrin gels as hemostatic sealant glue in surgical procedures

Fibrin glue has seen implementation in current surgical practices that involve the stemming of surgical bleeds and is also sometimes considered a replacement of sutures in some minor operative procedures. There are many commercially available fibrin sealants like Crosseal, Tisseel, Floseal, Surgiflo, and Surgicel, that are approved and currently being used for hemostatic applications in the colonic, cardiac, liver, and splenic procedures [31]. A few reported case series have found sutureless application of fibrin gels ineffective in sealing of ruptured left ventricular wall following acute myocardial infarction [32]. One study has reported the use of fibrin sealant in effective hemostatic sealing of suture holes in patients with femoral artery grafts and found accelerated wound closure time with a shorter duration of hospitalization [33]. Fibrin sealants have also been used in esophageal rupture repair and hernia repair and are more effective than the standard prosthetic mesh, with better mesh fixation capabilities than staples [34]. A case series has reported achievement of hemostasis with a significant decline in mean blood loss per patient undergoing resection of small renal lesions requiring no further blood transfusion [35]. All these clinical and research work in surgical settings emphasizes the highly versatile nature of fibrin gels in creating blood clots, sutureless sealing, and gluing of tissues together while providing mechanical support.

3.2 Fibrin gels in spinal cord regeneration and neuronal repair

The central nervous system (CNS) comprises the spinal cord responsible for controlling sensory and motor functions. Every year around 760,000 people suffer from a severe spinal cord injury due to traffic accidents and other incidents [36]. Paralysis of the lower extremities, incontinence, and sexual dysfunction are expected consequences of traumatic and nontraumatic Spinal Cord Injury. This points toward the urgent need to protect and regenerate the damaged nerves and connections by niche modification using tissue regeneration techniques.

Researchers have found that adult mammalian CNS axon regeneration is severely affected by Spinal Cord Injury. The major obstacle in neural regeneration is inhibition caused by the surrounding environment and the creation or deletion of a functional connection [37]. Multifunctional Scaffolds that can carry cells and medicinal compounds are suitable in neural tissue engineering for solving the issues outlined above.

In nerve regeneration, synthetic polymer scaffolds with high mechanical strength, fewer impurities, and manipulative flexibility have been widely used [38,39]. However, these polymer scaffolds have limitations, such as their toxic breakdown products and inadequate polymerization. Fibrin is an FDA-approved tissue sealant for wound healing and hemostasis. Fibrin-based hydrogels are biocompatible and possess numerous binding sites for ECM components, cells, and growth factors. Fibrin gels are also implemented in peripheral neuron regeneration. Studies point toward the potential of fibrin to control axonal regrowth and Schwann cell proliferation, both of which are critical for nerve regeneration. It has also previously been shown that a 3D-aligned layer of fibrin hydrogel formed by electrospinning provides an ideal microenvironment and serves as an intraluminal filler to speed up the axon regeneration by mimicking the original fiber architecture and function (Fig. 11.2) [40]. Fibrin glue is one such alternative to

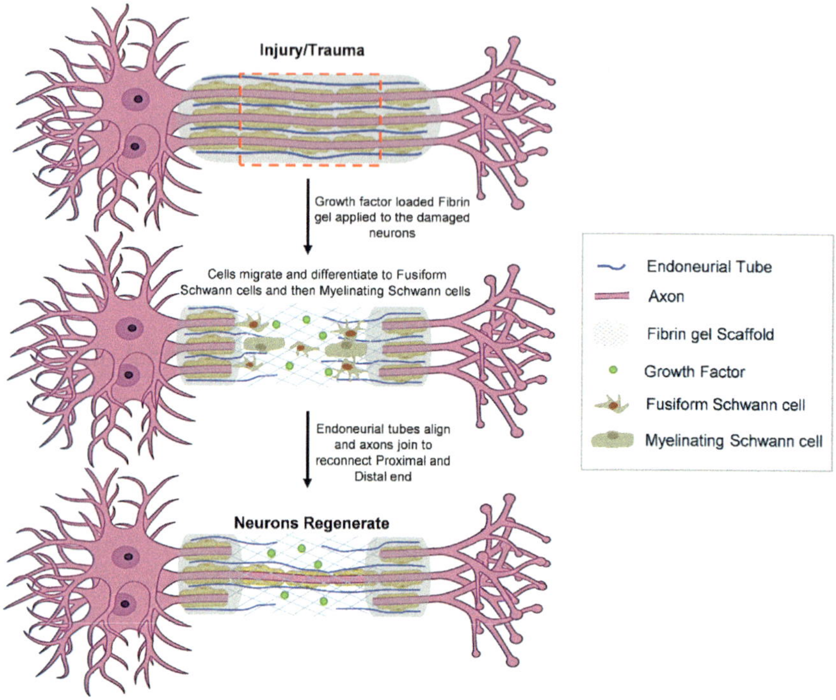

Figure 11.2 Figure showing the application of fibrin gel in nerve regeneration. At the site of damage, the growth factor-loaded fibrin gel mimics the physiological microenvironment of ECM, thereby promoting the migration of undifferentiated schwann cells, their differentiation into myelinating schwann cells, and the formation of functional axonal connection.

microsurgical suturing in nerve coaptation. Experiments were conducted on a sciatic nerve transplantation mice model to compare fibrin glue with microsuture coaptation in the wound repair time and gap size. It was determined that the gap size at the surgical site was the same in both groups, but surgical repair time was reduced by using fibrin glue [41]. Fibrin scaffolds are an effective substrate for creating tissues from pluripotent stem cells. Human pluripotent stem cell differentiation for tissue engineering applications is complicated by the rapid breakdown of fibrin. In a study, Genipin was used as a cross-linking agent to strengthen the scaffold stability in 2D culture and architecture in 3D culture. Genipin improved the differentiation of neural progenitors from human-induced pluripotent stem cells. Genipin cross-linked fibrin scaffold stimulated the neurite outgrowth and maintained neural aggregates while remaining stable for 2 weeks compared with 5 days in unmodified fibrin [42].

3.3 Fibrin gels in arterial and cardiac tissue repair

Coronary heart disease is one of the major problems worldwide. Permanent cardiac tissue damage caused by myocardial infarction ultimately results in heart failure. Heart transplantation is the only gold standard in these types of cases. Still, due to the scarcity of organ donors, researchers have turned to tissue engineering to regenerate functional heart tissue [43]. The therapeutic repair of the heart using stem cells and Platelet fibrin gel is thoroughly researched. Platelet fibrin gel and cardiac stem cells were found to have therapeutic benefits when put into the hearts of rats with myocardial infarction (MI). It was also shown that Matrix metalloproteinase is essential for the fibrin gel supplemented with stem cells to exert its beneficial effect. Inhibition of Metalloproteinase decreases the cellular engraftment and host angiogenesis in the Myocardial infarction model (Fig. 11.3) [44]. Researchers also used fibrin gel as a framework to create 3-D cardiovascular

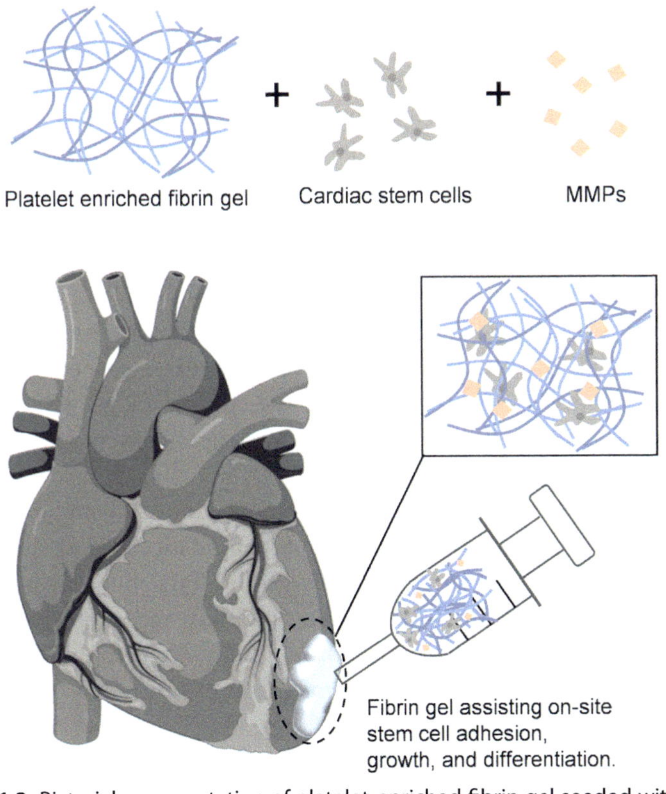

Figure 11.3 Pictorial representation of platelet-enriched fibrin gel seeded with cardiac stem cells and supplemented with MMPs to repair cardiac tissue.

structures such as arteries or valve conduits with as much as 3 mm thickness. In addition, the fibrin gel can be derived from the blood of patients, thus reducing the risk of immunogenic responses. The crucial drawback associated with the fibrin gel as a scaffold is its initial low mechanical rigidity and shrinkage, preventing new structures from being directly implanted [45]. Protease inhibitors like aprotinin and tranexamic acid may modulate the polymerization and breakdown of the fibrin gel to suit tissue [46].

In a study, polyvinylidene fluoride (PVDF) mesh was integrated into the fibrin gel containing carotid myofibroblast and then implanted into the patients. It was found that the fibrin matrix, which is surrounded by PVDF mesh, showed excellent cell proliferation and growth. These structures were also able to handle the pressure gradient and physiological flow because of the mechanical strength provided by the mesh structure [47]. The finding of a pilot study demonstrated that fibrin gel derived from the patient is a promising candidate for the development of an autologous heart valve. Autologous arterial cells derived from a sheep model were seeded on a molded fibrin gel which was further subjected to mechanical preconditioning. These valve conduits were then incorporated into the pulmonary trunk of the same model and extracted after 3 months. Surprisingly, these conduits were relatively stable, consistent (demonstrated original tissue properties), and showed a uniform monolayer of the vascular bed [48].

3.4 Fibrin gels in cartilage and bone repair

Cartilage damage has a limited healing tendency which can be traced to the absence of vascularization and innervation and a complete lack of progenitor cells [49,50]. It is composed of a fiber-reinforced composite with chondrocytes dispersed throughout a tissue-specific ECM with functional and glycoproteins arranged in a unique spatial arrangement [51]. Fibrin gel alone and in combination has been used for cartilage tissue repair and engineering. Alginate hydrogel is a highly biocompatible and non-immunogenic polymer with prominent hemostatic and wound healing properties [6,7], Frequently combined with fibrin to obtain hydrogels with enhanced cellular interaction promoting mobility and proliferation at the site for better vasculature in vivo [52]. In a study involving cartilage repair, fibrin gels supplemented with ECM microparticles, freshly isolated stromal stem cells, and transforming growth factor (TGF)-β3 have been used to detect effective deposition of cartilage and sulfated glycosaminoglycan (sGAG) with evidence of significantly improved chondrogenesis [53].

As opposed to cartilage, bones are highly vascularized with excellent mechanical strength and structural complexity. The bone ECM is incorporated with growth factors and cytokines that support chondrocyte and osteogenic growth and development while providing proper anchorage support [51]. Fibrin gels alone have limited application in bone defect repair, and supplementation with bone graft particles and osteogenic cells is often required to heal bone defects effectively. In a study on bone regeneration capabilities of fibrin gels combined with autologous bone fragments and enriched with platelets, a significant improvement in bone regeneration is observed with reduced time of hospitalization [54]. A similar platelet-enriched fibrin gel was also implemented successfully in repairing mandible-associated defects, vertical alveolar ridge repair, and sinus floor augmentation in mongrel dogs, where the platelet enrichment was achieved by the use of fibrinogen and thrombin derived from platelet-rich plasma [55–57].

4. Limitations of fibrin hydrogels

One of the significant limitations associated with fibrin-based hydrogels is their immunogenic capacity as the fibrinogen is derived from human plasma. This problem can be addressed by concentrating fibrinogen from the patient's plasma minimizing the possibility of any immunogenic reaction [58]. However, this also takes several hours to prepare and requires the patient to be free of any clotting-related disorders. Another shortcoming of fibrin is the rapid degradation/shrinkage rate and relatively weak mechanical stiffness. Surprisingly, in a study on neuronal repair, fibrin glue was shown to hinder neuron regeneration when used as a coating over a porous conduit. It was concluded that fibrin gel coating over the porous conduit attracts non-neural cells and enhances scar tissue penetration, thus compromising functional recovery [59]. The fibrin gels need to be combined with other synthetic/natural polymers to carry out complex procedures like on-site implantation. Multiple studies have also found that fibrin gels have a negative effect on bone healing, connecting it to higher concentrations of fibrinogen used in the study as well as immunogenic response to the xenogeneic proteins used for the gelation process (fibrinogen and thrombin from human plasma and aprotinin from bovine origin) [60,61].

5. Conclusion

Fibrin gels have shown immense potential in hemostatic clinical applications, including sutureless sealing of surgically incised tissues and even providing structural support to procedures involving arterial, esophageal, and hernia repair with accelerated wound healing. Fibrin gels and modified products are promising in soft tissue engineering due to their excellent biocompatibility, bioactivity, and self-assembling nature. The fibrin network ideally mimics the ECM for cellular attachment, migration, growth, and proliferation. The preparation of fibrin gels by combining fibrinogen and thrombin is also convenient as the fibrin and thrombin protein can be stored in lyophilized form and at ambient temperature without any loss of activity. These gels have a very high degree of compliance to deformations by external strains and forces, returning to a relaxed state once force is removed. This physically soft nature of fibrin gels makes them an excellent candidate for providing an ideal microenvironment to cells. Fibrin gels have shown much encouraging research evidence in the field of wound tissue repair and tissue engineering requiring further efforts to translate them into clinical application.

References

[1] Atala A. Regenerative medicine strategies. J Pediatr Surg 2012;47:17–28.
[2] Ahmed TAE, Dare E v, Hincke M. Fibrin: a versatile scaffold for tissue engineering applications. Tissue Eng Part B 2008;14:199–215.
[3] Jackson MR. Fibrin sealants in surgical practice: an overview. Am J Surg 2001;182:S1–7.
[4] Ciano PS, Colvin RB, Dvorak AM, McDonagh J, Dvorak HF. Macrophage migration in fibrin gel matrices. Lab Invest 1986;54:62–70.
[5] Ehrbar M, Metters A, Zammaretti P, Hubbell JA, Zisch AH. Endothelial cell proliferation and progenitor maturation by fibrin-bound VEGF variants with differential susceptibilities to local cellular activity. J Contr Release 2005;101:93–109.
[6] Kumar A, Bhatt AN, Singh LRK, Karim Z, Ansari MS. Alginate-based hydrogels for tissue engineering. Polysaccharide-based nanocomposites for gene delivery and tissue engineering. Elsevier; 2021. p. 59–69.
[7] Kumar A, Sah DK, Khanna K, Rai Y, Yadav AK, Ansari MS, et al. A calcium and zinc composite alginate hydrogel for pre-hospital hemostasis and wound care. Carbohydr Polym 2023;299:120186.
[8] Gupta I, Kumar A, Bhatt AN, Sapra S, Gandhi S. Green synthesis-mediated silver nanoparticles based biocomposite films for wound healing application. J Inorg Organomet Polym Mater 2022;32(8):1–18.
[9] Zheng W, Chen C, Zhang X, Wen X, Xiao Y, Li L, et al. Layer-by-layer coating of carboxymethyl chitosan-gelatin-alginate on cotton gauze for hemostasis and wound healing. Surf Coat Technol 2021;406:126644.

[10] Kalonia A, Sharma AK, Shaw P, Kumar A, Bhatt AN, Shukla A, et al. Ascorbate formulation improves healing efficacy in excisional wound mice model through interplay between pro and anti-inflammatory cytokines and angiogenic markers. Cytokine 2023;164:156158.
[11] Zhang S, Li J, Chen S, Zhang X, Ma J, He J. Oxidized cellulose-based hemostatic materials. Carbohydr Polym 2020;230:115585.
[12] Ma J, Li X, Bao Y. Advances in cellulose-based superabsorbent hydrogels. RSC Adv 2015;5:59745−57.
[13] Attalla R, Puersten E, Jain N, Selvaganapathy PR. 3D bioprinting of heterogeneous bi- and tri-layered hollow channels within gel scaffolds using scalable multi-axial microfluidic extrusion nozzle. Biofabrication 2018;11:15012.
[14] Yang W, Wang Z, Zhang J, Yang K, Lu C, Cui X, et al. Fibrin scaffolds embedded with sonic hedgehog/chitosan microspheres for recovery of spinal cord injury in rats. Materials Express 2020;10:437−45.
[15] Carriel V, Garrido-Gómez J, Hernández-Cortés P, Garzón I, García-García S, Sáez-Moreno JA, et al. Combination of fibrin-agarose hydrogels and adipose-derived mesenchymal stem cells for peripheral nerve regeneration. J Neural Eng 2013;10:26022.
[16] Wang ZH, Zhang J, Zhang Q, Gao Y, Yan J, Zhao XY, et al. Evaluation of bone matrix gelatin/fibrin glue and chitosan/gelatin composite scaffolds for cartilage tissue engineering. Genet Mol Res 2016;15:1−8.
[17] Katarivas LG, Ong J, Birch MA, Justin AW, Markaki AE. Albumin-enriched fibrin hydrogel embedded in active ferromagnetic networks improves osteoblast differentiation and vascular self-organisation. Polymers 2019;11:1743.
[18] Sarig-Nadir O, Seliktar D. Compositional alterations of fibrin-based materials for regulating in vitro neural outgrowth. Tissue Eng 2008;14:401−11.
[19] Yao S, Yang Y, Wang X, Wang L. Fabrication and characterization of aligned fibrin nanofiber hydrogel loaded with PLGA microspheres. Macromol Res 2017;25:528−33.
[20] Gamboa-Martínez TC, Gómez Ribelles JL, Gallego Ferrer G. Fibrin coating on poly (L-lactide) scaffolds for tissue engineering. J Bioact Compat Polym 2011;26:464−77.
[21] Schek RM, Wilke EN, Hollister SJ, Krebsbach PH. Combined use of designed scaffolds and adenoviral gene therapy for skeletal tissue engineering. Biomaterials 2006;27:1160−6.
[22] Gundy S, Manning G, O'Connell E, Ellä V, Harwoko MS, Rochev Y, et al. Human coronary artery smooth muscle cell response to a novel PLA textile/fibrin gel composite scaffold. Acta Biomater 2008;4:1734−44.
[23] Li Y, Meng H, Liu Y, Lee BP. Fibrin gel as an injectable biodegradable scaffold and cell carrier for tissue engineering. Sci World J 2015;2015.
[24] Bailey K, Astbury WT, Rudall KM. Fibrinogen and fibrin as members of the keratin-myosin group. Nature 1943;151:716−7.
[25] Mosesson MW. Dysfibrinogenemia and thrombosis. Semin Thromb Hemost 1999;25:311−9.
[26] Weisel JW, Litvinov RI. Fibrin formation, structure and properties. Fibrous Proteins: Struct Mechanism 2017:405−56.
[27] Wolfenstein-Todel C, Mosesson MW. Human plasma fibrinogen heterogeneity: evidence for an extended carboxyl-terminal sequence in a normal gamma chain variant (gamma). Proceed Nat Acad Sci 1980;77:5069−73.
[28] Mosesson MW, DiOrio JP, Siebenlist KR, Wall JS, Hainfeld JF. Evidence for a second type of fibril branch point in fibrin polymer networks, the trimolecular junction. Blood 1993;82:1517−21.
[29] Whitmore E. Preparation of autologous plasma and fibrin gel. Johnson Medical Inc.; 1999. United States Patent US 5935437.

[30] Blombäck B, Bark N. Fibrinopeptides and fibrin gel structure. Biophys Chem 2004;112:147–51.
[31] Spotnitz WD, Burks SG, Prabhu R. Fibrin-based adhesives and hemostatic agents. Tissue Adhes Clin Med 2005;6:126–42.
[32] Endo M, Kurosawa H. Left ventricular free wall rupture. Kyobu Geka 2004;57:690–7.
[33] Taylor LM, Mueller-Velten G, Koslow A, Hunter G, Naslund T, Kline R, et al. Prospective randomized multicenter trial of fibrin sealant versus thrombin-soaked gelatin sponge for suture-or needle-hole bleeding from polytetrafluoroethylene femoral artery grafts. J Vasc Surg 2003;38:766–71.
[34] Katkhouda N, Mavor E, Friedlander MH, Mason RJ, Kiyabu M, Grant SW, et al. Use of fibrin sealant for prosthetic mesh fixation in laparoscopic extraperitoneal inguinal hernia repair. Ann Surg 2001;233:18.
[35] Finley DS, Lee DI, Eichel L, Uribe CA, McDougall EM, Clayman R v. Fibrin glue-oxidized cellulose sandwich for laparoscopic wedge resection of small renal lesions. J Urol 2005;173:1477–81.
[36] Kumar R, Lim J, Mekary RA, Rattani A, Dewan MC, Sharif SY, et al. Traumatic spinal injury: global epidemiology and worldwide volume. World Neurosurg 2018;113:e345–63.
[37] Ahuja CS, Wilson JR, Nori S, Kotter M, Druschel C, Curt A, et al. Traumatic spinal cord injury. Nat Rev Dis Prim 2017;3:1–21.
[38] Boni R, Ali A, Shavandi A, Clarkson AN. Current and novel polymeric biomaterials for neural tissue engineering. J Biomed Sci 2018;25:1–21.
[39] Amani H, Kazerooni H, Hassanpoor H, Akbarzadeh A, Pazoki-Toroudi H. Tailoring synthetic polymeric biomaterials towards nerve tissue engineering: a review. Artif Cells, Nanomed Biotechnol 2019;47:3524–39.
[40] Du J, Liu J, Yao S, Mao H, Peng J, Sun X, et al. Prompt peripheral nerve regeneration induced by a hierarchically aligned fibrin nanofiber hydrogel. Acta Biomater 2017;55:296–309.
[41] Koulaxouzidis G, Reim G, Witzel C. Fibrin glue repair leads to enhanced axonal elongation during early peripheral nerve regeneration in an in vivo mouse model. Neural Regen Res 2015;10:1166.
[42] Robinson M, Douglas S, Michelle Willerth S. Mechanically stable fibrin scaffolds promote viability and induce neurite outgrowth in neural aggregates derived from human induced pluripotent stem cells. Sci Rep 2017;7:1–9.
[43] Christman KL, Fok HH, Sievers RE, Fang Q, Lee RJ. Fibrin glue alone and skeletal myoblasts in a fibrin scaffold preserve cardiac function after myocardial infarction. Tissue Eng 2004;10:403–9.
[44] Shen D, Tang J, Hensley MT, Li T, Caranasos TG, Zhang T, et al. Effects of matrix metalloproteinases on the performance of platelet fibrin gel spiked with cardiac stem cells in heart repair. Stem Cells Transl Med 2016;5:793–803.
[45] Jockenhoevel S, Zund G, Hoerstrup SP, Schnell A, Turina M. Cardiovascular tissue engineering: a new laminar flow chamber for in vitro improvement of mechanical tissue properties. Am Soc Artif Intern Organs J 2002;48:8–11.
[46] Cholewinski E, Dietrich M, Flanagan TC, Schmitz-Rode T, Jockenhoevel S. Tranexamic acid—an alternative to aprotinin in fibrin-based cardiovascular tissue engineering. Tissue Eng 2009;15:3645–53.
[47] Tschoeke B, Flanagan TC, Cornelissen A, Koch S, Roehl A, Sriharwoko M, et al. Development of a composite degradable/nondegradable tissue-engineered vascular graft. Artif Organs 2008;32:800–9.
[48] Flanagan TC, Sachweh JS, Frese J, Schnöring H, Gronloh N, Koch S, et al. In vivo remodeling and structural characterization of fibrin-based tissue-engineered heart valves in the adult sheep model. Tissue Eng 2009;15:2965–76.

[49] Vilela CA, Correia C, Oliveira JM, Sousa RA, Espregueira-Mendes J, Reis RL. Cartilage repair using hydrogels: a critical review of in vivo experimental designs. ACS Biomater Sci Eng 2015;1:726−39.
[50] Buckwalter JA. Articular cartilage: injuries and potential for healing. J Orthop Sports Phys Ther 1998;28:192−202.
[51] Benders KEM, van Weeren PR, Badylak SF, Saris DBF, Dhert WJA, Malda J. Extracellular matrix scaffolds for cartilage and bone regeneration. Trends Biotechnol 2013;31:169−76.
[52] Hwang CM, Ay B, Kaplan DL, Rubin JP, Marra KG, Atala A, et al. Assessments of injectable alginate particle-embedded fibrin hydrogels for soft tissue reconstruction. Biomed Mater 2013;8:14105.
[53] Almeida H v, Eswaramoorthy R, Cunniffe GM, Buckley CT, O'brien FJ, Kelly DJ. Fibrin hydrogels functionalized with cartilage extracellular matrix and incorporating freshly isolated stromal cells as an injectable for cartilage regeneration. Acta Biomater 2016;36:55−62.
[54] Giannini G, Mauro V, Agostino T, Gianfranco B. Use of autologous fibrin-platelet glue and bone fragments in maxillofacial surgery. Transfus Apher Sci 2004;30:139−44.
[55] Huh J-Y, Choi B-H, Zhu S-J, Jung J-H, Kim B-Y, Lee S-H. The effect of platelet-enriched fibrin glue on bone regeneration in autogenous bone grafts. Oral Surg Oral Med Oral Pathol Oral Radiol Endodontol 2006;101:426−31.
[56] Lee H-J, Choi B-H, Jung J-H, Zhu S-J, Lee S-H, Huh J-Y, et al. Vertical alveolar ridge augmentation using autogenous bone grafts and platelet-enriched fibrin glue with simultaneous implant placement. Oral Surg Oral Med Oral Pathol Oral Radiol Endodontol 2008;105:27−31.
[57] Lee H-J, Choi B-H, Jung J-H, Zhu S-J, Lee S-H, Huh J-Y, et al. Maxillary sinus floor augmentation using autogenous bone grafts and platelet-enriched fibrin glue with simultaneous implant placement. Oral Surg Oral Med Oral Pathol Oral Radiol Endodontol 2007;103:329−33.
[58] Durham LH, Willatt DJ, Yung MW, Jones I, Stevenson PA, Ramadan MF. A method for preparation of fibrin glue. J Laryngol Otol 1987;101:1182−6.
[59] Bhatnagar D, Bushman JS, Murthy NS, Merolli A, Kaplan HM, Kohn J. Fibrin glue as a stabilization strategy in peripheral nerve repair when using porous nerve guidance conduits. J Mater Sci Mater Med 2017;28:1−10.
[60] Karp JM, Sarraf F, Shoichet MS, Davies JE. Fibrin-filled scaffolds for bone-tissue engineering: an in vivo study. J Biomed Mater Res 2004;71:162−71.
[61] Pinholt EM, Solheim E, Bang G, Sudmann E. Bone induction by composites of bioresorbable carriers and demineralized bone in rats: a comparative study of fibrin-collagen paste, fibrin sealant, and polyorthoester with gentamicin. J Oral Maxillofac Surg 1992;50:1300−4.

CHAPTER 12

Elastin-based hydrogels for tissue engineering

Jacelyn Mohana Das[1], Khalid Umar[1], Mohd Jameel[2], H. Fadlullah[3] and Mohamad Nasir Mohamad Ibrahim[1]
[1]School of Chemical Sciences, Universiti Sains Malaysia, Penang, Malaysia; [2]Molecular Cancer Genetics & Translational Research Laboratory, Section of Genetics, Department of Zoology, Aligarh Muslim University, Aligarh, Uttar Pradesh, India; [3]Chemistry Education Department, Universitas Sultan Ageng Tirtayasa, Banten, Indonesia

1. Introduction

Tissue engineering has led to remarkable advancements in the development of viable substitutes that can compensate for the limitations of traditional medicine, including restoring, maintaining, or improving human tissue function. In recent years, it has gained increasing attention owing to millions of individuals who suffer from organ and tissue failure or loss annually. Although transplanted organs can be used to treat patients with sickness or wounded organs, the scarcity of organ donors continues to worsen as the aging population grows. Scientists in regenerative medicine and tissue engineering depend on cell transplantation, material science, and bioengineering to develop biological alternatives capable of repairing and maintaining normal function in tissues afflicted by disease or injury [1]. TE relies on the development of suitable scaffolds that can mimic the extracellular matrix (ECM). Scholars have explored and created various structures, including nanofibers, sponges, thin films, nanoparticles, composites, and hydrogels, with different properties and origins for fabricating scaffolds [2,3]. Hydrogels are among the most promising candidates because of their biomimetic and adjustable properties and various manufacturing methods [4,5].

Hydrogels are three-dimensional and hydrophilic and can absorb and hold large volumes of fluids [6] while maintaining their structure owing to chemical or physical cross-linked polymeric networks or chains [7]. because their high water content gives them a degree of elasticity similar to that of

Protein-Based Nanocomposites for Tissue Engineering
ISBN 978-0-323-99357-9
https://doi.org/10.1016/B978-0-323-99357-9.00005-3

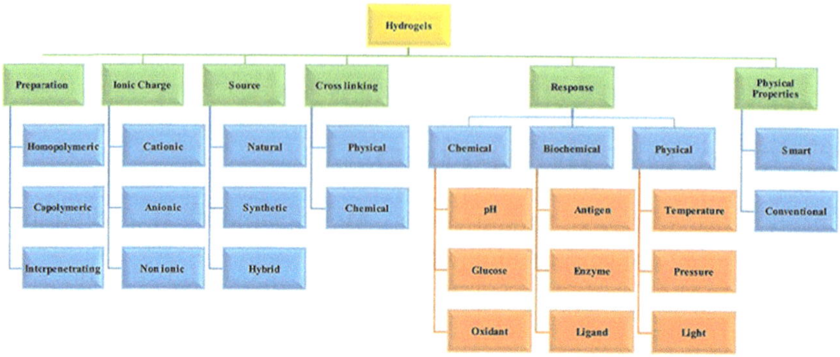

Figure 12.1 The classification of hydrogels is based on natural and synthetic polymers [8].

natural tissues, and their hydrophilicity is attributed to the presence of hydrophilic groups, such as $-NH_2$, $-COOH$, $-OH$, $-CONH_2$, $-CONH-$, and $-SO_3H$ [8,9]. Hydrogels undergo a significant volume or gel-sol phase transition in response to specific physical and chemical stimuli, but these conformational shifts are usually reversible. Hence, after a reaction, the hydrogels can return to their initial state after the trigger is withdrawn [8,9]. Hydrogels can be classified into two distinct categories: natural and synthetic polymers utilized in their fabrication, as depicted in Fig. 12.1. Among natural hydrogel varieties, protein-based hydrogels exhibit remarkable structural and functional properties, making them ideal for hydrogel production. These properties include biocompatibility, biodegradability, abundance, and reduced potential to trigger tissue inflammation [10,11]. In particular, elastin and its applications are examined as a promising protein-based hydrogel in tissue engineering.

2. Elastin possesses structural and biological properties

Cross-linked tropoelastin monomers form a durable, insoluble extracellular matrix protein called elastin. This protein is structured in a microfibrillar arrangement rich in fibrillin [1]. Elastin constitutes a significant portion of various tissues, including 30%–57% of the aorta, 50% of elastic ligaments, 28%–32% of major arterial vessels, 3%–7% of the lungs, 4% of tendons, and 2%–5% of the dry weight of the skin. Within elastic fibers, elastin plays a crucial role in providing extensibility and elastic recoil to diverse tissues

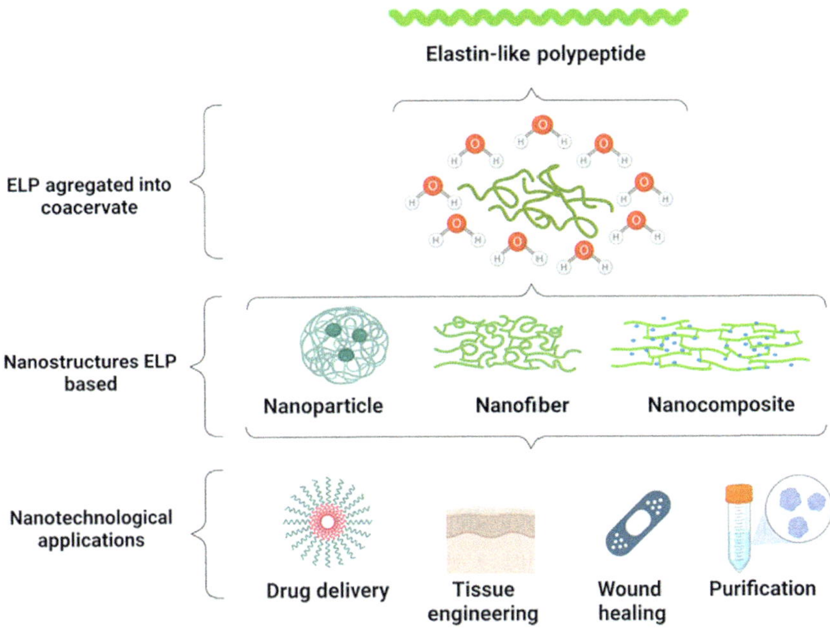

Figure 12.2 Aggregated coacervates of ELPs adopt diverse nanostructures in water, suitable for various nanotechnological applications [12].

such as arteries, ligaments, and lungs. Elastin shows biological properties and is used in nanotechnological applications such as drug delivery, wound healing purification, and tissue engineering, as illustrated in Fig. 12.2. These fibers are highly resilient and structurally stable, with a half-life of approximately 70 years in the aorta [13,14]. Elastin can undergo numerous cycles of transformation without losing its original properties or exhibiting memory effects [15]. It is mechanically essential and participates in various cell signaling activities. Elastin is formed during elastogenesis by crosslinking tropoelastin, a soluble precursor [16].

It is challenging to repair or replace damaged elastin without significantly altering the natural arrangement and organization of surrounding tissue [17]. Tropoelastin is a 60–70 kDA protein that is the main component of elastin and is primarily composed of nonpolar amino acids that form alternating hydrophobic and hydrophilic domains. The repeating sequence motifs within the hydrophobic domains provide flexibility to the protein and contribute to cell signaling [18]. Hydrophilic domains are characterized by lysine-rich regions, which are essential for cross-linking. In vivo, lysyl oxidase facilitates this process by converting lysine residues to produce allysine aldol, lysinonorleucine, desmosine, and isodesmosine bonds with surrounding modified and unmodified lysine residues [19,20], imparting stability to the protein array that mimics the specific regions of elastin.

Tropoelastin is a biologically active molecule that exists as a monomer in solution in two forms: an open spherical molecule and a stretched polypeptide chain [21]. It has multiple cell-interacting sites that facilitate various signaling events through glycosaminoglycans (GAGs), elastin-binding proteins (EBP), and integrins [1]. The increasing availability of accurate reproductions of the natural elastin precursor tropoelastin has enabled the handling of soluble components in aqueous solutions, leading to the development of increasingly sophisticated synthetic analogs of natural elastin. These synthetic analogs typically use elastin domains with hydrophobic segments for elasticity or temperature-dependent association or hydrophilic regions for amine-dependent cross-linking. It is important to note that elastin is not just a structural protein; its inherent signaling capabilities promote various responses, such as chemotaxis, cell proliferation, and tissue homeostasis [22].

3. Fabrication of elastin hydrogels

3.1 Formation of elastin hydrogel

The capacity of tropoelastin/elastin to self-assemble has generated enthusiasm for employing coacervation in producing elastin-based materials, including hydrogels and electrospun scaffolds, for tissue repair. However, obtaining substantial quantities of pure tropoelastin/elastin has consistently posed considerable challenges.

3.1.1 High-pressure CO_2

Processing elastin, a highly insoluble biopolymer, into new biomaterials is challenging due to its extensively polymerized state. To address this, researchers commonly utilize α-elastin, an oxalic acid-soluble derivative. The fabrication of α-elastin hydrogel involves two steps, similar to the formation of elastin from its precursor tropoelastin: coacervation and cross-linking. In aqueous solution [23], α-elastin molecules coacervate due to intermolecular hydrophobic associations, followed by chemical crosslinking to enhance mechanical integrity, forming hydrogels for tissue engineering applications.

However, traditional crosslinking methods exhibit drawbacks, such as small pore sizes and inadequate communication channels for nutrient exchange and cell infiltration. To overcome these challenges, dense gas carbon dioxide is introduced as an alternative to organic solvents and gas foaming agents for creating porous matrices [24] at high pressures ($\sim$60 bar) [1]. Operating close to the critical temperature, dense gases become supercritical fluids (SCF) beyond the critical point, possessing solvation strength and diffusivity similar to liquids and gases. Carbon dioxide, commonly used due to its low critical parameters ($Tc = 31.1°C$, $Pc = 73.8$ bar), affordability, and nontoxic nature [23], facilitates coacervation through interactions with hydrophobic tropoelastin domains and accelerates cross-linking within the polymer-rich phase [25]. A study by Annabi and the team confirmed that high-pressure CO_2 did not disrupt α-elastin coacervation and had no detrimental effects on its secondary structure. Under atmospheric pressure, hydrogels with thick-walled pores and limited interconnectivity are formed. In contrast, high-pressure synthesis results in a more rigid material with pores and a 10-fold reduction in wall thickness. The improved uniformity of the porous structure is attributed to the formation of microchannels within the hydrogels [23]. This structural enhancement alters the mechanical properties of the hydrogel, exemplified by a 1.5-fold increase in elastic modulus [26]. When fibroblasts are seeded, high-pressure elastin gels enhance cellular infiltration due to larger channels. In contrast, hydrogels formed under atmospheric conditions are constrained by solid surfaces, allowing cells to form a confluent monolayer but restricting their extension into the material [27].

3.1.2 Tropoelastin and solubilized elastin

In exploring alternatives to tropoelastin or elastin-based peptides, some researchers have undertaken chemical modifications of elastin samples derived from animals, resulting in the creation of "soluble elastin." Soluble elastins include α-elastin, an oxalic acid derivative of elastin, and κ-elastin, which is soluble through treatment with potassium hydroxide [28]. Circular dichroism and Raman spectroscopy were employed to establish that the secondary structure of κ-elastin is identical to that of the free monomer tropoelastin, validating its utility as a model system [28]. In a study by Tu et al. the intermediate stages of tropoelastin macro-assembly were elucidated using low concentrations of protein samples. This involved dissolving tropoelastin in phosphate-buffered saline and bis (sulfosuccinimidyl) suberate (BS3) [29]. Furthermore, the interaction between individual tropoelastin molecules is crucial in forming tropoelastin macro-assemblies. These assemblies do not randomly fuse but instead organize into intricate patterns resembling the geometry of fusing spheres, ultimately determining the final arrangement of synthetic elastin [29].

In the fabrication of micropatterned gels for aligning cardiomyocytes, microchannels with varying sizes and spacings on a silicon wafer were created, which form a master piece of material. Subsequently, the master was covered with a layer of PDMS prepolymer, cured it for 1 h at 80°C, and then removed the PDMS mold, cutting it into small molds (1 × 1 cm)—the resulting photoinitiator. Upon exposure to UV light for 35 s, the hydrogel crosslinked, producing a micropatterned MeTro gel. After soaking in PBS for 5 min, the PDMS mold was removed from the gel. In the next step, the hydrogel containing microchannels was seeded with cardiomyocytes isolated from neonatal rats to align cells within the channels, with an unpatterned MeTro gel used as a control [30].

3.2 Modified elastin

A novel approach to accelerate coacervation and enable chemical-free cross-linking involves modifying tropoelastin residues. Gel formation now takes seconds (less than a minute), a significant improvement from the standard 24-h incubation period. Addressing concerns about cytotoxicity involves eliminating harmful crosslinkers and organic solvents from the process [31]. In vivo, elastin-based gels gain improved stability and reduced leaching. This method is also cytocompatible, allowing three-dimensional cellular encapsulation within the hydrogel framework. The most studied method for tropoelastin modification involves the reaction of tropoelastin lysine residues with methacrylic anhydride [32,33]. This process minimally affects the overall protein, as evidenced by maintaining the secondary structure of tropoelastin in response to different degrees of methacrylation. In addition, this process increases tropoelastin's hydrophobicity, enhancing the coacervation rate. The degree of methacrylation significantly influences the gel characteristics [34]. Highly methacrylated monomers improve crosslinking density, reducing the hydrogel's pore size and swelling ratio. Depending on casting conditions, the swelling ratio of methacrylated tropoelastin (MeTro) gels was 1.5-fold lower than that of unmodified elastin hydrogels. Creating hydrogels from MeTro consistently establishes elastic benefits, with a 100-fold increase in the elastic modulus over similarly processed biological materials [35]. Furthermore, MeTro gels exhibit reduced energy losses in response to deformation and up to 400% extensibility, indicating robust elastic resilience three times that of native tropoelastin. MeTro gels actively stimulate cellular growth on their surface, significantly more than hydrogels manufactured from synthetic polymers like polyethylene glycol (PEG), which exhibit poor cellular adherence and growth. The ability of MeTro gels to support a diverse range of cell types suggests that cell-interactive portions of tropoelastin are present on the material surface in an active configuration. It has also been demonstrated that these manufactured gels can actively facilitate nutrition exchange throughout the gel structure, with embedded cells remaining alive for at least 7 days during casting [30]. This technology represents a significant advancement for elastin-based hydrogels and holds potential uses in cell-laden structures. Table 12.1 shows the mechanical properties and application of elastin hydrogels.

4. Fabrication of composite-based elastin hydrogels

4.1 Formation of composite elastin hydrogel

Researchers combine elastin with other proteins or polymers to enhance biomaterials' structural and functional qualities. They employ various methods, such as gas foaming and freeze-drying, to fabricate porous scaffolds (hydrogels) based on elastin with desirable characteristics for tissue engineering.

4.1.1 Gas foaming

Creating a porous structure involves forming and growing gas bubbles within a polymer [39]. One can generate these bubbles chemically, using a foaming blowing agent [40], or mechanically by expelling gas from a presaturated gas-polymer mixture at high pressure. To initiate the formation of gas bubbles, introduce a foaming or blowing agent into the prepolymer and chemically decompose it to produce gas. In producing porous hydrogels, sodium bicarbonate is a commonly employed foaming agent, as it generates CO_2 in mildly acidic solutions. Demonstrating this process, a highly porous hydrogel comprising PCL and elastin was fabricated. The PCL and NaCl particles were melded through melt mixing and subsequently gas-foamed using CO_2 at 65 bar and 70°C. The resulting PCL scaffolds were infused with an elastin solution containing glutaraldehyde [24].

Table 12.1 Mechanical properties and application of elastin hydrogels.

Material	Cross-linker	Swelling ratio (g PBS/g protein)	Tensile/compressive modulus (kPa)	Cells cultured	Applications	References
α-elastin	HMDI + high pressure CO2	4–9C	6.8	Vascular smooth muscle cells	Soft tissue repair; spinal replacement	[31]
α-elastin	HMDI	11–19C	4.8	Fibroblasts		[31]
α-elastin	EDGE	4–120E	10–25	–		[35]
Tropoelastin	BS3	220–280E	4–7	Epithelial cells	Elastic tissue repair	[36]
Tropoelastin	Lysyl oxidase	8–12E	5.4	–	–	[35]
Tropoelastin	MA	2.8–14.8E	–	Human umbilical vein endothelial cells	–	[37]
Topoelastin/α-elastin	GA + high pressure CO2	11E; 2C	7–18	Fibroblasts	Dermal replacement	[38]
Topoelastin/α-elastin	GA	8E; 2C	–	Fibroblasts	Dermal replacement	[38]

BS3, bis(sulfosuccinimidyl)suberate; *EGDE*, ethylene glycol diglycidyl ether; *GA*, glutaraldehyde; *HMDI*, Hexamethylene diisocyanate; *MA*, Methacrylic anhydride.

In another example, Sodium bicarbonate played a crucial role in creating a porous hydrogel by cross-linking acrylic acid and acrylamide with N, N′-methylenebisacrylamide in another instance [41]. The resulting hydrogel exhibited interconnected pores with sizes ranging from 100 to 250 mm and an equilibrium swelling ratio of 100% [41]. Recently, to enhance cell adhesion on the typically cell-repellant hydrogel material, researchers utilized sodium bicarbonate as a blowing agent to generate macroporous hydrogels from photocrosslinkable PEG diacrylate covalently bonded to the RGD peptide sequence. When human mesenchymal stem cells were exposed to osteogenic media on this scaffold, it was observed that the hydrogel supported their adhesion and long-term survival, ultimately stimulating mineralization [41]. Human mesenchymal stem cells could adhere to porous PEG-based gels without the RGD adhesion sequence, indicating that the scaffold structure is adequate for cell attachment [41]. Ammonium bicarbonate is another gas-blowing agent that induces linked pores within hydrogels, known for its decomposition into CO_2 and NH_3. In an illustrative case, researchers introduced ammonium bicarbonate during the irradiation of carboxymethylcellulose and polyacrylamide to facilitate porosity [42]. This addition enhanced the swelling ratio compared with hydrogels produced without a blowing agent. Due to the widespread availability of familiar foaming or blowing agents, this method is considered a cost-effective platform for incorporating porosity into hydrogel materials. The blowing agents employed are typically compatible with cells, and this technique can be implemented without organic solvents, making it well-suited for applications in tissue engineering.

4.1.2 Freeze drying

Freeze drying, also termed lyophilization, finds extensive application in tissue engineering to produce porous hydrogels [43]. This method rapidly condenses the system to induce thermodynamic instability and phase separation. Ice crystals form upon freezing a dispersion or solution, and subsequent removal during freeze-drying results in pores within the material. The pore size is inversely proportional to the freezing rate; for example, a tropoelastin-collagen solution frozen at 80°C yields porous disc-shaped or tubular scaffolds. Similarly, an elastin-glycosaminoglycan collagen composite hydrogel is created through gelation at 37°C, followed by lyophilization and cross-linking with 1-ethyl-3-(3 dimethylaminopropyl)

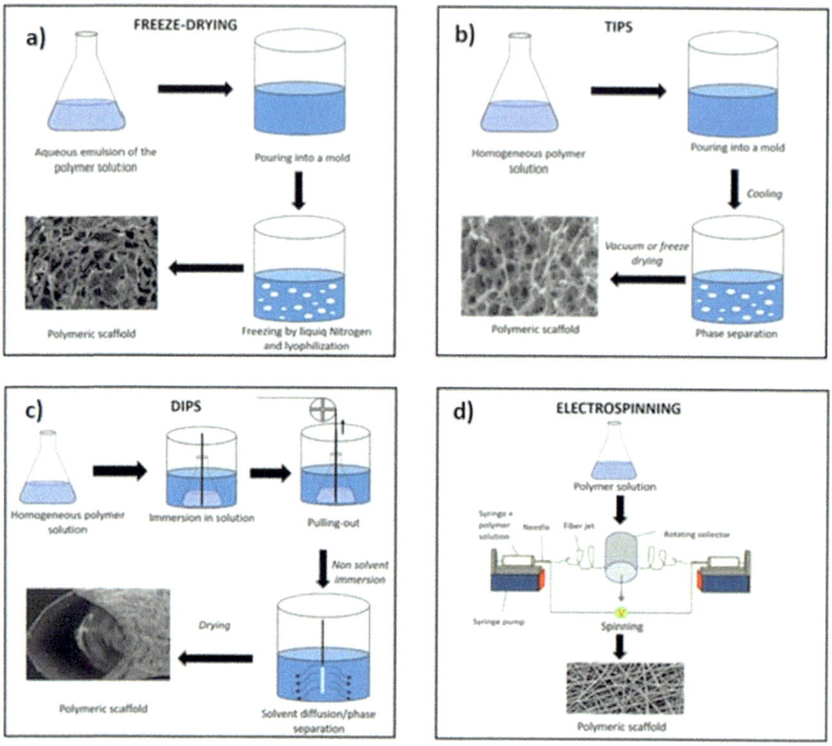

Figure 12.3 Shows the solution-based fabrication process of scaffolds by various techniques [45].

carbodiimide/N-hydroxysuccinimide (EDC/NHS) [44]. Freeze-drying genipin-crosslinked samples and stabilizing them with methanol immersion produces silk-elastin hydrogels. Tubular porous scaffolds are prepared by immersing a mandrill in a protein solution and freeze-drying. Employing multiple solution coating and freeze-drying cycles enables the formation of multilayered structures, such as those with an exterior collagen film and an interior tropoelastin-collagen sheet [43]. Fig. 12.3 illustrates the solution-based fabrication process of scaffolds through various techniques such as (a) freeze-drying, (b) thermally induced phase separation, (c) diffusion-induced phase separation, and (d) electrospinning.

While this method applies to various hydrogel materials, encompassing natural and synthetic hydrophilic polymers [46], it possesses drawbacks regarding precise pore size control. The kinetics of the heat quenching process influences the hydrogel architecture created by this technique. Moreover, the approach results in low structural stability and poor mechanical properties of the fabricated hydrogel materials. During freeze-drying, the matrix may collapse at the scaffold-air contact, forming surface skin due to interfacial tension induced by solvent evaporation [3,47]. In addition, freeze-drying consumes substantial energy and requires an extended period for solvent removal. Table 12.2 shows mechanical properties and application of composite-based elastin hydrogels.

5. Elastin nanocomposite

5.1 Elastin-like peptide

Self-assembling biopolymers known as ELPs are constructed from repeating amino acid sequences inspired by natural elastin. These polypeptides, with unique mechanical and biological properties, offer the advantage of controlling their physicochemical characteristics through sequence design, making them attractive building blocks for designing artificial protein polymers with specific functionalities. Various modular polymers based on ELPs have been created, including diblock or triblock copolymers composed of multiple ELPs exhibiting distinct self-assembling tendencies. In addition, ELPs have been fused with other self-assembling proteins or peptides such as silk-like, collagen-like, and viral coat proteins [51].

These ELPs exhibit self-assembly into diverse nanostructures like nanoparticles, nanofibers, and hydrogels, showcasing potential drug delivery and tissue engineering applications. Recent advancements involve using ELP conjugates in sophisticated nanobiosystems. ELPs can regulate the spatiotemporal distribution of target proteins, act as self-sorting machinery within cells, and serve as molecular switches. The prevalent elastin-based repeat motif is the pentapeptide sequence Val-Pro-Gly-X-Gly (VPGXG), as depicted in Fig. 12.4, where X can be any naturally occurring amino acid except proline [51]. This short repeating sequence (VPGXG)n displays temperature-dependent self-assembly behavior, known as coacervation, akin to tropoelastin [53]. Each ELP possesses a lower critical solution temperature (LCST) or transition temperature (Tt). Below Tt, ELPs exist as extended random-coiled structures, with hydrophobic side chains hydrated by ordered water molecules, rendering the proteins soluble in aqueous

Table 12.2 Mechanical properties and application of composite-based elastin hydrogels.

Material	Cross-linker	Mechanical properties	Pore size/ porosity	Cells cultured	Applications	References
PCL/α-elastin	GA	1.30 MPAC	540 μm/91%	Chondrocytes	Cartilage repair	[48,49]
Silk fibroin/Elastin	Genipin	—	78%–88%	Human dermal fibroblasts	Wound dressing	[50]
Collagen/Elastin/ Glycosaminoglycans	EDC/NHS	4.16 kPAC	—	Human adipose-derived stem cells	Nucleus pulposus regeneration	[51]
		0.54–0.76 MPAE	20–100 μm	Fibroblasts	Tissue engineering/ slow release vehicle for growth factor release	[43]
Collagen/Elastin	EDC/NHS	0.25–5.3 MPAE	130 μm	Smooth muscle cells	Small-diameter blood vessels	[26]
		1.12 MPAE	300 μm	—	Vascular graft	[26]

EDC/NHS, 1-ethyl-3-(3 dimethylaminopropyl)carbodiimide/*N* -hydroxysuccinimide; *GA*, glutaraldehyde.

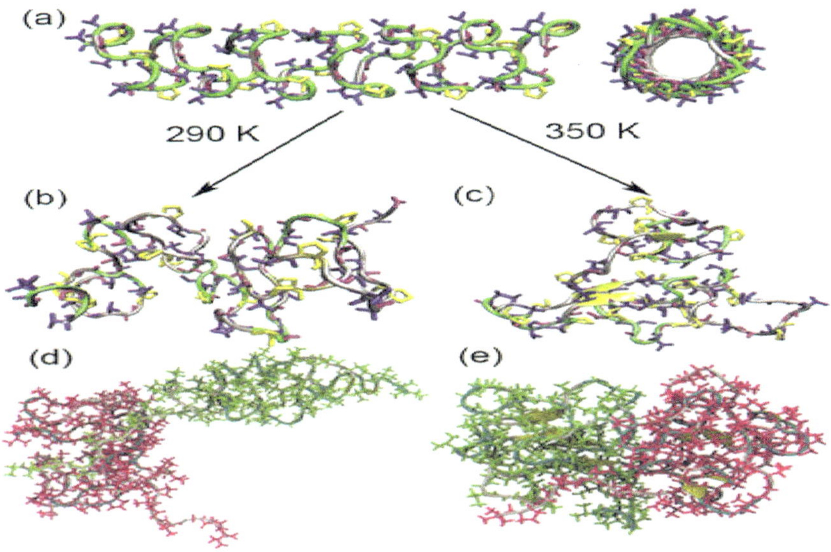

Figure 12.4 Illustrates the (A) side and front view of the β-spiral structure for (VPGVG) 18. The final simulation snapshots depict (B, C) a single (VPGVG)18 structure and (D, E) the interaction between two ELPs at temperatures (B, D) 290 K and (C, E) 350 K. The secondary structure ribbons represent the backbone, with the turn motif in green, β-sheet in yellow, and coil in silver. Sticks depict all heavy atoms. In panels (A–C), the side chains are color-coded by amino acid (Gly in purple, Pro in yellow, and Val in blue). In panels D and E, the side chains are color-coded by molecule [52].

solutions [52]. Upon dehydration, hydrophobic ELPs aggregate to form particulates through hydrophobic contact. The process's advantage lies in compensating for the increase in structured ELPs through the decrease in structured water. It is important to note that recent research has challenged the idealistic β-spiral model of ELPs, revealing that ELPs, such as (VPGXG) n, primarily exist as random coil polymers. Each repeat can temporarily adopt β-turn and polyproline type II (PPII) structures [54]. Nonapeptide LGAGGAGVL and pentapeptides KGGVG, GVGVP, and VGGVG [55] have been employed in constructing ELPs. A well-known ELP comprises repeats of the VPVXG motifs derived from bovine tropoelastin. Recently developed human elastin-like polypeptides (HELPs) utilize the VAPGVG motif, the most prevalent sequence in the human tropoelastin homolog, to enhance polypeptide characteristics [56]. Fig. 12.4 shows the representation of different behaviors of ELP.

ELPs, utilizing reversible stimuli-response via thermal triggers, find various applications, including their utilization in ELP-based nanoparticles for drug delivery. For instance, a sequence (VPGXG)160 (where X is V, A, or G) was fused to a C-terminal sequence containing eight cysteines (GGC) 8 to enable drug conjugation, such as with DOX, through a maleimide—thiol coupling reaction [57]. The resulting ELP—DOX molecule spontaneously assembles into micellar structures with an ELP corona, owing to its amphiphilic structure comprising the hydrophilic ELP (with a transition temperature Tt >> 37°C) and the hydrophobic drug domain. The formation of ELP-based nanoparticles is achieved by heating to 37°C, causing the ELP to coacervate and generate the hydrophobic core. Simultaneously, TRAIL (tumor necrosis factor-related apoptosis-inducing ligand) is displayed on the nanoparticle surface for interaction. Despite some reported challenges, (VPGXG)n-based nanoparticle systems generally face difficulties achieving precise control over their sizes or stabilities.

Proline-rich domain-inspired ELPs present an attractive option for generating hydrogels for artificial scaffolds in tissue engineering. Utilizing ELP-based hydrogels offers several advantages. First, optimizing production through bacterial systems allows for the synthesis of (VPGXG)n-based ELPs with high yields (up to subgram scale per liter culture), excellent purities, and remarkable monodispersities [52]. Second, the precision in designing ELPs is achieved through genetic engineering, highlighting a third benefit: the ability to exert precise control over their structures and functions. Lastly, these hydrogels demonstrate biocompatibility, biodegradability, and nonimmunogenicity.

5.2 ELP block copolymer forming nanoparticles

To produce nanoparticles, ELP block copolymers can be crafted as diblock amphiphiles, connecting a hydrophilic ELP block to a hydrophobic ELP block, as illustrated in Fig. 12.5. Determining "hydrophobicity" or "hydrophilicity" involves comparing the two block components. The hydrophobic ELP possesses a lower transition temperature (Tt) than the hydrophilic ELP, which has a higher Tt. Amphiphilic block structures and thermal triggers can be utilized to create micelles. At temperatures below both Tts, the diblock ELP remains a soluble unimer while being hydrated by water molecules [52,53]. At elevated temperatures between the lower and higher Tt, the hydrophobic block selectively dehydrates and aggregates, forming a dense hydrophobic core, while the hydrophilic block remains

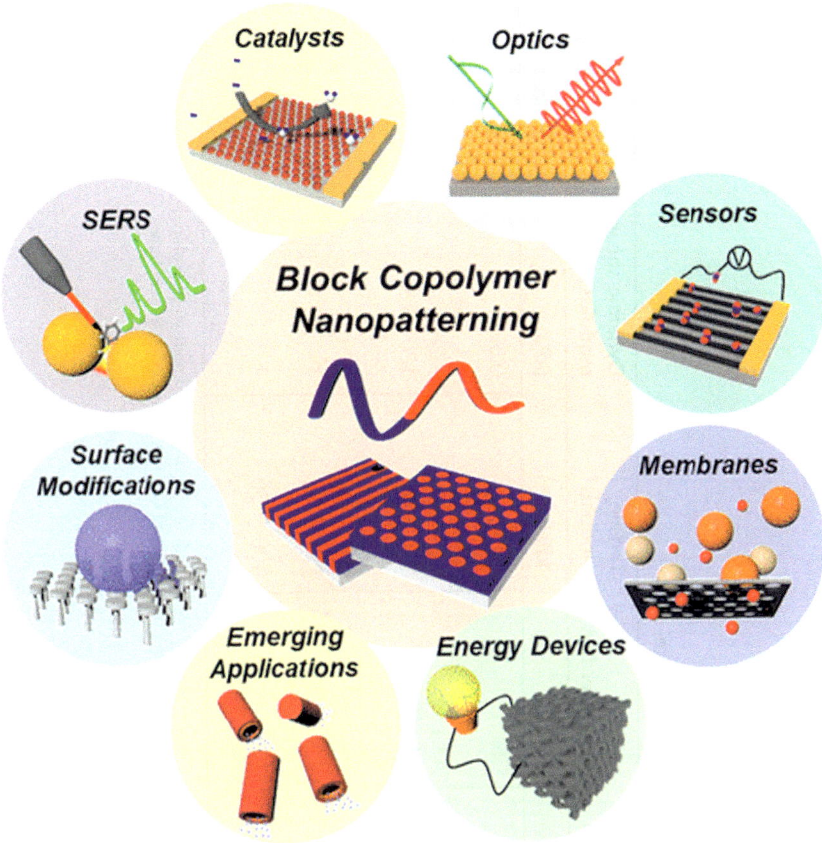

Figure 12.5 Block copolymer nanopatterning finds applications in nonsemiconductor devices [58].

solvated and exposed to solvents, resulting in the corona of the formed micelles. With increasing temperature, the hydrophilic block undergoes dehydration, leading to the aggregation of micelles into submicron particles. The temperatures at which unimers transform into micelles and micelles aggregate into larger particles are known as the critical micelle temperature (CMT) and aggregation temperature (Taggregation), respectively. By selecting optimal ELP sequences, micelle parameters such as CMTs, diameters, and aggregation counts (number of ELP chains per particle) can be precisely adjusted [53,56]. In response to heat, an amphiphilic block ELP actively assembles into nanoparticles, as depicted in Fig. 12.5 (Table 12.3).

Table 12.3 Mechanical properties and application elastin nanocomposite.

Material	Cross-linker	Concentration (mg/mL)	Monomer MW (kDa)	Tensile modulus (kPa)	Dynamic shear modulus (kPa)	References
ELP	None (coacervate)	324	36	–	0.08	[59]
ELP	tTG	100	47.1	–	0.26	[60]
ELP	DSS	NA	37.1	350–970	120–320	[61]
ELP	TSAT	180	42.7, 47.1		8–10	[62]
ELP	THPP	200	31, 28.3	–	5.8–45.8	[62]
ELP fusion polypeptide	BS3	200–400	37.1	80–700	22–60	[61]
ELP fusion polypeptide	HMDI	100	14–59	400–930	–	[63]

ELP stands for elastin-like polypeptide; *HMDI* represents hexamethylene diisocyanate; *THPP* stands for β-[tris(hydroxymethyl)-phosphine]-propionic acid; *BS3* is bis(sulfosuccinimidyl) suberate; *TSAT* is an abbreviation for tris-succinimidyl aminotriacetate; *tTG* refers to tissue transglutaminase.

6. Conclusions

Elastin and its derivatives possess inherent structural, biological, and assembly qualities that allow the creation of a diverse range of materials that guide and respond to cells. As discussed earlier, the biomaterial potential of these elastin-based structures is enhanced by incorporating additional synthetic or natural polymers and sequence motifs. The various engineering processes available for elastin-based materials offer precise control over the resulting architectural elements, meeting the specific mechanical and functional requirements for various applications, particularly in tissue engineering. This includes serving as a biomimetic bioactive scaffold with improved biocompatibility, reduced cytotoxicity, enhanced crosslinking, and high production levels.

Although the advantages and disadvantages of these materials have been thoroughly studied, a comprehensive understanding of elastin fabrication is crucial to adopting these procedures on a commercial scale in a reproducible manner. In summary, ELPs exhibit remarkable tunable features such as precise control over the peptide sequence, molecular weight, and thermal responsiveness. Overall, ELPs have promising potential for biomedical applications, particularly in tissue engineering. They can be utilized as cross-linked biomaterials to repair tissue injuries, treat damaged knees, regenerate nerves and dermal tissues, and as alternatives to coronary bypass surgery through vascular grafts. The aspiration is to inspire scientific researchers to explore novel ideas for incorporating more elastin-based proteins/peptides, providing a fascinating and practical approach for advancing future frontier research in tissue engineering.

Acknowledgments

The authors are thankful to Universiti Sains Malaysia for providing a financial support (short-term grant; 304/PKIMIA/6315580).

References

[1] Grumezescu A, editor. Nanobiomaterials in soft tissue engineering: applications of nanobiomaterials. William Andrew; February 23, 2016.

[2] Davari N, Bakhtiary N, Khajehmohammadi M, Sarkari S, Tolabi H, Ghorbani F, Ghalandari B. Protein-based hydrogels: promising materials for tissue engineering. Polymers February 28, 2022;14(5):986.

[3] Khan MA, Ahmad A, Umar K, Nabi SA. Synthesis, characterization, and biological applications of nanocomposites for the removal of heavy metals and dyes. Ind Eng Chem Res January 14, 2015;54(1):76–82.

[4] Afridi SK, Umar K, Parveen T, Razali MR. Nanocomposites in the degradation of organic pollutants. Nanocomp Advan Mater Energy Environ Asp January, 2023;1:321–47.

[5] Shin H, Jo S, Mikos AG. Biomimetic materials for tissue engineering. Biomaterials November 1, 2003;24(24):4353–64.

[6] Mancha Sánchez E, Gómez-Blanco JC, López Nieto E, Casado JG, Macías-García A, Díaz Díez MA, Carrasco-Amador JP, Torrejón Martín D, Sánchez-Margallo FM, Pagador JB. Hydrogels for bioprinting: a systematic review of hydrogels synthesis, bioprinting parameters, and bioprinted structures behavior. Front Bioeng Biotechnol August 6, 2020;8:776.

[7] Wichterle O, Lim D. Hydrophilic gels for biological use. Nature January 9, 1960;185(4706):117–8.

[8] Bahram M, Mohseni N, Moghtader M. An introduction to hydrogels and some recent applications. In: Emerging concepts in analysis and applications of hydrogels. IntechOpen; August 24, 2016.

[9] Haseen U, Umar K, Ahmad H, Parveen T, Mohamad Ibrahim MN. Graphene and its composites: applications in environmental remediation. Mod Age Waste Water Prob Solut Using Appl Nanotechnol 2020:85–91.

[10] Umar K. Water contamination by organic-pollutants: TiO_2 photocatalysis. Modern Age Environm Probl Remediat 2018:95–109.

[11] Silva R, Fabry B, Boccaccini AR. Fibrous protein-based hydrogels for cell encapsulation. Biomaterials August 1, 2014;35(25):6727–38.

[12] Lima LF, Sousa MG, Rodrigues GR, de Oliveira KB, Pereira AM, da Costa A, Machado R, Franco OL, Dias SC. Elastin-like polypeptides in development of nanomaterials for application in the medical field. Front Nanotechnol April 25, 2022;4:874790.

[13] Powell JT, Vine N, Crossman M. On the accumulation of D-aspartate in elastin and other proteins of the ageing aorta. Atherosclerosis December 1, 1992;97(2–3):201–8.

[14] Gonzalez de Torre I, Alonso M, Rodriguez-Cabello JC. Elastin-based materials: promising candidates for cardiac tissue regeneration. Front Bioeng Biotechnol June 30, 2020;8:657.

[15] Vindin H, Mithieux SM, Weiss AS. Elastin architecture. Matrix Biol November 1, 2019;84:4–16.

[16] Rodríguez-Cabello JC, de Torre IG, Ibañez-Fonseca A, Alonso M. Bioactive scaffolds based on elastin-like materials for wound healing. Adv Drug Deliv Rev April 1, 2018;129:118–33.

[17] Vrhovski B, Weiss AS. Biochemistry of tropoelastin. Eur J Biochem November 15, 1998;258(1):1–8.

[18] Gerber GE, Anwar RA. Structural studies on cross-linked regions of elastin. J Biol Chem August 25, 1974;249(16):5200–7.

[19] Toonkool P, Regan DG, Kuchel PW, Morris MB, Weiss AS. Thermodynamic and hydrodynamic properties of human tropoelastin: analytical ultracentrifuge and pulsed field-gradient spin-echo NMR studies. J Biol Chem July 27, 2001;276(30):28042–50.

[20] Abdullah A, Abdullah AZ, Ahmed M, Khan J, Shahadat M, Umar K, Alim MA. A review on recent developments and progress in sustainable acrolein production through catalytic dehydration of bio-renewable glycerol. J Clean Prod March 20, 2022;341:130876.

[21] Almine JF, Bax DV, Mithieux SM, Nivison-Smith L, Rnjak J, Waterhouse A, Wise SG, Weiss AS. Elastin-based materials. Chem Soc Rev 2010;39(9):3371–9.

[22] Annabi N, Mithieux SM, Weiss AS, Dehghani F. The fabrication of elastin-based hydrogels using high pressure CO_2. Biomaterials January 1, 2009;30(1):1–7.

[23] Tai H, Popov VK, Shakesheff KM, Howdle S. Putting the fizz into chemistry: applications of supercritical carbon dioxide in tissue engineering, drug delivery and synthesis of novel block copolymers. Bio Chem Trans 2007;35.
[24] Dehghani F, Annabi N, Valtchev P, Mithieux SM, Weiss AS, Kazarian SG, Tay FH. Effect of dense gas CO_2 on the coacervation of elastin. Biomacromolecules April 14, 2008;9(4):1100–5.
[25] Annabi N, Mithieux SM, Weiss AS, Dehghani F. Cross-linked open-pore elastic hydrogels based on tropoelastin, elastin and high pressure CO_2. Biomaterials March 1, 2010;31(7):1655–65.
[26] Yeo GC, Aghaei-Ghareh-Bolagh B, Brackenreg EP, Hiob MA, Lee P, Weiss AS. Fabricated elastin. Adv Healthcare Mater November, 2015;4(16):2530–56.
[27] Wise SG, Mithieux SM, Weiss AS. Engineered tropoelastin and elastin-based biomaterials. Advan Prot Chem Struct Biol January 1, 2009;78:1–24.
[28] Debelle L, Alix AJ, Wei SM, Jacob MP, Huvenne JP, Berjot M, Legrand P. The secondary structure and architecture of human elastin. Eur J Biochem December 1, 1998;258(2):533–9.
[29] Tu Y, Wise SG, Weiss AS. Stages in tropoelastin coalescence during synthetic elastin hydrogel formation. Micron April 1, 2010;41(3):268–72.
[30] Annabi N, Tsang K, Mithieux SM, Nikkhah M, Ameri A, Khademhosseini A, Weiss AS. Functional biomaterials: highly elastic micropatterned hydrogel for engineering functional cardiac tissue. Adv Funct Mater October 18, 2013;23(39):4949.
[31] Annabi N, Mithieux SM, Zorlutuna P, Camci-Unal G, Weiss AS, Khademhosseini A. Engineered cell-laden human protein-based elastomer. Biomaterials July 1, 2013;34(22):5496–505.
[32] Nichol JW, Koshy ST, Bae H, Hwang CM, Yamanlar S, Khademhosseini A. Cell-laden microengineered gelatin methacrylate hydrogels. Biomaterials July 1, 2010;31(21):5536–44.
[33] Safian MT, Umar K, Ibrahim MN. Synthesis and scalability of graphene and its derivatives: a journey towards sustainable and commercial material. J Clean Prod October 10, 2021;318:128603.
[34] Hasan A, Memic A, Annabi N, Hossain M, Paul A, Dokmeci MR, Dehghani F, Khademhosseini A. Electrospun scaffolds for tissue engineering of vascular grafts. Acta Biomater January 1, 2014;10(1):11–25.
[35] Quirk RA, France RM, Shakesheff KM, Howdle SM. Supercritical fluid technologies and tissue engineering scaffolds. Curr Opin Solid State Mater Sci June 1, 2004;8(3–4):313–21.
[36] Rubis BA, Danikas D, Neumeister M, Williams WG, Suchy H, Milner SM. The use of split-thickness dermal grafts to resurface full thickness skin defects. Burns December 1, 2002;28(8):752–9.
[37] Fung YC. Biomechanics: mechanical properties of living tissues. Springer Science and Business Media; March 14, 2013.
[38] Lips PA, Velthoen IW, Dijkstra PJ, Wessling M, Feijen J. Gas foaming of segmented poly (ester amide) films. Polymer October 24, 2005;46(22):9396–403.
[39] Caykara T, Küçüktepe S, Turan E. Swelling characteristics of thermo- sensitive poly [(2-diethylaminoethyl methacrylate)-co-(N,N-dimethylacrylamide)] porous hydrogels. Polym Int 2007;56(4):532–7.
[40] Huh KM, Baek N, Park K. Enhanced swelling rate of poly (ethylene glycol)-grafted superporous hydrogels. J Bioact Compat Polym May, 2005;20(3):231–43.
[41] El-Rehim HA, Hegazy ES, Diaa DA. Characterization of super absorbent material based on carboxymethylcellulose sodium salt prepared by electron beam irradiation. J Macromol Sci Part A January 1, 2006;43(1):101–13.

[42] Annabi N, Mithieux SM, Boughton EA, Ruys AJ, Weiss AS, Dehghani F. Synthesis of highly porous crosslinked elastin hydrogels and their interaction with fibroblasts in vitro. Biomaterials September 1, 2009;30(27):4550–7.

[43] Mercuri J, Addington C, Pascal IIIR, Gill S, Simionescu D. Development and initial characterization of a chemically stabilized elastin glycosaminoglycan collagen composite shape memory hydrogel for nucleus pulposus regeneration. J Biomed Mater Res December, 2014;102(12):4380–93.

[44] Lv Q, Hu K, Feng Q, Cui F. Fibroin/collagen hybrid hydrogels with crosslinking method: preparation, properties, and cytocompatibility. J Biomed Mater ResOffic J Soci Biomat Jap Soc Biomater Austral Soc Biomater Korean Soc Biomater January, 2008;84(1):198–207.

[45] Capuana E, Lopresti F, Carfì Pavia F, Brucato V, La Carrubba V. Solution-based processing for scaffold fabrication in tissue engineering applications: a brief review. Polymers June 22, 2021;13(13):2041.

[46] Lin WC, Yu DG, Yang MC. Blood compatibility of novel poly (γ-glutamic acid)/ polyvinyl alcohol hydrogels. Coll Surf B Biointerf January 15, 2006;47(1):43–9.

[47] Hu X, Park SH, Gil ES, Xia XX, Weiss AS, Kaplan DL. The influence of elasticity and surface roughness on myogenic and osteogenic-differentiation of cells on silk-elastin biomaterials. Biomaterials December 1, 2011;32(34):8979–89.

[48] Hu X, Wang X, Rnjak J, Weiss AS, Kaplan DL. Biomaterials derived from silk–tropoelastin protein systems. Biomaterials November 1, 2010;31(32):8121–31.

[49] Dehghani F, Annabi N. Engineering porous scaffolds using gas-based techniques. Curr Opin Biotechnol October 1, 2011;22(5):661–6.

[50] Trabbic-Carlson K, Meyer D, Liu L, Piervincenzi R, Nath N, LaBean T, Chilkoti A. Effect of protein fusion on the transition temperature of an environmentally responsive elastin-like polypeptide: a role for surface hydrophobicity? Protein Eng Des Sel 2004;17(1):57–66.

[51] Luan CH, Harris RD, Prasad KU, Urry DW. Differential scanning calorimetry studies of the inverse temperature transition of the polypentapeptide of elastin and its analogues. Biopolym Orig Res Biomole December, 1990;29(14):1699–706.

[52] Li NK, Quiroz FG, Hall CK, Chilkoti A, Yingling YG. Molecular description of the LCST behaviour of an elastin-like polypeptide. Biomacromolecules October 13, 2014;15(10):3522–30.

[53] Le DH, Sugawara-Narutaki A. Elastin-like polypeptides as building motifs toward designing functional nanobiomaterials. Mole Syst Des Eng 2019;4(3):545–65.

[54] Spezzacatena C, Perri T, Guantieri V, Sandberg LB, Mitts TF, Tamburro AM. Classical synthesis of and structural studies on a biologically active heptapeptide and a nonapeptide of bovine elastin. Eur J Org Chem January, 2002;2002(1):95–103.

[55] Ciofani G, Genchi GG, Liakos I, Athanassiou A, Mattoli V, Bandiera A. Human recombinant elastin-like protein coatings for muscle cell proliferation and differentiation. Acta Biomater February 1, 2013;9(2):5111–21.

[56] Andrew MacKay J, Chen M, McDaniel JR, Liu W, Simnick AJ, Chilkoti A. Self-assembling chimeric polypeptide–doxorubicin conjugate nanoparticles that abolish tumours after a single injection. Nat Mater December, 2009;8(12):993–9.

[57] Costa RR, Custódio CA, Arias FJ, Rodríguez-Cabello JC, Mano JF. Nanostructured and thermoresponsive recombinant biopolymer-based microcapsules for the delivery of active molecules. Nanomed Nanotechnol Biol Med October 1, 2013;9(7):895–902.

[58] Yang GG, Choi HJ, Han KH, Kim JH, Lee CW, Jung EI, Jin HM, Kim SO. Block copolymer nanopatterning for nonsemiconductor device applications. ACS Appl Mater Interf March 1, 2022;14(10):12011–37.

[59] Du A, Zhou B, Xu W, Yu Q, Shen Y, Zhang Z, Shen J, Wu G. Reaction-induced microsyneresis in oxide-based gels: the assembly of hierarchical microsphere networks. Langmuir September 10, 2013;29(36):11208–16.

[60] Gowda DC, Parker TM, Harris RD, Urry DW. Synthesis, characterizations, and medical applications of bioelastic materials. In: Peptides: design, synthesis, and biological activity. Boston, MA: Birkhäuser Boston; 1994. p. 81–111.

[61] Lin CC, Metters AT. Hydrogels in controlled release formulations: network design and mathematical modeling. Adv Drug Deliv Rev November 30, 2006;58(12–13):1379–408.

[62] Amruthwar SS, Janorkar AV. In vitro evaluation of elastin-like polypeptide–collagen composite scaffold for bone tissue engineering. Dent Mater February 1, 2013;29(2):211–20.

[63] Chow D, Nunalee ML, Lim DW, Simnick AJ, Chilkoti A. Peptide-based biopolymers in biomedicine and biotechnology. Mater Sci Eng R Rep September 1, 2008;62(4):125–55.

CHAPTER 13

Silk-based hydrogels for tissue engineering

Mohammad Amir Qureshi[1,2], Nahid Nishat[1], Yasser Azim[3], Basree[3] and Mohammad Shahadat[4,5]

[1]Department of Chemistry, Faculty of Science, Jamia Millia Islamia (Central University), New Delhi, India; [2]Department of Applied Sciences and Humanities, KCC Institute of Technology and Management, Knowledge Park III, Greater Noida, Uttar Pradesh, India; [3]Department of Applied Chemistry, Zakir Husain College of Engineering & Technology, Faculty of Engineering and Technology, Aligarh Muslim University, Aligarh, Uttar Pradesh, India; [4]School of Chemical Sciences, Universiti Sains Malaysia USM, Penang, Malaysia; [5]Department of Textile and Fiber Engineering, Indian Institute of Technology, New Delhi, India

1. Introduction

Since last 30 years, tissue implants have been searched as permanent cure for many problems [1], decellularized matrix [2] and biomaterials positively preparing new tissues. Although former one is fruitful in copying desired tissues, laboratory-prepared biomaterials may still be a best option for tissue implants. Hydrogels are very good in copying the tissue due to high viscoelastic and nutrient transfer properties [3]. Hydrogels are the 3D porous polymeric network that can absorb high amount of water [4–7]. Interconnected porous network of hydrogels gives free way for water, nutrients, drugs, and proliferation of cells [8–10]. Bio-polymeric hydrogels mostly used for biomedical applications. Silk is a hugely studied biopolymer that serves in various medical applications [11]. It can be processed to make thin films, microsphere, gel, scaffold, etc [12–15]. Its hydrogels are broadly utilized as drug delivery vehicle, research matrix, etc, [16,17]. Silk hydrogels specially received great attention in tissue engineering. Silk hydrogel preparation depends on the protein concentrations, temperature, ions, and pH [18,19]. It is been hugely analyzed that silk showed good biocompatibility and mechanical strength in biomedical applications [13,20]. Biocompatible silk showed promising applications as a scaffold for bone, cartilage, skin, nerve, and blood vessel due to the minimum inflammation and tunable biodegradability [21–25]. Silk hydrogels are available for these

Protein-Based Nanocomposites for Tissue Engineering
ISBN 978-0-323-99357-9
https://doi.org/10.1016/B978-0-323-99357-9.00011-9

applications because of their simulation with extracellular cell matrix (ECM).

This book chapter is design to highlight current progress in the types of silk-based hydrogels with focus on its synthesis by different methods. The chemistry of silk structure was also mentioned to understand its changes during the applications. This book chapter has collective information of recent work on silk-based hydrogels in tissue engineering as tissue implants for different organs impairments.

2. Silk-based hydrogels

Hydrogels have high capability to hold large amount of H_2O through cross-linked fibers [26], and they have been broadly utilizing in tissue engineering because they can mimic the native tissues atmosphere. The conventional silk fibroin hydrogels (SFH) have plain structure of cross-linking. Since, the working atmosphere of hydrogels is frequently complex and SFH with simple network are usually unable to fulfill the real needs of applications. However, the advancement of functional SFH has given the chance to overcome the constraints of SFH. Functional design of SFH has fascinated the awareness of researchers worldwide.

The growth of cells, their division, performance, communication, and migration are supported by the ECM which gives mechanical support to the cells. ECM consists of laminin, collagen, fibronectin, and proteoglycans. These protein chains weave a mesh-like structure to give mechanical assistance [27]. Hydrogels have been broadly recognized as close representative of ECM and have been establish as preferable 3D matrix for cell growth [28,29]. The earlier hydrogels, a passive 3D base for cell growth, have important characteristics like mechanical rigidity to promote physiological activity [30]. Thus, the focus has now tilted to develop SF-based hydrogels that consider the essence of cellular environment for cell attachment and its growth [31]. The superior mechanical strength of SFH may offer chance to surpass the barriers that are usually faced while preparing hydrogels of other bio-polymers [32].

2.1 Silk fibroin hydrogels

Several barriers connected with individual polymers can be surpass and important characteristics can be incorporated by making composite hydrogels of silk fibroin (SF). Composite hydrogel of silk prepared by blending and cross-linking improved the strength, porosity, swelling, and biocompatibility [33]. While developing a composite hydrogel, it is important to guarantee that effort while improving a specific property would not affect other aspects of the hydrogels. Production of genetically engineered SF hydrogels is in practice to tune the material properties of hydrogels. This regenerated SF (RSF) has been cross-linked with synthetic polymers to improve the mechanical features. In one work by Mandal et al. polyacrylamide (PAAM) combined with SF to obtain hydrogels which has high mechanical strength and cytocompatibility after changing the ratios of components [34]. Composite hydrogels of poly (vinyl alcohol)-SF in 50:50 ratios possess three fold increases in young's modulus as compared to SF gel only prepared by photo cross-linking [35]. Kang et al. studied the incorporation of poloxamer 407 which evolved as temperature-responsive SF composite hydrogels [36]. Silk on combination with collagen and gelatin can also make composite hydrogels [37–39]. SF has been used to make composite hydrogel with hyaluronan (HA) to slow down the degradation of HA hydrogel [40,41]. HA was chemically cross-linked by PEG-diacrylate. Several ratios of fibrin-based covalent or noncovalent interpenetrating networks (IPNs) and semi-IPNs have been prepared to make cross-linked interlocking networks of composite hydrogels [42,43]. The IPN hydrogels of PVP/SF have probably 100% light transmission and good mechanical strength to open new opportunities in tissue engineering, cell encapsulation, bioprinting, etc. [44]. Gil et al. have also prepared temperature-sensitive semi-IPNs of hydrogels that have poly (N-isopropyl acrylamide) (pNIPAm) and SF. Incorporation of fibroin in pNIPAm changes its micro-network, which leads to an increase its deswelling rate [33].

Functionalized SF and multiwall carbon nanotube (CNT) hydrogels developed by acrylamide and N,N′-methylenebisacrylamide polymerization in SF solution possess carboxylated multiwall CNT. CNT notably increases the mechanical strength of blended hydrogel for their use as SF-based biomaterials [45]. The composite hydrogels of gelatin/SF exhibited a low swelling capacity, low degradation rate, and high compressive strength than gelatin methacrylate hydrogels [38]. A biocompatible hydrogel of RSF and hydroxypropyl methyl cellulose (HPMC) developed with great mechanical properties. The exploration of gelation phenomenon exhibit the uniform distribution of cross-links network that dominated by smaller β-sheet, which is ascribed to the synergistic effects hydrophobic bonding between HPMC and RSF [46].

2.2 Silk-elastin hydrogel

Silk-elastin has obtained a good amount of recognition because of its eye-catching self-assembling nature. Silk-elastin-like proteins (SELPs) were developed by Cappello et al. [47]. Degradation of SELPs hydrogels can be evidently controlled by environmental signals like expression of matrix metalloproteinase [48,49]. Dinerman et al. [50] studied the effect of solute hydrophobicity and charge on diffusion behavior in physically cross-linked SELPs.

2.3 Sericin hydrogels

Sericin, silk protein contains many hydrophilic amino acids, is an auspicious natural source for making protein-based hydrogels [51]. We expected that sericin hydrogel would be a useful in view of special properties [52]. Hu et al. prepared a hydrogel by having cross-linking graft copolymerization of acrylamide (AAm) and acrylic acid onto silk sericin chains. Cross-linker N,N′-methylenebisacrylamide and initiator system $K_2S_2O_8{-}Na_2SO_3$, were used. A composite hydrogel of sericin with pAAm prepared for dermal reconstruction and with N-isopropylacrylamide for cell culture [53].

3. Other important silk hydrogels

3.1 3D and 4D printed silk hydrogels

The use of this technique is to exactly generate biomimetic scaffolds that match the cellular environment, and it has seen an oozing shift in biomedical applications. The procedure needs the synthesis of biocompatible, biodegradable, and bio-printable hydrogel inks. Zheng et al. [54] synthesized an injectable SF-based hydrogel bio-ink scaffold that mixed with PEG and hMSC for mice implantation. After 6 weeks, the developed scaffold showed shape stability with huge number of cells proliferated on to it. Various ratios of SFH synthesized by normal gelation with sodium tetradecyl sulfate and dimyristoyl glycerol-phosphoryl-glycerol. The 4-layer box network of all 2SF-based hydrogel could be printed without structural break. Both above hydrogels showed a good capability to use as a 3D-printing material due to its rheological nature and structural stability [55]. A 4D bio-printing system is a shape-controllable tool in cellular atmosphere to access in vivo application. This method is based on digital light processing 3D bioprinting technology and photo-polymerizable SF bioink [56,57].

3.2 Genetically engineered silk hydrogel

Progress in science of silk at genetic levels has offered a big plan for genetic engineering of SF. One of the unequal powers of this is to accurately modify the network and function according to the particular requirements. Therefore, we can make biomaterials with desirable characteristics by employing huge chemical variations that present in the building blocks of protein [58]. One more cause for cloning the silk genes is to get huge amount of protein in an economic way. Although the protein can also be extracted in a big quantity from *B. mori* and other spiders, the extracted amount of protein is not enough for number of applications. Continuous efforts, by generating variants of the repeated order of *N. clavipes* and *B. mori*, have resulted in fortunate synthesis of RSF [48,59]. Number of plans and host cells like insect cells [60], *E. coli* [61], microbes [62], mammalian cells [63], goats [64], and potato and tobacco plants [65] have been attempted to maximize the production of protein, to enhance the solubility of SF, to modify SF, and to allow its definite folding. Not only proteins obtain in huge amount but also new characteristics also integrated [59]. The prime operational modalities that have been integrated in these RSF are directed in making self-assembling proteins, stimuli responsive, mechanically strong, etc., so that they could acquire a particular embodiment for cell attachment and signaling assistance. Integration of these properties finally targeted to make genetically modified protein-based hydrogels that are suitable for tissue engineering [66].

3.3 High-strength hydrogels

The biocompatible silk protein hydrogels (SPHs) are frequently used in tissue repair. The subordinate mechanical characteristics restrict the applications of SPHs, particularly in tissue repair. Increasing the mechanical characteristics of SPHs to match surrounding tissues is important to spread their scope. To keep these points in mind, different high-strength hydrogels of SF discussed below.

3.4 Self-healing hydrogels

Self-healing SFHs have fascinated significant awareness to enhance the life duration, protection, and strength in the course of applications [67]. If these damaged in certain limit while working, the dynamic nature of non-covalent and reversible covalent bonds in the hydrogel allow them to fast restore [68,69]. It can be noticed in the several studies that these hydrogels have been developing and in use since long period but studies on SF-based self-healing hydrogels has only kick off in the past years. At present, SF self-healing hydrogels are usually prepared through different interactions but host-guest connectivity showed the most classic method for these hydrogels synthesis. Liu et al. [70], grafted β-cyclodextrin (β-CD) onto side chains on SF by photo-chemical method. This host-guest interaction between β-CD and SF leads to the formation of these hydrogels. These hydrogels were actually noticed through metal-coordination bonds.

3.5 Adhesive hydrogels

The synthesis of adhesive hydrogels is important as hemostatic agents, medical adhesives, heart patches, and epidermal sensors. The preparation of SFHs with adhesive characteristics has been investigated by Monica et al. [71]. The researchers utilized SF and PEG to synthesize SF-based cross-linked tissue adhesives hydrogels. Afterward, Yuan et al. [72] used HCl in the SF and PEG blend to induce the gelation. The developed hydrogels exhibited adhesive characteristics.

4. Methods of silk hydrogel preparation

4.1 Reverse dialysis

SFHs are in center for vast studies because of their biocompatibility, biodegradability, and capability to make hierarchical structures. However, the poor mechanical strength and long gelation time limit SFHs actual applications. This method is put in to develop robust and composite SFHs that were totally H-bonded. The explained mechanism of this method gave an easy perspective to make a physically cross-linked SFHs with exceptional mechanical properties [73]. Silk hydrogels and silk-pectin hydrogels synthesized through this method against CH_3OH to have high SF concentrated hydrogels. The available observations propose that pectin connect with silk when its amount is more than 15wt% to make heterogeneous network of hydrogel, which is different from IPNs and DNHs, high-strength hydrogels in respect of biocompatibility and biodegradability [74].

4.2 Bioprinting

Various new methodologies are being discussed to synthesize SFHs. 4D bio-printing in combination with the fourth dimension, "time," with 3D bio-printing is recently coming out as the next generation bio-fabrication method. This new method may not only overcome the usual barriers of

3D bio-printing but also copy the experienced dynamics of local tissues [75], better the response of newly generated tissues [76], and allow minimum invasive surgery [77]. In 4D bio-printing, osmotic pressure [78], magnetic stimulation [79], heat [80], electrical current, and light [81] are vital factors to develop the planar output structure which printed by 3D printer. 4D printing usually needs shape memory materials which are favorable for optimizing 3D printers so that their physico-chemical characteristics can be alter with the desired properties. This method is based on digital light processing (DLP) 3D bio-printing technique and photo-polymerizable SF bioink [56,57,82]. DLP use photo-curing based bio-printing process and prints a complete single layer at once. DLP has fast printing speed and higher cell viability [83,84]. Common DLP 3D printing has limits to make ovulate network with two or more components.

4.3 Physical methods

Gelation is initially prompted by weak bonding which does not include vital 2 degrees changes. Weak changes are followed by irreversible virtual strong β-sheet formation. These treatments can be divided into three categories: the modulation of physiochemical environment, physical methods, and chemical methods.

4.3.1 By increasing temperature

It is one of the most important factors connected with protein precipitation [85]. This effect is conducive to cross-link SF chains and this cross-linking is increased with increase in temperature. Temperature increase affects the vibrational motion of molecules thereby directly influences the diffusion coefficients, increase the collisions frequency, and enhance the precipitation of SF [86,87]. SF precipitation at high temperature depends on variation in the hydration of the system [88]. Upon increasing the temperature, the hydrated SF becomes free of H_2O. The disordering of the densely packed water overcomes the protein at high temperature and it has two 1 degree effects on protein aggregation, first is the local dehydration of hydrophobic chains that resulted in high hydrophobic exposure and high hydrophobic interactions; second is the changing in free energy of SF that leads to protein unfolding and high hydrophobic portion exposure. The result of these effects motivates the assembly formation [89]. In a study by Kim et al. [87], On increasing the temperature within a definite limit: the gelation time become short, pore size become smaller after freeze-drying, and mechanical strength increased.

4.3.2 Low pH

It is an important factor that has a good impact on protein solubility. It directly affects the distribution of surface charge on proteins which finally regulate protein-protein aggregation. Solubility of proteins is very low, because of minimum protein charge repulsion, as the pH of solution approaches to isoelectric point (pI). So, sheer adjustment of solution pH to near pI of protein can be a schematic tool to induce a hydrogel formation. Nagarkar et al. [90] reported the effect of pH on SF gelation. The authors reported that the addition of HCl to the freshly prepared SF solution led to the instant generation of a weak gel as the pH of solution decreased to 2 from 8.2, thus, this process reduces the gelation time. Protonation of silk solutions leads to a net deduction in repulsive forces between silk chains, an increase in collisions, and, thereby, facilitates the physical cross-linking [91]. Reversible SF gelation was observed by changing the solution pH with acidic or basic vapors for a short time [92]. This process was ascribe to short exposure to acidic environments, which resulted in weak gel synthesis. The acidic pH can also be adjusted by CO_2 mediation in SF solution for the gel formation. The whole process is bio-friendly, and no cross-linkers are used [93]. Floren et al. first showed this method to make SF hydrogels by using high-pressure CO_2 as a volatile acid. The simple and high amount recovery of CO_2, after processing, led to an exceptional clean synthesis which offers great benefits in biomedical engineering. This method decreases complexity, no use of cross-linkers, increase in rate of stable SF hydrogel synthesis, and avoid negative biological effects [93].

4.3.3 Self-assembly

This simple method is time-taking for making the SFHs. In solution form, SF is particularly exist as random coil. SF attain a low energy β-sheet network which followed by hydrogel synthesis under self-aggregation due to thermodynamic instability at room temperature [86]. Chouhan et al. [94] incubated a mixture of *A. assama* SF and *B. mori* SF at 37.1°C. During this synthesis, the hydrophobic bonding and synergistic effect of H-bond between both types of SF increased the bonding between polymeric chains which leads to a self-assembly of an opaque hydrogel formation. By having deep observation, it was a self-assembly process of amorphous regions of SF and SA molecules. The amount of β-sheet in the SFHs becomes decreased on increasing the SA amount. Fig. 13.1, Showed the schematic representation of the self-healing silk hydrogel preparation. Fig. 13.1a exhibit the hydrogel formation by host–guest interaction between SF and β-CD,

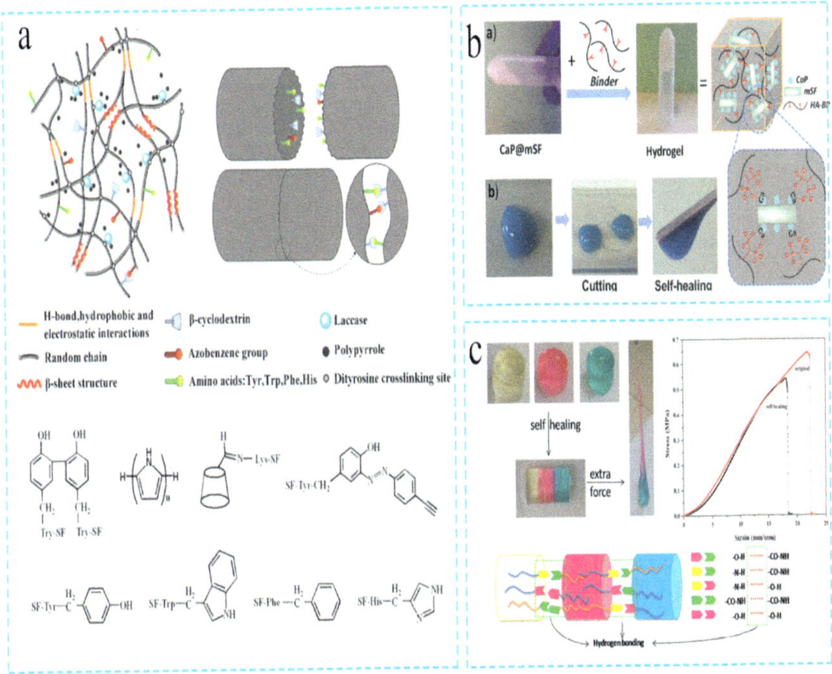

Figure 13.1 Different ways of preparing self-healing silk hydrogel. (a) Synthesis of self-healing silk protein functional hydrogel by the host–guest interaction between SF and β-cyclodextrin (β-CD). (b) Self-healing silk-based hydrogel prepared by the introduction of metal coordination bonds. (c) Same hydrogel prepared by hydrogen bonds. *(Obtained from Ref. [95].)*

Fig. 13.1b exhibit the hydrogel formation by introducing the metal co-ordination bonds and Fig. 13.1c exhibit the self-healing silk hydrogel formation by H-bonding [95].

4.3.4 Ultrasonication

The application of high-frequency sound waves to a protein solutions results in gel formation. Sonication is the input of energy to the system. Silk protein sonication explores the control protein precipitation and hydrogel formation. It is a fast and productive technique for SFH synthesis. When sound waves directed toward a solution then generate locally expanded and compressed regions which resulted in cavitation and bubble formation [96]. Collapsing of bubbles accelerate the solution greatly to induce collisions which resulted in local extreme increase in temperature and pressure. The cumulative effect of this process finally resulted in dehydration and polymer precipitation [97]. Silk protein gelation could be further adjusted by adding

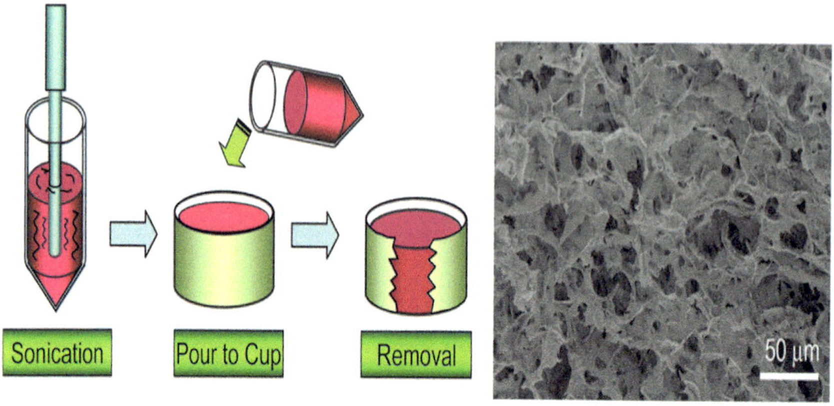

Figure 13.2 Process to form sonication-induced hydrogels. *(Obtained from Ref. [99].)*

K^+ ions and pH adjustment. Gorenkova et al. [98] sonicated the SF solution for 15–45 s to instigate the gelation for hydrogel formation. Fig. 13.2, showed the sonication method for hydrogel preparation. A fix amount of silk solution and DMEM powder sonicated for 30 s and then added to a cup made from ABS plastic. The side walls of the mold are subsequently broken and the gel removed (left). The SEM images showed the micrograph of 8% gel solution that has been flash-frozen and freeze-dried prior to imaging (right) [99].

4.3.5 Vortexing

This method alters the network of SF from coil to a β-sheet [100]. It involved subjecting the high-speed vortexing, imposes both extensional and rotational forces on to SF solution which resulted in the visible gelation of SF [101]. These variations to the molecular landscape can affect the end-to-end distances and distribution of polymer chain, enhance the amount oscillation, and increase the intermolecular interactions [102]. The gelation kinetics could be managed from minutes to hours by tuning the time, temperature, and/or component concentration. Chen et al. [103] blended the SF with sodium surfactin solution and followed by the synthesis of SFHs by vortexing at speeds of 75, 145, and 245 rpm. The studies analyzed that the given process decreased the gelation time.

4.4 Electrolysis methods

The structure of SF can also be modified under electric field. Under an electric current, the electrogelation includes the transformation of protein from coil to helical structure, where reversibility is possible. Nevertheless, additional transformation to β-sheet is one directional. Until now, here are three methods which include principles like electro-gelation, electrophoretic deposition, and electro-polymerization.

4.4.1 Electro-gelation

The use of electric field, to manage the gelation, has just gain the interest in silk hydrogel synthesis. Aqueous SF solution goes through a sol-to-gel transformation at low voltage. This method generates a soft gel with fair adhesive qualities. Leisk et al. exhibited that the prepared e-gel can be turned back to the solution form by supplying back electrical process. When polarity of the electrode reversed and 25 VDC was reapplied; the e-gel disappeared, whereas the new gel developed at the new positive electrode [104]. Kojic et al. were the first to make a system that allowed a pH change under electric field and the observation of e-gel growth [105]. In electro-gelation, the random coil structure transforms to α-helix rather than β-sheet, and the transformation process get reversed by changing the polarity of applied potential [106].

4.4.2 Electro-phoretic deposition

This process has gained huge amount of attention due to low process time and simple handling method [107]. SF can change the metal by coating onto their surface by this method. Zhang et al. used this method to deposit positively charged chitosan (CS)/SF coatings on titanium. CS experienced a high pH at cathode where CS and $-NH_2$ groups deprotonated and became insoluble; after applying voltage. Hence, CS/SF simultaneously deposited onto titanium surface which acted as cathode [108].

4.4.3 Electro-polymerization

Recently, the authors reported a process for the synthesis of electro-polymerized SFHs which are developed at the barrier of nano-porous film. When an RSF solution in tris buffer mixed into the reservoir with negative charge and the SF moved toward the positive charge at a higher DC voltage; the SFHs developed onto the barrier film [109].

4.5 Chemical methods

In this section, SF chains connect with each other via chemical bonds. The hydrogels usually showed superior stability as compared to physical hydrogels. Recently chemical methods include photo-polymerization, irradiation, use of cross linker, and enzyme cross-linking.

4.5.1 Photo-polymerization

Photo-polymerized hydrogels are developed by starting the polymerization by using UV-visible light with photo-initiator. Photo-initiator absorbs the UV light to generate the free radicals of molecules in the excited state. Free radicals afterward start the formation of unsaturated bonds in the monomer for free radical polymerization and hydrogel synthesis takes place after cross-linking. Photo-polymerized hydrogels are becoming famous because their synthesis is simple; Cells and bioactive molecules can preserve their activity by managing the intensity of UV light with the favorable selection of photo-initiator [110]. Kundu et al. showed the synthesis of photo-polymerized hydrogel based on SIPNs network of PVA-methacrylate-SF which possesses modifiable network [35].

4.5.2 γ-Irradiation

The highly intense penetrating γ-radiation frequently used for sterilization but they also instigate cross-linking and gel formation [111]. This process was used to make SFHs, since cross-linking and co-polymerization usually happen on irradiation to instigate hydrogel formation in a control and cost-effective way; without having initiator and cross-linkers [112]. These radiation triggers huge number of free radical in the aqueous solutions. These free radicals rearrange themselves to form new bonds which resulted in entanglement of polymer chains and synthesis of hydrogel takes place subsequently. Kim et al. [113] targeted γ-rays to different concentrated solution of SF to start cross-linking between the chains. Nevertheless of SF and radiation amount, the SFHs were synthesized quickly after imparting radiation. Kim et al. [113] prepared SFHs by using γ-ray. Mechanical analysis exhibited that the elasticity and rigidity of γ-ray irradiated SFHs enhanced while its compressive strength decreased due to low crystallinity and intermolecular cross-linking; in comparison with physically cross-linked SFHs.

4.5.3 Chemical cross-linking agents

The nature of gel is affected by cross-linker and reaction condition. The frequently used cross-linkers are glutaraldehyde [114], N,N′-methylene bisacrylamide, carbodiimide [115], genipin [116], and 1-(3-dimethylaminopropyl)23-ethylcarbodiimide, etc. Genipin, low toxic, frequently used in the synthesis of SFHs. Zhou et al. [117] synthesized the PVA/SF/nanohydroxyapatite hydrogel by using genipin. Besides genipin; glutaraldehyde and carbodiimide were also the most widely used cross-linkers [39,118]. Li et al. [119] studied a SFHs which is covalently synthesized and cross-linking by glutaraldehyde. Lv et al. [39] applied carbodiimide to cross-link SF and collagen for hybrid hydrogel formation. Covalent cross-linking of tyrosine of silk, by using horseradish peroxidase and H_2O_2, has just been explored [120]. Stabilization of SFHs via covalent di-tyrosine bonds resulted in robust network, lack crystalline domains, and exhibit elasticity and resilience. It is also keep in mind that cross-linkers may impart toxicity onto the cells. Therefore, the utilization of cross-linkers should be reduced [32].

4.5.4 Salt effect

The effect of salts in a polymeric solution is a complex process but it is usually accepted that the effect of ions on protein agglomeration is because of competition given by each constituents' that desire to bind with H_2O. This competition can result either in some hardship of solvent interaction with the protein (salting out) or some inclusion of the solvent to the protein (salting in). It is thought that ions that can efficiently instigate the protein aggregation may be thought to dehydrate the protein hydration shell to motivate the protein-protein aggregation [121]. Kim et al. [87] analyzed the effect of Ca^{2+} and K^+ ions on the gelation of SF solution. The authors observed noteworthy reduction in gelation time in case of Ca^{2+} with SF solution but low effect observed with K^+. Lammel et al. [122], performed a salting out method with K_3PO_4 to generate silk hydrogel particles with modifiable characteristics like 2 degrees structure.

4.5.5 Solvent effect

Organic solvents can be applied to affect the aggregation of proteins. Alcohols are frequently used to start local dehydration of α-helices and motivate the transformation to β-sheet [123]. Organic solvents reduce the dielectric constant of the medium that would in turn decrease the electric fields of solution which arbitrate macromolecular precipitation. Addition of organic solvent decreases the solvating capacity of H_2O, hence increase the gelation [121]. Rammensee et al. developed spider silk hydrogels by adding CH_3OH [124]. Ribeiro et al. [87] add C_2H_5OH to induce the quick synthesis of SF/nano-hydroxyapatite hydrogels.

4.5.6 Use of surfactants

Surfactant can also play an important solvating role in gelation. It can either enhance or stop protein precipitation which depends on the nature of using surfactant and silk. It is usually recognized that the attachment of surfactant to protein results in protein unfolding and evolvement of a precipitation-susceptible state. This method is based on the amphiphilic property of surfactant so that it can fold the hydrophobic parts of SF. Consequently, it decreases the surface tension of SF solution, forms H-bonds with SF, and encourages the making of β-sheets to increase the preparation of hydrogels. Surfactants like sodium lauroyl sarcosinate [125], sodium lauryl sulfate [126], poloxamer [127], and sodium dodecyl sulfate [126] can be mixed with SF to increase the SFH induction.

4.5.7 Enzyme cross-linking

This method particularly utilizes the catalytic activity of enzymes to functionalize particular groups of SF side chains thereby encourage the cross-linking in the chains. This biocompatible process uses light reaction parameters to keep away toxic matters [11]. Regularly used enzymes are horseradish peroxidase (HRP), glutamine transferase, carbonic anhydrase (CA), alcohol oxidase (AOX) [128–130], etc. In addition, in different analysis, HRP and H_2O_2 were utilized as an enzyme catalyzed cross-linker to provide high elasticity and modifiable rigidity in SFHs [120,131,132]. Raia et al. [133] added HRP to cross-link SF and tyramine-substituted hyaluronic acid (HA) to prepare hydrogels. The enzyme catalyzed the cross-linking of tyrosine-containing SF and tyramine-substituted HA to make tyramine-tyrosine bond. Wang et al. [134] used laccase to cross-link tyramine-modified HA with SF to make SFHs that possess good stability and optimized formability.

5. Structure of silk hydrogels

Silk proteins, extracted from cocoons, obtained from various silkworms showed changes in their structures [16,135,136]. It primarily consists of two proteins, fibroin and sericin. *B. mori* SF composed of P25 (26 kDa) glycoprotein and a heavy chain (325 kDa), linked by S—S bond [137]. On the contrary, SF of *A. mylitta* consist of two equal-sized polypeptides chains (197 kDa) each of which are bonded by S—S bond [138]. Sericin (10—300 kDa) act as glue to keep the fibroin chains together. These proteins composed of (a) repetitive amino acids pattern of *B. mori* (Gly-Ala-Gly-Ala-Gly-Ser) to give stability and (b) elastin amino acids pattern (Gly-Val-Gly-Val-Pro) that give flexibility, enhance solubility, and determine the cross-link density [47,139]. These predominant hydrophobic amino acids blocks lead to extensive hydrogen and hydrophobic bonding to all over the protein which resulted in a uniform 2 degrees network. These highly crystalline portions, have repetitive Ala or Gly patterns, connect with low organized portions of 34−40 amino acids chains which are distributed between the crystalline portions [140].

SF is extensively judged because of its biological response, modifiable biodegradability, and desired mechanical qualities [141−143]. SF is an FDA-accepted biopolymer for applications like sutures, tissue regeneration, and drug delivery system [144,145]. The actual network of SF is composed of Silk I, Silk II, and weak Silk III, which exists in air/water interface of SF solution.

Silk I, metastable network with a zigzag hydrophobic conformation, belongs to orthorhombic system. Silk I has the lowest crystallinity due to the presence of random coils and α-helix in majority which resulted in its weak strength and water-solubility [146]. Silk II (β-sheets/β-turns) belongs to monoclinic system and has the highest crystallinity which leads to its stability, water-insolubility, and mechanical stability [145]. Silk III is a crystalline polymorph with a 3-fold helical crystal. It has a metastable network that possesses crystallinity between Silk I and Silk II [145]. SF has hydrophilic (Tyr, Ser) and hydrophobic (Gly, Ala) amino acids sequence placed alternately [147]. H-bonds between adjacent segments resulted in the rigidity of SF. Silk I can be easily transformed into Silk II by soaking in CH_3OH and UV radiation [141,147,148]. In Silk III, the free −OH groups of Ser faces toward H_2O make it hydrophilic, while Ala protrude to the air phase makes it hydrophobic [145]. The network transformations and crystallinity amount of SF affect its physicochemical, mechanical, and biological properties [141]. Fig. 13.3. Is the representation of silk protein that comprises of Fig. 13.3a heavy chains (i.e., N-terminal, β-sheets, amorphous, and C-terminal) and light chains linked through s-s bonds (Fig. 13.3b) Silkworm thread, fibril overall structure, and silk fibroin polypeptide chains [149].

6. Overview of silk hydrogel application in tissue engineering

Recently, in addition to the attempts to make SPHs with superior mechanical properties, the progress in such hydrogels has also been carried out to achieve other targets like injectability, self-healing, adhesion, and 3D

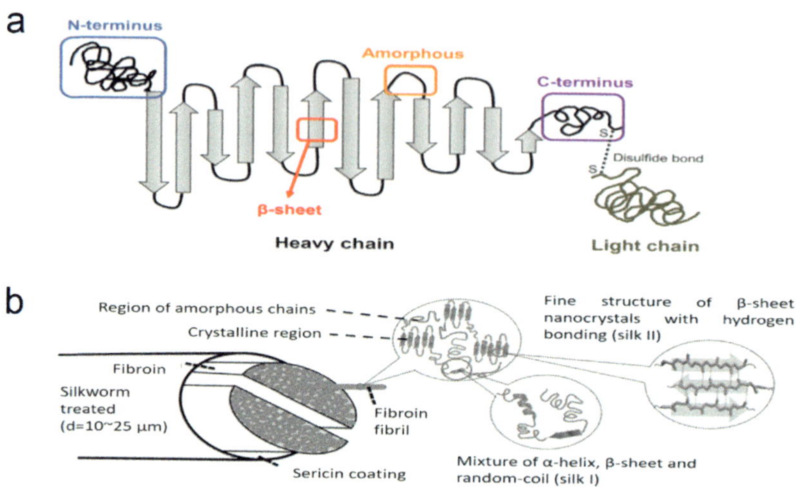

Figure 13.3 Schematic presentation of the silk structure. (a) Heavy chain (i.e., N-terminus, β-sheets, Amorphous and C-terminus) and light chain which linked via s-s bonds. (b) Silkworm thread, fibril overall structure and silk fibroin polypeptide chains. *(Obtained from Ref. [149].)*

printing. The supportive plan of various components and synergy of functionalities make it possible to have new applications of SFHs. It is analyzed that different functions of SPHs are recently used in tissue engineering, drug release, wound repair, etc. and they have discussed below.

6.1 Tissue engineering

Making/modifying the biopolymer to replace/repair a malfunctioned tissue is one of the most vital recent progresses. The success of hydrogel as tissue engineering material lies in the fact that their composition and qualities like water absorption, viscoelasticity, and stability can be prepared to copy various types of tissues. Resemblance of hydrogels to tissues and their capability to assist the transport of hormones, growth factors, and amino acid patterns while keeping the conformational integrity [150]. Hydrogels have the ability to entangle the cells within it during synthesis. Give light reaction conditions for synthesis so that the cell viability not affected [151]. Cell entanglement during preparation resulted in a more homogenous dispersal of cells, as compared to populating the matrix after gelation which resulted in higher cell numbers onto the gel surface [152] (Fig. 13.4). Showed schematic way of applications of silk hydrogels in tissue engineering and controlled drug release [153].

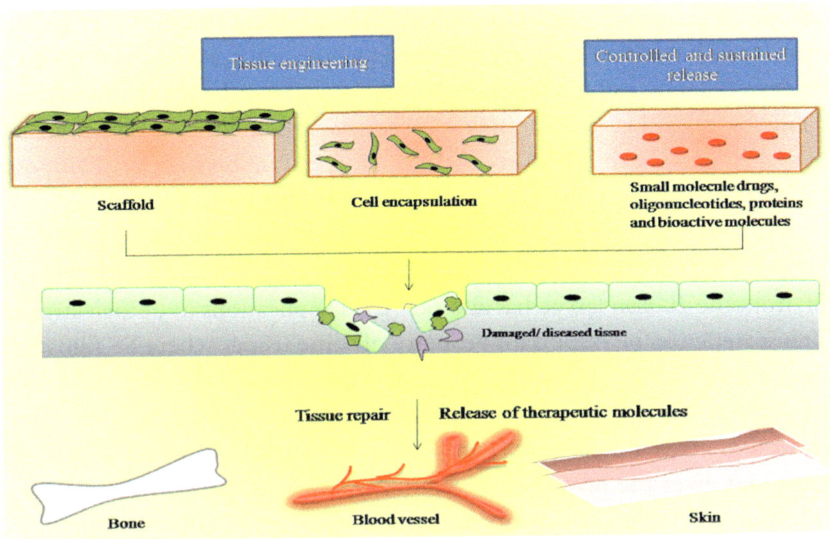

Figure 13.4 Schematic way of silk hydrogel applications in tissue engineering and controlled release. *(Obtained from Ref. [153].)*

6.2 Bone tissue engineering

Silk proteins can be customized to prepare a bioactive bone implants to instigate direct bone synthesis and finally osteo-integration. SFHs have exhibited superior ability to assist cell metabolism and bone remodeling [154,155]. Bone graft use for speeding up the bone regeneration suffers notable shortcomings like disease communication risk and donor site morbidity. These barriers have pushed the analysts to evaluate the effects of scaffolds with biochemical cues to increase bone repair. Recently, SF has been put forward as an implant and as a scaffold that able to assist tissue regeneration [156]. Diab et al. studied the effectiveness of a delivery vehicle that consists of an electrospun polycaprolactone nanofiber mesh with SFHs that contain bone morphogenetic protein-2 (BMP-2). The results conclude that the developed material showed a productive scheme for repair of large bone injuries and were equal to age-matched intact femurs [157].

6.3 Cartilage tissue engineering

Cartilaginous tissues inherently lack regenerative power. Available curing protocols for osteoarthritis have barriers like autologous donor material and suboptimal integration with the defect zone. A biocompatible and mechanically stable material is required for fruitful results. SFH scaffolds can encourage the accumulation of cartilage in a rigid and uniform way because of delayed biodegradation as compared to collagen scaffolds, and they can be developed by using aqueous method [158]. To enhance the mechanical stabilities of SFHs, just a new process has been utilized, wherein silk hydrogel has been reinforced with silk microfibers. The composite hydrogel showed stabilities comparable to agarose hydrogels [159].

6.4 Corneal tissue engineering

SF from the *B. mori* larvae has also powerful applications in optoelectronics. Transparency is the important property of some tissues where SF films have shown the stamina as scaffold material, but it needs hydration and fruitful attachment of cells without functionalization. The shortage of donor corneal grafts is a big and existing problem in corneal disease. Tissue engineering gives the power of generating transplants that can be utilized to take place of native malfunctioned corneas. Guan et al. cultured keratocytes on SF/CS hydrogels. The cells showed stellate morphology and a noteworthy enhancement in the appearance of keratocan compared with identical cultures. The acellular membrane was transplanted into the rabbit corneal stromal pockets, and there was no inflammatory problems observed at major level [160].

6.5 Artificial skin

Artificial skin, not cost effective, is a human skin substitute that is prepared in vitro to repair or replace defective skin. Scientists have prepared a number of artificial leather. The medical professionals have fortunately utilized composite skin for huge burn area. In the clinical treatment of skin problems, SF is known to instigate reepithelialization and collagen making. In addition, SF is considered to be favorable for the preparation of biomedical materials because of its low negative effects [161]. Sawitree et al. analyzed the performance of silk hydrogels on wound compared with a Cutinova hydro dressing. The results clearly showed that the regeneration of the dermis and epidermis of the wound beds covered with the silk hydrogel was faster than with a Cutinova hydro dressing [162].

7. Conclusion

This book chapter discusses different silk hydrogels with their preparation methods and application as tissue scaffold for different body parts of living beings. The structure and basic components of silk also discussed to understand its chemistry for hydrogel preparation and application in tissue engineering. Hydrogels of silk fibroin, silk elastin, and silk sericin give broad range of dimensions for optional applications as scaffold. The preparation methods of silk-based hydrogels include reverse dialysis, bioprinting, physical, chemical, and electrolysis. The information regarding other types of silk hydrogels like bioprinted hydrogels, genetically modified silk hydrogels, high-strength hydrogels, etc., also included. The application of silk-based hydrogels explored in this chapter for tissue engineering like bone tissue, cartilage, corneal tissue, and artificial skin. Due to economic and mechanical strength issues, low-cost natural silk must be on the line to prepared desired product for application as scaffold with minimal side effects. This book chapter will be helpful to prepare silk-based hydrogels as an implant for different impaired body tissues. The other silk-based hydrogels can be prepared for the same purposes. The information given about the structure of silk will be helpful to increase or decrease the mechanical properties of silk for desired applications. The detailed discussion on several methods for silk hydrogel synthesis will be helpful for the researcher to choose best possible methods for best productive results. The information about different types of silk hydrogels will give idea about best possible implants for impaired tissue.

Abbreviations

CS Chitosan
ECM Extra cellular matrix
HRP Horseradish peroxidase
IPN Interpenetrating networks
pI Isoelectric point
SF Silk fibroin
SFH Silk fibroin hydrogels
SPHs Silk protein hydrogels
β-CD β-cyclodextrin

Acknowledgments

Mohammad Amir Qureshi sincerely thanks my colleagues for helping me to sort out some problem while writing this book chapter. This research did not receive any specific grant from funding agencies in the public, commercial, or not for profit sectors.

References

[1] van der Lei B, Wildevuur CRH, Nieuwenhuis P, Blaauw EH, Dijk F, Hulstaert CE, et al. Regeneration of the arterial wall in microporous, compliant, biodegradable vascular grafts after implantation into the rat abdominal aorta. Cell Tissue Res 1985;242:569–78.

[2] Badylak SF, Nerem RM. Progress in tissue engineering and regenerative medicine. Proc Natl Acad Sci U S A 2010;107:3285–6.

[3] Vepari C, Kaplan DL. Silk as a biomaterial. Prog Polym Sci 2007;32:991–1007.

[4] Qureshi MA, Khatoon F. In vitro study of temperature and pH-responsive gentamycin sulphate-loaded chitosan-based hydrogel films for wound dressing applications. Polym Plast Technol Eng 2015. https://doi.org/10.1080/03602559.2014.974186.

[5] Hamidi M, Azadi A, Rafiei P. Hydrogel nanoparticles in drug delivery. Adv Drug Deliv Rev 2008;60:1638–49.

[6] Numata K, Katashima T, Sakai T. State of water, molecular structure, and cytotoxicity of silk hydrogels. Biomacromolecules 2011;12:2137–44.

[7] Das A, Ghosh S, Ray AR. Unveiling the self-assembly behavior of copolymers of AAc and DMAPMA in situ to form smart hydrogels displaying nanogels-within-macrogel hierarchical morphology. Polymer 2011;52:3800–10.

[8] Nuttelman CR, Mortisen DJ, Henry SM, Anseth KS. Attachment of fibronectin to poly (vinyl alcohol) hydrogels promotes NIH3T3 cell adhesion, proliferation, and migration. J Biomed Mater Res An Off J Soc Biomater Japanese Soc Biomater Aust Soc Biomater Korean Soc Biomater 2001;57:217–23.

[9] Tan J, Gemeinhart RA, Ma M, Saltzman WM. Improved cell adhesion and proliferation on synthetic phosphonic acid-containing hydrogels. Biomaterials 2005;26:3663–71.

[10] Singh A, Bhattacharya R, Shakeel A, Sharma AK, Jeevanandham S, Kumar A, et al. Hydrogel nanotubes with ice helices as exotic nanostructures for diabetic wound healing. Mater Horiz 2019;6:274–84.

[11] Hennink WE, van Nostrum CF. Novel crosslinking methods to design hydrogels. Adv Drug Deliv Rev 2012;64:223–36.

[12] Gupta AC, Chawla S, Hegde A, Singh D, Bandyopadhyay B, Lakshmanan CC, et al. Establishment of an in vitro organoid model of dermal papilla of human hair follicle. J Cell Physiol 2018;233:9015–30.

[13] Kundu B, Kurland NE, Bano S, Patra C, Engel FB, Yadavalli VK, et al. Silk proteins for biomedical applications: bioengineering perspectives. Prog Polym Sci 2014;39:251–67.

[14] Rajkhowa R, Levin B, Redmond SL, Li LH, Wang L, Kanwar JR, et al. Structure and properties of biomedical films prepared from aqueous and acidic silk fibroin solutions. J Biomed Mater Res, Part A 2011;97:37–45.

[15] Zhao H, Heusler E, Jones G, Li L, Werner V, Germershaus O, et al. Decoration of silk fibroin by click chemistry for biomedical application. J Struct Biol 2014;186:420–30.

[16] Rockwood DN, Preda RC, Yücel T, Wang X, Lovett ML, Kaplan DL. Materials fabrication from *Bombyx mori* silk fibroin. Nat Protoc 2011;6:1612–31.

[17] Midha S, Chameettachal S, Dey E, Ghosh S. Nonmulberry silk braids direct terminal osteocytic differentiation through activation of wnt-signaling. ACS Biomater Sci Eng 2017;3:1062–74.

[18] Dubey P, Murab S, Karmakar S, Chowdhury PK, Ghosh S. Modulation of self-assembly process of fibroin: an insight for regulating the conformation of silk biomaterials. Biomacromolecules 2015;16:3936–44.

[19] Yin Z, Kuang D, Wang S, Zheng Z, Yadavalli VK, Lu S. Swellable silk fibroin microneedles for transdermal drug delivery. Int J Biol Macromol 2018;106:48–56.
[20] Kundu B, Rajkhowa R, Kundu SC, Wang X. Silk fibroin biomaterials for tissue regenerations. Adv Drug Deliv Rev 2013;65:457–70.
[21] Ko E, Lee JS, Kim H, Yang SY, Yang D, Yang K, et al. Electrospun silk fibroin nanofibrous scaffolds with two-stage hydroxyapatite functionalization for enhancing the osteogenic differentiation of human adipose-derived mesenchymal stem cells. ACS Appl Mater Interf 2017;10:7614–25.
[22] Shi W, Sun M, Hu X, Ren B, Cheng J, Li C, et al. Structurally and functionally optimized silk-fibroin–gelatin scaffold using 3D printing to repair cartilage injury in vitro and in vivo. Adv Mater 2017;29:1701089.
[23] Xie S-Y, Peng L-H, Shan Y-H, Niu J, Xiong J, Gao J-Q. Adult stem cells seeded on electrospinning silk fibroin nanofiberous scaffold enhance wound repair and regeneration. J Nanosci Nanotechnol 2016;16:5498–505.
[24] Xue C, Zhu H, Tan D, Ren H, Gu X, Zhao Y, et al. Electrospun silk fibroin-based neural scaffold for bridging a long sciatic nerve gap in dogs. J Tissue Eng Regen Med 2018;12:e1143–53.
[25] Zhan K, Bai L, Wu Q, Lei D, Wang G. Fractal characteristics of the microvascular network: a useful index to assess vascularization level of porous silk fibroin biomaterial. J Biomed Mater Res, Part A 2017;105:2276–90.
[26] Qureshi MA, Nishat N, Jadoun S, Ansari MZ. Polysaccharide based superabsorbent hydrogels and their methods of synthesis: a review. Carbohydr Polym Technol Appl 2020;1:100014.
[27] Naba A, Clauser KR, Ding H, Whittaker CA, Carr SA, Hynes RO. The extracellular matrix: tools and insights for the "omics" era. Matrix Biol 2016;49:10–24.
[28] Qureshi MA, Khatoon F. Different types of smart nanogel for targeted delivery. J Sci Adv Mater Dev 2019;4:201–12. https://doi.org/10.1016/j.jsamd.2019.04.004.
[29] Tibbitt MW, Anseth KS. Hydrogels as extracellular matrix mimics for 3D cell culture. Biotechnol Bioeng 2009;103:655–63.
[30] Discher DE, Janmey P, Wang Y. Tissue cells feel and respond to the stiffness of their substrate. Science 2005;310:1139–43.
[31] Minoura N, Aiba S, Gotoh Y, Tsukada M, Imai Y. Attachment and growth of cultured fibroblast cells on silk protein matrices. J Biomed Mater Res 1995;29:1215–21.
[32] Wang H, Zhang Y. Processing silk hydrogel and its applications in biomedical materials. Biotechnol Prog 2015;31:630–40.
[33] Gil ES, Hudson SM. Effect of silk fibroin interpenetrating networks on swelling/deswelling kinetics and rheological properties of poly (N-isopropylacrylamide) hydrogels. Biomacromolecules 2007;8:258–64.
[34] Mandal BB, Kapoor S, Kundu SC. Silk fibroin/polyacrylamide semi-interpenetrating network hydrogels for controlled drug release. Biomaterials 2009;30:2826–36.
[35] Kundu J, Poole-Warren LA, Martens P, Kundu SC. Silk fibroin/poly (vinyl alcohol) photocrosslinked hydrogels for delivery of macromolecular drugs. Acta Biomater 2012;8:1720–9.
[36] Kang G, Nahm J, Park J, Moon J, Cho C, Yeo J. Effects of poloxamer on the gelation of silk fibroin. Macromol Rapid Commun 2000;21:788–91.
[37] Sun W, Incitti T, Migliaresi C, Quattrone A, Casarosa S, Motta A. Genipin-crosslinked gelatin–silk fibroin hydrogels for modulating the behaviour of pluripotent cells. J Tissue Eng Regen Med 2016;10:876–87.
[38] Xiao W, He J, Nichol JW, Wang L, Hutson CB, Wang B, et al. Synthesis and characterization of photocrosslinkable gelatin and silk fibroin interpenetrating polymer network hydrogels. Acta Biomater 2011;7:2384–93.

[39] Lv Q, Hu K, Feng Q, Cui F. Fibroin/collagen hybrid hydrogels with crosslinking method: preparation, properties, and cytocompatibility. J Biomed Mater Res Part A An Off J Soc Biomater Japanese Soc Biomater Aust Soc Biomater Korean Soc Biomater 2008;84:198–207.
[40] Elia R, Newhide DR, Pedevillano PD, Reiss GR, Firpo MA, Hsu EW, et al. Silk–hyaluronan-based composite hydrogels: a novel, securable vehicle for drug delivery. J Biomater Appl 2013;27:749–62.
[41] Hu X, Lu Q, Sun L, Cebe P, Wang X, Zhang X, et al. Biomaterials from ultrasonication-induced silk fibroin– hyaluronic acid hydrogels. Biomacromolecules 2010;11:3178–88.
[42] Myung D, Koh W, Ko J, Hu Y, Carrasco M, Noolandi J, et al. Biomimetic strain hardening in interpenetrating polymer network hydrogels. Polymer 2007;48:5376–87.
[43] Schmolka IR. A comparison of block copolymer surfactant gels. J Am Oil Chem Soc 1991;68:206–9.
[44] Wen Z, Jiang F, Wu F, Yin Z, Kaur K, Chakraborty J, et al. Photocurable silk fibroin-polyvinylpyrrolidone hydrogel. Materialia 2020;9:100525.
[45] Zaharia C, Tudora M-R, Damian CM, Vasile E, Stanescu PO. Silk fibroin and functionalized multiwall carbon nanotubes hydrogels and their biomineralization potential. Mater Plast 2013;50:159–62.
[46] Luo K, Yang Y, Shao Z. Physically crosslinked biocompatible silk-fibroin-based hydrogels with high mechanical performance. Adv Funct Mater 2016;26:872–80.
[47] Cappello J, Crissman J, Dorman M, Mikolajczak M, Textor G, Marquet M, et al. Genetic engineering of structural protein polymers. Biotechnol Prog 1990;6:198–202.
[48] Price R, Poursaid A, Cappello J, Ghandehari H. Effect of shear on physicochemical properties of matrix metalloproteinase responsive silk-elastinlike hydrogels. J Contr Release 2014;195:92–8.
[49] Price R, Poursaid A, Cappello J, Ghandehari H. In vivo evaluation of matrix metalloproteinase responsive silk–elastinlike protein polymers for cancer gene therapy. J Contr Release 2015;213:96–102.
[50] Dinerman AA, Cappello J, El-Sayed M, Hoag SW, Ghandehari H. Influence of solute charge and hydrophobicity on partitioning and diffusion in a genetically engineered silk-elastin-like protein polymer hydrogel. Macromol Biosci 2010;10:1235–47.
[51] Teramoto H, Nakajima K, Takabayashi C. Chemical modification of silk sericin in lithium chloride/dimethyl sulfoxide solvent with 4-cyanophenyl isocyanate. Biomacromolecules 2004;5:1392–8.
[52] Teramoto H, Nakajima K, Takabayashi C. Preparation of elastic silk sericin hydrogel. Biosci Biotechnol Biochem 2005;69:845–7.
[53] Zhang Q, Dong P, Chen L, Wang X, Lu S. Genipin-cross-linked thermosensitive silk sericin/poly (N-isopropylacrylamide) hydrogels for cell proliferation and rapid detachment. J Biomed Mater Res Part A An Off J Soc Biomater Japanese Soc Biomater Aust Soc Biomater Korean Soc Biomater 2014;102:76–83.
[54] Zheng Z, Wu J, Liu M, Wang H, Li C, Rodriguez MJ, et al. 3D bioprinting of self-standing silk-based bioink. Adv Healthc Mater 2018;7:1701026.
[55] Pudkon W, Laomeephol C, Damrongsakkul S, Kanokpanont S, Ratanavaraporn J. Comparative study of silk fibroin-based hydrogels and their potential as material for 3-dimensional (3D) printing. Molecules 2021;26:3887.
[56] Hong H, Seo YB, Lee JS, Lee YJ, Lee H, Ajiteru O, et al. Digital light processing 3D printed silk fibroin hydrogel for cartilage tissue engineering. Biomaterials 2020;232:119679.

[57] Kim SH, Lee YJ, Chao JR, Kim DY, Sultan M, Lee HJ, et al. Rapidly photocurable silk fibroin sealant for clinical applications. NPG Asia Mater 2020;12:1–16.
[58] Chow D, Nunalee ML, Lim DW, Simnick AJ, Chilkoti A. Peptide-based biopolymers in biomedicine and biotechnology. Mater Sci Eng R Reports 2008;62:125–55.
[59] Hardy JG, Scheibel TR. Silk-inspired polymers and proteins. Biochem Soc Trans 2009;37:677–81.
[60] Huemmerich D, Scheibel T, Vollrath F, Cohen S, Gat U, Ittah S. Novel assembly properties of recombinant spider dragline silk proteins. Curr Biol 2004;14:2070–4.
[61] Fahnestock SR, Irwin SL. Synthetic spider dragline silk proteins and their production in *Escherichia coli*. Appl Microbiol Biotechnol 1997;47:23–32.
[62] Fahnestock SR, Yao Z, Bedzyk LA. Microbial production of spider silk proteins. Rev Mol Biotechnol 2000;74:105–19.
[63] Lazaris A, Arcidiacono S, Huang Y, Zhou J-F, Duguay F, Chretien N, et al. Spider silk fibers spun from soluble recombinant silk produced in mammalian cells. Science 2002;295:472–6.
[64] Williams D. Sows' ears, silk purses and goats' milk: new production methods and medical applications for silk. Med Device Technol 2003;14:9–11.
[65] Scheller J, Gührs K-H, Grosse F, Conrad U. Production of spider silk proteins in tobacco and potato. Nat Biotechnol 2001;19:573–7.
[66] Rammensee S, Slotta U, Scheibel T, Bausch A. Assembly mechanism of recombinant spider silk proteins. Proc Natl Acad Sci U S A 2008;105:6590–5.
[67] Taylor DL, in het Panhuis M. Self-healing hydrogels. Adv Mater 2016;28:9060–93.
[68] Talebian S, Mehrali M, Taebnia N, Pennisi CP, Kadumudi FB, Foroughi J, et al. Self-healing hydrogels: the next paradigm shift in tissue engineering? Adv Sci 2019;6:1801664.
[69] Deng Z, Wang H, Ma PX, Guo B. Self-healing conductive hydrogels: preparation, properties and applications. Nanoscale 2020;12:1224–46.
[70] Liu L, Han Y, Lv S. Design of self-healing and electrically conductive silk fibroin-based hydrogels. ACS Appl Mater Interf 2019;11:20394–403.
[71] Serban MA, Panilaitis B, Kaplan DL. Silk fibroin and polyethylene glycol-based biocompatible tissue adhesives. J Biomed Mater Res, Part A 2011;98:567–75.
[72] Yuan M, Yan S, Liu H, Kundu SC, Cai Y, Yao J. Performance of water-immiscible silk fibroin based hydrogel as underwater biomedical adhesive. Fibers Polym 2019;20:2032–41.
[73] Chang H, Meng L, Shao C, Cui C, Yang J. Physically cross-linked silk hydrogels with high solid content and excellent mechanical properties via a reverse dialysis concentrated procedure. ACS Sustain Chem Eng 2019;7:13324–32.
[74] Numata K, Yamazaki S, Katashima T, Chuah J, Naga N, Sakai T. Silk-pectin hydrogel with superior mechanical properties, biodegradability, and biocompatibility. Macromol Biosci 2014;14:799–806.
[75] Kirillova A, Maxson R, Stoychev G, Gomillion CT, Ionov L. 4D biofabrication using shape-morphing hydrogels. Adv Mater 2017;29:1703443.
[76] Morouço P, Lattanzi W, Alves N. Four-dimensional bioprinting as a new era for tissue engineering and regenerative medicine. Front Bioeng Biotechnol 2017;61.
[77] Kutikov AB, Reyer KA, Song J. Shape-Memory Performance of Thermoplastic Amphiphilic Triblock Copolymer Poly (d, l-lactic acid-co-ethylene glycol-co-d, l-lactic acid)(PELA)/Hydroxyapatite Composites. Macromol Chem Phys 2014;215:2482–90.
[78] Raviv D, Zhao W, McKnelly C, Papadopoulou A, Kadambi A, Shi B, et al. Active printed materials for complex self-evolving deformations. Sci Rep 2014;4:1–8.

[79] Kokkinis D, Schaffner M, Studart AR. Multimaterial magnetically assisted 3D printing of composite materials. Nat Commun 2015;6:1–10.
[80] Teoh JEM, An J, Chua CK, Lv M, Krishnasamy V, Liu Y. Hierarchically self-morphing structure through 4D printing. Virtual Phys Prototyp 2017;12:61–8.
[81] Leist SK, Zhou J. Current status of 4D printing technology and the potential of light-reactive smart materials as 4D printable materials. Virtual Phys Prototyp 2016;11:249–62.
[82] Kim SH, Yeon YK, Lee JM, Chao JR, Lee YJ, Seo YB, et al. Precisely printable and biocompatible silk fibroin bioink for digital light processing 3D printing. Nat Commun 2018;9:1–14.
[83] Zhu W, Ma X, Gou M, Mei D, Zhang K, Chen S. 3D printing of functional biomaterials for tissue engineering. Curr Opin Biotechnol 2016;40:103–12.
[84] Gu Z, Fu J, Lin H, He Y. Development of 3D bioprinting: from printing methods to biomedical applications. Asian J Pharm Sci 2020;15:529–57.
[85] Wang W, Nema S, Teagarden D. Protein aggregation—pathways and influencing factors. Int J Pharm 2010;390:89–99.
[86] Aigner TB, DeSimone E, Scheibel T. Biomedical applications of recombinant silk-based materials. Adv Mater 2018;30:1704636.
[87] Kim U-J, Park J, Li C, Jin H-J, Valluzzi R, Kaplan DL. Structure and properties of silk hydrogels. Biomacromolecules 2004;5:786–92.
[88] Urry DW. Molecular machines: how motion and other functions of living organisms can result from reversible chemical changes. Angew Chem Int Ed Engl 1993;32:819–41.
[89] Nagarkar S, Nicolai T, Chassenieux C, Lele A. Structure and gelation mechanism of silk hydrogels. Phys Chem Chem Phys 2010;12:3834–44.
[90] Nagarkar S, Patil A, Lele A, Bhat S, Bellare J, Mashelkar RA. Some mechanistic insights into the gelation of regenerated silk fibroin sol. Ind Eng Chem Res 2009;48:8014–23.
[91] Matsumoto A, Chen J, Collette AL, Kim U-J, Altman GH, Cebe P, et al. Mechanisms of silk fibroin sol– gel transitions. J Phys Chem B 2006;110:21630–8.
[92] Terry AE, Knight DP, Porter D, Vollrath F. pH induced changes in the rheology of silk fibroin solution from the middle division of Bombyx m ori silkworm. Biomacromolecules 2004;5:768–72.
[93] Floren ML, Spilimbergo S, Motta A, Migliaresi C. Carbon dioxide induced silk protein gelation for biomedical applications. Biomacromolecules 2012;13:2060–72.
[94] Lohe CDTu, Samudrala PK, Mandal BB. Situ form inject silk fibroin hydrogel promot ski regen full thick burn wounds. Adv Healthc Mater 2018;7:1801092.
[95] Zheng H, Zuo B. Functional silk fibroin hydrogels: preparation, properties and applications. J Mater Chem B 2021;9:1238–58.
[96] Paulusse JMJ, Sijbesma RP. Ultrasound in polymer chemistry: revival of an established technique. J Polym Sci Part A Polym Chem 2006;44:5445–53.
[97] Wang X, Kluge JA, Leisk GG, Kaplan DL. Sonication-induced gelation of silk fibroin for cell encapsulation. Biomaterials 2008;29:1054–64.
[98] Gorenkova N, Osama I, Seib FP, Carswell HVO. In vivo evaluation of engineered self-assembling silk fibroin hydrogels after intracerebral injection in a rat stroke model. ACS Biomater Sci Eng 2018;5:859–69.
[99] Kluge JA, Rosiello NC, Leisk GG, Kaplan DL, Dorfmann AL. The consolidation behavior of silk hydrogels. J Mech Behav Biomed Mater 2010;3:278–89.
[100] Davis NE, Beenken-Rothkopf LN, Mirsoian A, Kojic N, Kaplan DL, Barron AE, et al. Enhanced function of pancreatic islets co-encapsulated with ECM proteins and mesenchymal stromal cells in a silk hydrogel. Biomaterials 2012;33:6691–7.

[101] Rangel-Nafaile C, Metzner AB, Wissbrun KF. Analysis of stress-induced phase separations in polymer solutions. Macromolecules 1984;17:1187–95.
[102] Yucel T, Cebe P, Kaplan DL. Vortex-induced injectable silk fibroin hydrogels. Biophys J 2009;97:2044–50.
[103] Chen D, Yin Z, Wu F, Fu H, Kundu SC, Lu S. Orientational behaviors of silk fibroin hydrogels. J Appl Polym Sci 2017;134:45050.
[104] Leisk GG, Lo TJ, Yucel T, Lu Q, Kaplan DL. Electrogelation for protein adhesives. Adv Mater 2010;22:711–5.
[105] Kojic N, Panzer MJ, Leisk GG, Raja WK, Kojic M, Kaplan DL. Ion electrodiffusion governs silk electrogelation. Soft Matter 2012;8:6897–905.
[106] Lu Q, Huang Y, Li M, Zuo B, Lu S, Wang J, et al. Silk fibroin electrogelation mechanisms. Acta Biomater 2011;7:2394–400.
[107] Boccaccini AR, Keim S, Ma R, Li Y, Zhitomirsky I. Electrophoretic deposition of biomaterials. J R Soc Interface 2010;7:S581–613.
[108] Zhang Z, Jiang T, Ma K, Cai X, Zhou Y, Wang Y. Low temperature electrophoretic deposition of porous chitosan/silk fibroin composite coating for titanium biofunctionalization. J Mater Chem 2011;21:7705–13.
[109] Wang H-Y, Zhang Y-Q. Processing and characterisation of a novel electropolymerized silk fibroin hydrogel membrane. Sci Rep 2014;4:1–11.
[110] Mathews DT, Birney YA, Cahill PA, McGuinness GB. Vascular cell viability on polyvinyl alcohol hydrogels modified with water-soluble and-insoluble chitosan. J Biomed Mater Res Part B Appl Biomater An Off J Soc Biomater Japanese Soc Biomater Aust Soc Biomater Korean Soc Biomater 2008;84:531–40.
[111] Davison L, Themistou E, Buchanan F, Cunningham E. Low temperature gamma sterilization of a bioresorbable polymer, PLGA. Radiat Phys Chem 2018;143:27–32.
[112] Tavakol M, Vasheghani-Farahani E, Mohammadifar MA, Dehghan-Niri M. Effect of gamma irradiation on the physicochemical and rheological properties of enzyme-catalyzed tragacanth-based injectable hydrogels. J Polym Eng 2019;39:442–9.
[113] Kim MH, Park WH. Chemically cross-linked silk fibroin hydrogel with enhanced elastic properties, biodegradability, and biocompatibility. Int J Nanomed 2016;11:2967.
[114] Mandal BB, Ghosh B, Kundu SC. Non-mulberry silk sericin/poly (vinyl alcohol) hydrogel matrices for potential biotechnological applications. Int J Biol Macromol 2011;49:125–33.
[115] Park S-H, Gil ES, Cho H, Mandal BB, Tien LW, Min B-H, et al. Intervertebral disk tissue engineering using biphasic silk composite scaffolds. Tissue Eng 2012;18:447–58.
[116] Chiono V, Pulieri E, Vozzi G, Ciardelli G, Ahluwalia A, Giusti P. Genipin-crosslinked chitosan/gelatin blends for biomedical applications. J Mater Sci Mater Med 2008;19:889–98.
[117] Zhou H, Wang Z, Cao H, Hu H, Luo Z, Yang X, et al. Genipin-crosslinked polyvinyl alcohol/silk fibroin/nano-hydroxyapatite hydrogel for fabrication of artificial cornea scaffolds—a novel approach to corneal tissue engineering. J Biomater Sci Polym Ed 2019;30:1604–19.
[118] Ferrero F, Periolatto M, Burelli S, Carletto RA. Silk grafting with chitosan and crosslinking agents. Fibers Polym 2010;11:185–92.
[119] Lin Y, Xia X, Shang K, Elia R, Huang W, Cebe P, et al. Tuning chemical and physical cross-links in silk electrogels for morphological analysis and mechanical reinforcement. Biomacromolecules 2013;14:2629–35.
[120] Partlow BP, Hanna CW, Rnjak-Kovacina J, Moreau JE, Applegate MB, Burke KA, et al. Highly tunable elastomeric silk biomaterials. Adv Funct Mater 2014;24:4615–24.

[121] McPherson A. Introduction to protein crystallization. Methods 2004;34:254–65.
[122] Lammel AS, Hu X, Park S-H, Kaplan DL, Scheibel TR. Controlling silk fibroin particle features for drug delivery. Biomaterials 2010;31:4583–91.
[123] Stevenson CL. Characterization of protein and peptide stability and solubility in non-aqueous solvents. Curr Pharmaceut Biotechnol 2000;1:165–82.
[124] Rammensee S, Hümmerich D, Hermanson KD, Scheibel T, Bausch AR. Rheological characterization of hydrogels formed by recombinantly produced spider silk. Appl Phys 2006;82:261–4.
[125] Zhang F, Li JJ, Jiang R, Zhang SS, Zhu T, Lu SZ. Excellent cell compatibility in time controlled silk fibroin hydrogels. Mater Sci Forum 2015;815:407–11.
[126] Wu X, Hou J, Li M, Wang J, Kaplan DL, Lu S. Sodium dodecyl sulfate-induced rapid gelation of silk fibroin. Acta Biomater 2012;8:2185–92.
[127] Deng C, Zhong T, Xu Y, Yue X, Ming J, Zuo B. Influences of poloxamer on structure and morphology of regenerated silk fibroin gelation. Silk 2013;21.
[128] Hasturk O, Jordan KE, Choi J, Kaplan DL. Enzymatically crosslinked silk and silk-gelatin hydrogels with tunable gelation kinetics, mechanical properties and bioactivity for cell culture and encapsulation. Biomaterials 2020;232:119720.
[129] Han Y, Yu S, Liu L, Zhao S, Yang T, Yang Y, et al. Silk fibroin-based hydrogels as a protective matrix for stabilization of enzymes against pH denaturation. Mol Catal 2018;457:24–32.
[130] Burrs SL, Vanegas DC, Bhargava M, Mechulan N, Hendershot P, Yamaguchi H, et al. A comparative study of graphene–hydrogel hybrid bionanocomposites for biosensing. Analyst 2015;140:1466–76.
[131] Zhou B, Wang P, Cui L, Yu Y, Deng C, Wang Q, et al. Self-crosslinking of silk fibroin using H_2O_2-horseradish peroxidase system and the characteristics of the resulting fibroin membranes. Appl Biochem Biotechnol 2017;182:1548–63.
[132] Chirila TV, Suzuki S, Papolla C. A comparative investigation of *Bombyx mori* silk fibroin hydrogels generated by chemical and enzymatic cross-linking. Biotechnol Appl Biochem 2017;64:771–81.
[133] Raia NR, Partlow BP, McGill M, Kimmerling EP, Ghezzi CE, Kaplan DL. Enzymatically crosslinked silk-hyaluronic acid hydrogels. Biomaterials 2017;131:58–67.
[134] Wang L, Xu B, Nong Y, Wang P, Yu Y, Deng C, et al. Laccase-mediated construction of flexible double-network hydrogels based on silk fibroin and tyramine-modified hyaluronic acid. Int J Biol Macromol 2020;160:795–805.
[135] Craig CL, Hsu M, Kaplan D, Pierce NE. A comparison of the composition of silk proteins produced by spiders and insects. Int J Biol Macromol 1999;24:109–18.
[136] Kundu B, Kurland NE, Yadavalli VK, Kundu SC. Isolation and processing of silk proteins for biomedical applications. Int J Biol Macromol 2014;70:70–7.
[137] Valluzzi R, Winkler S, Wilson D, Kaplan DL. Silk: molecular organization and control of assembly. Philos Trans R Soc London Ser B Biol Sci 2002;357:165–7.
[138] Datta A, Ghosh AK, Kundu SC. Purification and characterization of fibroin from the tropical Saturniid silkworm, Antheraea mylitta. Insect Biochem Mol Biol 2001;31:1013–8.
[139] Dandu R, Von Cresce A, Briber R, Dowell P, Cappello J, Ghandehari H. Silk–elastinlike protein polymer hydrogels: influence of monomer sequence on physicochemical properties. Polymer 2009;50:366–74.
[140] Craig CL, Riekel C. Comparative architecture of silks, fibrous proteins and their encoding genes in insects and spiders. Comp Biochem Physiol, Part B: Biochem Mol Biol 2002;133:493–507.
[141] Wang Y, Kim BJ, Peng B, Li W, Wang Y, Li M, et al. Controlling silk fibroin conformation for dynamic, responsive, multifunctional, micropatterned surfaces. Proc Natl Acad Sci U S A 2019;116:21361–8.

[142] Hu L, Han Y, Ling S, Huang Y, Yao J, Shao Z, et al. Direct observation of native silk fibroin conformation in silk gland of *Bombyx mori* silkworm. ACS Biomater Sci Eng 2020;6:1874–9.
[143] Zhu Z, Ling S, Yeo J, Zhao S, Tozzi L, Buehler MJ, et al. High-strength, durable all-silk fibroin hydrogels with versatile processability toward multifunctional applications. Adv Funct Mater 2018;28:1704757.
[144] Numata K, Kaplan DL. Silk-based delivery systems of bioactive molecules. Adv Drug Deliv Rev 2010;62:1497–508.
[145] Pham DT, Tiyaboonchai W. Fibroin nanoparticles: a promising drug delivery system. Drug Deliv 2020;27:431–48.
[146] Pham DT, Saelim N, Tiyaboonchai W. Crosslinked fibroin nanoparticles using EDC or PEI for drug delivery: physicochemical properties, crystallinity and structure. J Mater Sci 2018;53:14087–103.
[147] Qi Y, Wang H, Wei K, Yang Y, Zheng R-Y, Kim IS, et al. A review of structure construction of silk fibroin biomaterials from single structures to multi-level structures. Int J Mol Sci 2017;18:237.
[148] Bessonov I, Moysenovich A, Arkhipova A, Ezernitskaya M, Efremov Y, Solodilov V, et al. The mechanical properties, secondary structure, and osteogenic activity of photopolymerized fibroin. Polymers 2020;12:646.
[149] Sun W, Gregory DA, Tomeh MA, Zhao X. Silk fibroin as a functional biomaterial for tissue engineering. Int J Mol Sci 2021;22:1499.
[150] Varghese S, Elisseeff JH. Hydrogels for musculoskeletal tissue engineering. Polym Regen Med 2006:95–144.
[151] Tsang VL, Bhatia SN. Three-dimensional tissue fabrication. Adv Drug Deliv Rev 2004;56:1635–47.
[152] Chan BP, Leong KW. Scaffolding in tissue engineering: general approaches and tissue-specific considerations. Eur Spine J 2008;17:467–79.
[153] Kapoor S, Kundu SC. Silk protein-based hydrogels: promising advanced materials for biomedical applications. Acta Biomater 2016;31:17–32.
[154] Venkatesan J, Nithya R, Sudha PN, Kim S-K. Role of alginate in bone tissue engineering. Adv Food Nutr Res 2014;73:45–57.
[155] Gentile P, Chiono V, Carmagnola I, Hatton PV. An overview of poly (lactic-co-glycolic) acid (PLGA)-based biomaterials for bone tissue engineering. Int J Mol Sci 2014;15:3640–59.
[156] Meinel L, Karageorgiou V, Fajardo R, Snyder B, Shinde-Patil V, Zichner L, et al. Bone tissue engineering using human mesenchymal stem cells: effects of scaffold material and medium flow. Ann Biomed Eng 2004;32:112–22.
[157] Diab T, Pritchard EM, Uhrig BA, Boerckel JD, Kaplan DL, Guldberg RE. A silk hydrogel-based delivery system of bone morphogenetic protein for the treatment of large bone defects. J Mech Behav Biomed Mater 2012;11:123–31.
[158] Bueno EM, Glowacki J. Biologic foundations for skeletal tissue engineering. Synth Lect Tissue Eng 2011;3:1–220.
[159] Yodmuang S, McNamara SL, Nover AB, Mandal BB, Agarwal M, Kelly T-AN, et al. Silk microfiber-reinforced silk hydrogel composites for functional cartilage tissue repair. Acta Biomater 2015;11:27–36.
[160] Guan L, Tian P, Ge H, Tang X, Zhang H, Du L, et al. Chitosan-functionalized silk fibroin 3D scaffold for keratocyte culture. J Mol Histol 2013;44:609–18.
[161] Wang Y, Kim H-J, Vunjak-Novakovic G, Kaplan DL. Stem cell-based tissue engineering with silk biomaterials. Biomaterials 2006;27:6064–82.
[162] Suwannasing S. Comparison of the efficacy of hydrogel biomaterial preparation from silk waste protein and commercial product (sutinovahysro) for deep wound healing in Guinea pigs. 2007.

Index

Note: 'Page numbers followed by *f* indicate figures and *t* indicate table.'

9780323993579